Guidelines for Air and Ground Transport of Neonatal and Pediatric Patients

■ ■ ■ ■ ■ ■

Author:
Section on Transport Medicine
American Academy of Pediatrics

George A. Woodward, MD, MBA, FAAP
Editor-in-Chief

Robert M. Insoft, MD, FAAP
Associate Editor

Monica E. Kleinman, MD, FAAP
Associate Editor

AAP Staff
S. Niccole Alexander, MPP

American Academy of Pediatrics
141 Northwest Point Boulevard
Elk Grove Village, IL 60007

Library of Congress Control Number: 2006927641
ISBN-10: 1-58110-219-4
ISBN-13: 978-1-58110-219-2
MA0353

The recommendations in this publication do not indicate an exclusive course of treatment or serve as a standard of care. Variations, taking into account individual circumstances, may be appropriate.

Statements and opinions expressed are those of the authors and not necessarily those of the American Academy of Pediatrics.

Product and brand names are furnished for identification purposes only. No endorsement of the manufacturers or products listed is implied.

3-123/0606

Contributors

Thomas J. Abramo, MD, FAAP, FACEP
Children's Hospital at Vanderbilt
Nashville, TN

Paula M. Agosto, RN, MHA, CCRN
Children's Hospital of Philadelphia
Philadelphia, PA

Linda S. Arapian, MSN, RNC, CEN,
     EMT-B
Children's National Medical Center
Washington, DC

Tamara Bleak, RN, BSN
Intermountain Health Care Life Flight
Sandy, UT

Ira J. Blumen, MD, FACEP
University of Chicago Hospitals
Chicago, IL

S. Louise Bowen, RNC, CMTE,
     MSN, ARNP
All Children's Hospital
St. Petersburg, FL

Jan Cody, RN, BSN, LP, CMTE
Children's Medical Center
Dallas, TX

Kimberly A. Cox, RN, CCRN
Children's Hospital Boston
Boston, MA

Karen Cremin, EMT
Children's Hospital Boston
Boston, MA

Douglas S. Diekema, MD, MPH, FAAP
Children's Hospital and Regional
     Medical Center
Seattle, WA

Eileen Frazer, RN, CMTE
Commission on Accreditation of
     Medical Transport Systems
Anderson, SC

Andrew L. Garrett, MD, EMT, FAAP
National Center for Disaster
     Preparedness at Columbia
     University
New York, NY

Mary Astor Gomez, RN, MSN, CPNP
Children's Memorial Hospital
Chicago, IL

Robert M. Insoft, MD, FAAP
Massachusetts General Hospital
Boston, MA

David Jaimovich, MD, FAAP
Advocate Hope Children's Hospital
Oak Lawn, IL

Patricia J. Jason, RN, BSN, CCRN
Children's Hospital and Regional
     Medical Center
Seattle, WA

Brent R. King, MD, FACEP, FAAEM,
     FAAP
The University of Texas Houston
     Medical School
Houston, TX

Bruce Lawrence Klein, MD, FAAP
Children's National Medical Center
Washington, DC

Monica E. Kleinman, MD, FAAP
Children's Hospital Boston
Boston, MA

Nadine Levick, MD, MPH
Maimonides Medical Center
New York, NY

Jeffrey Linzer, Sr., MD, MICP, FACEP, FAAP
Emory University School of Medicine
Atlanta, GA

Calvin Glen Lowe, MD, FAAP
Children's Hospital Los Angeles
Los Angeles, CA

Gary McAbee, DO, JD, FAAP
Robert Wood Johnson School of Medicine
Camden, NJ

Anthony Wade Minge, MBA
Children's Medical Center Dallas
Dallas, TX

Pamela C. Moore, RN
Intermountain Health Care Life Flight
Salt Lake City, UT

Lisa Rachel Morlitz, PharmD
Massachusetts General Hospital
Boston, MA

Richard A. Orr, MD, FAAP
Children's Hospital of Pittsburgh
Pittsburgh, PA

Anthony L. Pearson-Shaver, MD, MHSA, FAAP, FCCM
Medical College of Georgia
Augusta, GA

Janice Romito, MSN, RNC, NNP
Texas Children's Hospital
Houston, TX

Robert Shields, RN, CCRN, CEN, NREMT-P
Children's Hospital Boston
Boston, MA

Michael Stone Trautman, MD, FAAP
Indiana University School of Medicine
Indianapolis, IN

Nicholas Tsarouhas, MD, FAAP
Children's Hospital of Philadelphia
Philadelphia, PA

Francine J. Westergaard, RN, BSN
Advocate Hope Children's Hospital
Oak Lawn, IL

Abigail Williams, RN, JD, MPH
Abigail Williams & Associates PC
Worcester, MA

George A. Woodward, MD, MBA, FAAP, FACEP
Children's Hospital and Regional Medical Center
Seattle, WA

B. Robert Young, RPh
Massachusetts General Hospital
Boston, MA

Section on Transport Medicine Executive Committee 2004–2005

Robert M. Insoft, MD, FAAP, *chair*
Monica E. Kleinman, MD, FAAP
Calvin Glen Lowe, MD, FAAP
Bruce Lawrence Klein, MD, FAAP

Anthony L. Pearson-Shaver, MD, MHSA, FAAP, FCCM
Michael Stone Trautman, MD, FAAP
David Jaimovich, MD, FAAP, *immediate past chair*

Acknowledgment

The editors thank the following Academy groups for their thoughtful review and consideration of this manual: Committee on Bioethics, Committee on Child Health Financing, Committee on Fetus and Newborn, Committee on Hospital Care, Committee on Injury, Violence, and Poison Prevention, Committee on Medical Liability, Committee on Pediatric Emergency Medicine, Committeeon Pediatric Workforce, Committee on Practice and Ambulatory Medicine, Section on Critical Care, Section on Emergency Medicine, Section on Hospital Medicine, Section on Neurological Surgery, Section on Perinatal Pediatrics, Section on Transport Medicine, and the Council on Clinical Information Technology. They also thank the Ambulatory Pediatric Association, American Association for Respiratory Care, American College of Emergency Physicians, Commission on Accreditation of Medical Transport Systems, Emergency Nurses Association, National Association of EMS Physicians, the National Association of Neonatal Nurses, Zsolt Somogyvári MD, PhD, MSc, from the National Institute of Child Health in Hungary, and Paul Sirbaugh, DO from Texas Children's Hospital.

Dedication

The editorial team is proud to have been able to represent the
transport community with their involvement in this text. We are
greatly indebted to the contributors, reviewers, and staff who have
worked diligently during the past two years to bring this text to print.
We would like to recognize the men and women who perform at
their best on a daily basis, sometimes with limited resources, to
train, become educated, and provide optimal care for those in need
of critical care transport. This relatively new field of medicine has
already had its share of champions, heroes, and superstars. We have
also experienced our share of tragedy and loss. To those who have
worked so hard to build our field and to those who have endured
loss personally or within their team, we dedicate this text.

Mission Statement

The goal of neonatal and pediatric interfacility transport is to enable each patient in need to benefit from available advanced and specialized care. Advances in the critical care of neonates, infants, and older children, as well as regionalization of specialty and critical care personnel, capabilities, and services underscore the need for safe, expert, and efficient interfacility patient transport.

Transport medicine is an integral part of medical care. Optimal initial medical evaluation and stabilization, timely and appropriate transport care, and specialized referral center management will improve outcomes in critically ill or injured neonates, infants, and older children. Transport providers have an opportunity to influence each step in this continuum. Throughout this text, information, education, and guidelines are provided for health care professionals who provide and/or supervise interfacility transport of children. We hope that this material enables the readers to better identify best and standard practices and to optimize their vital activities.

Table of Contents

Introduction to the Third Edition

Twenty years have passed since the first American Academy of Pediatrics publication titled "Guidelines for Air and Ground Transportation of Pediatric Patients." The Task Force on Transport Medicine was organized shortly thereafter and served as a forum for professionals with a common interest in improving the outcome of infants and children who must travel between facilities for specialized pediatric care. The group published a free-standing manual that included updated transport guidelines for both pediatric and neonatal patients. By 1990, the Task Force was elevated to the status of a Section within the American Academy of Pediatrics, which served as an acknowledgment of the growing specialized field of pediatric and neonatal transport medicine.

The modern era of transport medicine incorporates specific practices and principles from the various fields from which it evolved: neonatology, pediatric critical care and emergency medicine, pediatric surgery, trauma, and emergency medical services (EMS) for children. Neonatal and pediatric transport programs permit hospitals to extend critical care services into the community, so that patients will benefit from earlier initiation of essential therapies that would ordinarily not be available until after arrival at a tertiary care facility. The mobile environment has inherent risks and limitations that can be balanced by pretransport stabilization, the presence of qualified professionals, and the use of equipment and monitoring devices that have been adapted for use during transport.

The third edition of the Guidelines represents the collaborative work of authors from a multitude of backgrounds, analogous to the diverse team of professionals who may be involved in neonatal or pediatric transport. Topics of interest to hospital administrators, clinicians, communications personnel, and policy makers are included. In particular, all topics have been significantly updated and revised, while new chapters have been added to further address quality improvement, reimbursement, ethical considerations, legal issues, research, international transport, stress management, integration with EMS, accreditation, family-centered care, and unique clinical transport issues. Although the editors recognize that the document relies heavily on expert opinion and consensus, whenever possible, available evidence has been referenced to support recommendations. Opportunities for research to fill gaps in knowledge have been highlighted in the hopes that our understanding of transport systems and practices will be further advanced by the next generation of providers.

■ ■ ■ ■ ■ ■

■ Organization of a Neonatal-Pediatric ■ Interfacility Transport Service

Outline
■ Background and principles of neonatal-pediatric transport systems
■ Essential components of a neonatal-pediatric transport service
■ Impact of a neonatal-pediatric specialty team

Background and Principles of Neonatal-Pediatric Interfacility Transport

Neonatal-pediatric interfacility transport programs are part of the continuum of care in a system of emergency medical services for children. Specifically, they provide a safe, therapeutic environment for pediatric patients who must be transferred between health care institutions under urgent or emergency circumstances. Regionalization of neonatal and pediatric intensive care has also necessitated the development of specialized interfacility transport services. In the United States, hospital-based neonatal transport programs were created in the 1960s and 1970s, and similar programs for older infants and children emerged in the 1980s. For many critically ill or injured pediatric patients—particularly those being treated at institutions that are unable to provide the level of care required—access to a skilled transport team is essential.

The main goals of a neonatal-pediatric transport team are early stabilization and initiation of advanced care at the referring institution, with continuation of critical care therapies and monitoring en route, so as to improve safety of the transport and patient outcome. The patient's condition should not deteriorate owing to preventable issues during transport and, ideally, is improved by arrival at the receiving hospital. Initial contact with the transport service should allow critical history and physical information to be shared with the appropriate medical control physician (medical control officer [or MCO] or medical command physician [or MCP]; the physician often at the receiving hospital who directs care for the person being transported) and recommendations for care to be provided until the transport team arrives. The transport team continues treatment and monitoring with the expected expertise and capabilities of the tertiary care center while the patient is still in the referring facility. Transition of care from referring hospital to transport team to receiving center should be seamless, without compromise in the level of care or monitoring. This approach differs from the "swoop and scoop" (limited evaluation at the scene, with the goal of the rapid stabilization and transport to an advanced care environment) practice that may be appropriately applied during the prehospital transport of a patient from an accident scene to an emergency department (ED). Most neonatal and pediatric patients will benefit more from an anticipated, coordinated, and organized transport than from one that prioritizes speed over optimal stabilization and care, with the potential exception of patients whose outcomes will be compromised without rapid access to care not available at the referring hospital or in the transport environment, for example, a patient with an expanding intracranial hemorrhage admitted to the ED of an institution without neurosurgical capability.

Essential Components of a Neonatal-Pediatric Transport Service

Interfacility transfer should be performed expeditiously and safely by qualified personnel, with appropriate training and equipment. In this text, the logistical, operational, educational, and care information applies to transport teams providing services to potentially critically ill or injured neonatal and/or pediatric patients. Like other parts of the emergency medical and critical care systems, a neonatal-pediatric transport program must be tailored to the specific needs and resources of the region served. Nevertheless, most larger transport services have certain organizational features in common. The most important is a dedicated team of health care professionals proficient at providing neonatal and/or pediatric critical care, depending on the scope of their mission and patient populations, during transport. In addition, there must be a sufficient volume of critically ill and injured patients to enable team members to maintain their skills and to permit staff to be utilized optimally. Other key components include the following: (1) online (real-time) medical control by qualified medical physicians, (2) ground and/or air ambulance capabilities, (3) communications and dispatch capability, (4) prospectively written clinical and operational guidelines, (5) a comprehensive database allowing for quality and performance improvement activities, (6) medical and nursing direction, (7) administrative resources, and (8) institutional endorsement and support. Subsequent chapters discuss these components and other clinical and organizational factors in more detail.

In most programs, the transport team's composition depends on the patient's anticipated needs and is usually determined in consultation with the team members and medical control physician. Dedicated transport staff can come from a pool of qualified physicians, nurses, nurse practitioners, paramedics, and respiratory therapists. A team member's professional degree is less vital than his or her ability to provide the level of care required in a mobile environment. Providing critical care under transport conditions is significantly different from practicing in an intensive care unit or ED. It should not be assumed that a health care professional who is competent in the intensive care unit will function equally well in the patient compartment of an ambulance or in an unfamiliar hospital ED. In addition to their clinical expertise, team members should have excellent interpersonal skills and the ability to solve problems. Moreover, additional training in transport medicine is mandatory. A senior member of the program who is experienced in transport and talented at teaching should oversee the training. The transport curriculum should include didactic and practical instruction in the clinical and operational aspects of transport medicine.

The referring physician is responsible for determining the type of resources needed during interfacility transport, according to federal regulations that govern the transfer of patients with emergency medical conditions (see Chapter 7). However, it is advisable that those decisions be made after consultation and in conjunction with the neonatal-pediatric transport team, the medical control physician, and the vehicle operator. Ideally, a transport program should have the ability to provide or arrange for transport by ground ambulance, helicopter, and/or fixed-wing aircraft. The recommendation for a

████████████████████████████████████

specific mode of transport should be based on factors such as patient condition, current and available levels of medical care delivery, number of transport staff required, distance to the referring institution, traffic congestion, and weather conditions. Although speed might be a priority, the safety of the crew and patient is of paramount importance.

The number of team members dispatched for a transport is directed by the patient's current and projected needs and is governed by the size and spatial configuration of the vehicle used. Ground ambulances can typically carry up to 3 to 4 caregivers, helicopters 2 to 4, and fixed-wing aircraft 2 to 5, although these may not be the desired or required personnel numbers for any particular transport. Whenever possible, the mode of transport should allow the presence of a family member during the transport. Regardless of mode, the team must be able to mobilize and depart from its origin (base facility, base of operations) quickly. Teams may be stationed at hospitals or strategic off-site locations. A clear distinction of tasks performed by non–health care transport team members (pilots, drivers) from those performed by health care personnel optimizes safety and response time and is cost-effective.

The health care professionals on the team must be able to provide medical care without inordinate concern for the technical aspects of the transport. Similarly, the pilot or ambulance operator must be permitted to function free of distractions or emotive patient data that might impair his or her judgment. At the same time, adequate understanding of each team member's role can improve communication and teamwork, thus improving efficiency and safety.

Providing intensive care in a mobile environment is challenging. Transport teams must function despite potential constraints in staff, equipment, mobility, and space. In addition, it may be difficult—sometimes impossible—to assess a patient or perform certain procedures while working in a moving vehicle, especially a smaller helicopter. Therefore, major therapies needed to stabilize the patient's condition or to ensure against decompensation en route should be considered and/or performed before departure from the referring facility. The team member's threshold for performing interventions such as airway management may be lower than if the patient were already at the tertiary care center owing to the differences in environment and resources during the transport.

"Reverse" (back or return) transport involves return of the patient to the referring hospital when clinically appropriate; this practice encourages efficient use of the region's neonatal and pediatric critical care resources and promotes cooperation among institutions. Consideration should be given to policies encouraging the transport of infants and children back to the referring facility if further inpatient care remains necessary and can be safely managed by the institution and its personnel. Transfer agreements specific to each referring institution are useful, especially if they include criteria for patient acceptance and return transport. One potential issue with this practice is that third-party payers might question the necessity or benefit of back transport and hospitalization at the referring hospital and challenge payment for the transport or hospital components. Lack of flexibility for this process can put undue stress on the family and can affect care and capacity at the referring and receiving hospitals.

Impact of a Neonatal-Pediatric Specialty Team

Specialized and regionalized intensive care services for infants and children improve patient outcome. Likewise, there is a potential benefit to patients from transport by teams with pediatric and neonatal training, experience, and specific supervision. As with other areas of pediatric health care, not all institutions or regions have access to specialized neonatal-pediatric transport services. In locations where the available transport team primarily serves an adult patient population, it may be desirable to have hospital-based neonatal or pediatric specialists accompany the team to provide additional expertise. Hospital-based providers should be oriented to equipment and should understand safety considerations before the transport. This type of cooperative relationship should be extended proactively to include educational activities and case reviews for the benefit of all parties involved.

In other areas, there may be multiple neonatal-pediatric transport services within a region. In these areas, it is beneficial to all to ensure that the services communicate and cooperate with each other. Merging individual services into a regional transport program should be considered, with the expectation that a regional program could be more effective and efficient.

■■■■■■■■■■■■■■■■■■■■■■■■■■■■■■■

Selected Readings

Hatherill M, Waggie Z, Reynolds L, Argent A. Transport of critically ill children in a resource-limited setting. *Intensive Care Med.* 2003;29:1414–1416

MacDonald MG, Ginzburg HM, eds. *Guidelines for Air and Ground Transport of Neonatal and Pediatric Patients.* 2nd ed. Elk Grove Village, IL: American Academy of Pediatrics; 1999

Warren J, Fromm RE Jr, Orr RA, Rotello LC, Horst HM. Guidelines for the inter- and intrahospital transport of critically ill patients. *Crit Care Med.* 2004;32:256–262

Woodward GA, Insoft RM, Pearson-Shaver AL, et al. The state of pediatric interfacility transport: consensus of the second National Pediatric and Neonatal Interfacility Transport Medicine Leadership Conference. *Pediatr Emerg Care.* 2002;18:38–43

Questions

1. Which of the following statements about neonatal-pediatric interfacility transport is *true?*
   a. The concept of "swoop and scoop" is optimal for prehospital emergency care and interfacility transport of infants and children.
   b. The level of care and monitoring always decreases because of the need to transfer the patient between institutions.
   c. There are significant differences between taking care of pediatric patients in the intensive care unit as compared with the transport environment.
2. Which factors influence the decision to transport by ground ambulance vs rotor-wing aircraft?
   a. Patient condition
   b. Distance to the referring institution
   c. Weather
   d. Terrain
   e. All of the above
3. All of the following are true of neonatal-pediatric transport teams *except:*
   a. Specialized training and equipment are essential.
   b. Team composition should always include a physician.
   c. Online medical control and written protocols guide practice.
   d. Team members should have excellent communication and teamwork skills.

Answers

1. c
2. e
3. b

Transport Program Administration

Outline

- What is a mission statement? Will it help?
- Effective administration
- A word on how to manage
- Cost, quality of care, and staff education and how they interact
- Scope of practice and licensure and certification requirements
- Transport in support of resident education
- Insurance needs and options
- Relationships with referral personnel
- Patient condition for transfer
- Communication between facilities

Like other organizations, transport teams require a clear vision to achieve objectives and enable managers and administration to meet important organizational goals. Within this framework, administrators who are part of the team, within the sponsoring organization but not part of the team, and from referring hospitals must all understand the team structure and function. As with many businesses, transport systems must operate within justifiable and often relatively fixed budgets. In the chapter, we describe administrative issues important to successful administration of a transport team.

This chapter makes reference in general to transport team leadership, hospital administrators, and transport administration. Administrative roles, leadership qualifications, and responsibilities are discussed more specifically in Chapter 4. Reference to transport team administrative leadership in this chapter refers to titles such as *transport team program director, transport team medical director,* and *transport team coordinator.* Hospital or institutional administrative leadership refers to members of the hospital administrative leadership team responsible for program coordination, development, and monitoring.

What Is a Mission Statement? Will it Help?

Business authors suggest that mission statements are plans that allow an organization to direct efforts that address critical strategic objectives.[1-4] In other words, a mission statement helps an organization stay on track by creating a template for goals and objectives and a measure by which to judge success. Unlike vision statements that describe an organization's philosophy and aspirations, mission statements help an organization develop short-term objectives to meet immediate goals. The best mission statements are developed as part of a strategic planning process, and input is solicited from all stakeholders, perhaps even competitors. Ideally, a mission statement is created after an environmental or SWOT (Strengths, Weakness, Opportunities, and Threats) analysis has been performed and goals and objectives have been stated. The product of a logical planning process, the mission statement should be clear and concise. It will be a more valuable tool if it is simple enough to be understood, real enough to be practical, and able to be recited by all members of the organization. Ideally, the statement is short enough to be memorized and sincere enough to be believed by all levels of the organization. As a tool, the mission focuses organizational efforts on the tasks at hand. The mission statement not only should reflect the transport team goals, but also should incorporate and support the institutional goals as the two relate to each other. Once developed, the statement must be disseminated widely to reach all stakeholders. Because its scope is short-term, a mission statement requires frequent revision.

Because organizations are unique, mission statements will reflect the unique aspects of the organizations that develop them. Similar to other organizations, transport teams can benefit from strong mission statements that reflect the goals of the institutions they represent. Although teams could develop independent statements, they would be less meaningful if not in concert with the mission of the sponsoring organization. Practically, proposals for additional resources or programs should reference the sponsoring organization's mission statement and describe how the proposed change will help the sponsoring hospital meet its objectives. Similarly, core services must be consistent with the organization's and the team's mission.

Effective Administration

Although the transport team members might serve in administrative and clinical roles, the team also requires support from the sponsoring organization's administrators. Ideally, one person will be assigned as the administrative liaison to the transport program and will be responsible for managing and monitoring issues related to team functions that are under the purview of hospital administration. The administrative liaison supervises contracts, the financial impact of the transport team on the sponsoring institution, and other issues of institutional interest. Because the liaison often does not have extensive clinical transport experience, it becomes important for the transport team leadership (ie, transport team program director and transport team medical director) to educate and partner with the liaison concerning issues related to the provision of care during transports. Effective communication with institutional administrators will improve the transport team's ability to gain additional resources when the need arises.

In many hospitals, nursing resources are evaluated and allocated by nursing supervisors on a shift-to-shift basis. When transport team members also serve as staff nurses in the hospital, their patient assignments should be flexible enough to be easily and efficiently transferred should a call for transport be received. When staffing is limited and a transport nurse is without a current patient assignment, justifying the down time to nontransport personnel or managers can be challenging, but reassignment without planning for a potential transport need can be problematic as well. Asking or expecting a transport nurse to take a patient assignment that cannot be easily transferred can cause delays in departure when an urgent medical need and transport request arises. There may be opportunities, however, to use the procedural skills of the transport team elsewhere in the facility (eg, ancillary intravenous team), with the caveat that they should not be expected to be present at all times. If these services are vital and expected by the hospital, the transport team can offer staffing assistance but should not assume total responsibility.

■■■■■■■■■■■■■■■■■■■■■■■■■■■■■■■■■

It is important for the transport team's leadership personnel to have knowledge of the financial health of the program and its impact on the financial status of the sponsoring institution. They should be conversant about the team's finances and have recent data that describe the team's activity, referral base, and costs. Because the transport team's direct costs might be high, it is imperative that the team's leadership maintain an understanding of financial issues related to team operation and how the team affects the hospital's margin. Active involvement of the hospital's finance department can prove valuable. Appropriate financial information should be available to leadership of the hospital and the transport team, if these are separate entities, to enable them to make the most appropriate fiscal decisions.

It is important to cultivate relationships with referral facilities to improve market share and the quality of patient care. In the current financial climate, many smaller hospitals are decreasing pediatric subspecialty services and referring more children to tertiary pediatric facilities. Transfer agreements that define the responsibilities of the referring and receiving hospital are being more frequently used. Typically, transfer agreements establish policies that clearly define administrative procedures, professional responsibilities, and patient care goals. Many transfer agreements determine the level of care expected at each facility and might also address reimbursement issues. These agreements might also guarantee or streamline acceptance of acutely ill patients by the receiving hospital and establish the expectation that chronically ill and recuperating patients will return to the referring facility in a timely manner. Transfer agreements must, however, comply with local, state, and federal mandates.

Effective relationships between the administrative staffs of referring and receiving hospitals will improve the ability of each facility to monitor transfer activity and intervene when problems are at a manageable stage. Because negotiating authority might rest with nontransport administrative and legal staffs of referring and receiving hospitals, it is the responsibility of transport team leadership to educate and partner with those participants about neonatal-pediatric transport team services.

A Word on How to Manage

Management texts suggest that leaders identify and communicate a vision consistent with the direction of the organization. They understand where the organization is going and work to move the organization in an appropriate direction. Managers are responsible for implementing the leader's vision through a clearly articulated mission that is supported by goals and objectives. All managers must also be leaders and direct subordinates to accomplish goals and objectives that satisfy the organization's mission. An important feature of an organization's leadership is the degree to which managers and leaders are accountable for their performance. Both should be accountable to stakeholders for accomplishment of goals and objectives.

Adults are intrinsically motivated and invest in that which is valuable to them. The effective manager understands that employees seek work that is valuable, sustains an important self-image, and allows individual aspirations to be met. To negotiate successful assignments, managers must clearly communicate expectations, define the expected quality and quantity of the finished assignment, identify a deadline, and identify available resources. When justified, the manager may need to make additional resources available. An effective manager monitors progress and offers appropriate feedback. The successful manager is a good coach who supports and encourages team members while holding them accountable for their performance.

Cost, Quality of Care, and Staff Education and How They Interact

Transport teams are expensive. The cost to provide the service includes vehicle maintenance and repairs (significant even if the need is met by a vendor contract), the cost of durable equipment (eg, monitors, infusion pumps), the cost of disposable supplies (eg, syringes, tubing), medication costs, the expense to maintain a communications center (possibly its own cost center with component costs), marketing costs, and personnel salaries and benefits. As in other areas of health care, personnel costs remain the largest share of a transport team's budget. Transport team staff might be more expensive than some hospital department staff because they tend to be more experienced and have greater seniority.

Transport team staff require additional education to provide the level of care required in the field. Recent work published in the nursing literature suggests that the increased cost to educate transport staff members is a worthy investment. Prowse and Lyne[5] suggest that knowledge gained from literature and lectures becomes effective and clinically useful when placed into context by practice. Regardless of their personal knowledge base, the participants in that study were noted to improve effective (practical) knowledge through exposure to new information (study of the literature or participation in discussions regarding a topic of interest) and practical application. Furthermore, participants were motivated to improve knowledge by a significant clinical event and the desire to improve their personal practice.

Other work suggests that in addition to improving personal and effective knowledge, the level of staff education and the caliber of educational programs are associated with improved clinical outcomes. Aiken et al[6] noted that the risk of mortality was lower and patient outcomes improved in surgical units staffed by bachelor-prepared nurses. White[7] demonstrated the ability of a nursing intervention program to directly impact patient care by improving pain assessment management by nursing staff for postoperative patients.

Given these findings, it becomes apparent that time and money invested in transport team staff education is well spent. Orientation programs must develop a basic level of knowledge required to allow staff to independently care for patients in the field. Continuing education is clearly important to increase referential knowledge that will become effective knowledge with increased experience. In the final analysis, improved education of transport staff translates into improved patient outcomes.

Scope of Practice and Licensure and Certification Requirements

Licensure and certification are requirements used to encourage advanced education among staff members. Many transport teams require various certifications as a method of improving staff competence and ensuring a core knowledge base. Available courses include the following:

- Advanced Cardiac Life Support (ACLS)
- Basic Life Support (BLS)

- Pediatric Advanced Life Support (PALS)
- Advanced Pediatric Life Support (APLS)
- Neonatal Resuscitation Program (NRP)
- Trauma Nursing Core Course (TNCC)
- Emergency Nurses Pediatric Course (ENPC)
- Critical Care Emergency Medical Transport Program (CCEMTP)
- S.T.A.B.L.E. (Sugar, Temperature, Artificial breathing, Blood pressure, Lab work, and Emotional support)
- Advanced Care of the Resuscitated Newborn (ACoRN)
- Critical Care Registered Nurse (CCRN)
- Neonatal/Pediatric Specialist Credential (NPS) (respiratory therapy)
- Pediatric Education for Prehospital Professionals (PEPP)
- Advanced Trauma Life Support (ATLS)
- Basic Trauma Life Support (BTLS)

Each course exposes participants to issues important to the assessment, stabilization, and management of critically ill and/or injured pediatric and neonatal patients. Because the causes and manifestations of respiratory failure, shock, cardiopulmonary arrest, and arrhythmias in children differ from those in adults, it is imperative that teams transporting neonates, infants, and children thoroughly understand the principles of neonatal and pediatric resuscitation. One should not assume, or promote, competency in neonatal-pediatric transport based solely on personnel attendance and successful completion of certification courses. These courses must be accompanied by significant additional and ongoing education, exposure, and experience to maximize clinical competence and quality of care.

Transport team leadership should determine educational and certification requirements for team members. Teams that transfer only neonatal patients might require certifications specific to their patient population, whereas teams that transfer neonatal patients, pediatric patients, and adults will have additional requirements. Each organization and team member must be committed to the care of critically ill patients. Further education and certifications will provide team members with the necessary knowledge to provide the required care for critically ill children. Registered nurses, respiratory therapists, and paramedics enter their professional life through various educational routes (associate's degree, bachelor's degree, or master's degree); many teams are requiring staff to be bachelor's or master's prepared.

██

Attending physicians who provide medical control to the team must be licensed to practice medicine in the state where the base facility is located, and, ideally, they will be trained and certified in pediatric emergency medicine, pediatric critical care medicine, or neonatology. If physicians in training (fellows or residents) are part of the transport team, requirements for participation must be developed. Many programs require fellows who participate in transport to have advanced clinical experience in resuscitation and advanced airway skills. Compliance with training requirements and preparation for clinical transport experience should be documented by the fellowship training director.

Licensure to practice is a state requirement, and transport team members must be licensed for their profession according to the regulations of the state in which they work. Individual states might require that health care professionals retrieving and treating patients in a state other than that of their base of operations maintain the same credentials as health care professionals practicing in that state or might request a copy of the credentials for the same health care professionals. Paramedics have the option of national certification, but local licensure is still required. It is optimal for the base hospital to maintain records of licensure and certification as part of employment files. Similarly, physician-credentialing files should include evidence that medical licenses, board certifications, and other required endorsements are current.

Standard operating guidelines, protocols, and scope of practice should be defined for transport team members by the team's leadership. Protocols allow the team to function if there is a change in a patient's condition and the medical control physician cannot be immediately contacted. Because changes in condition can occur that require treatment but are not covered by a physician's orders, standard operating protocols provide consistent guidance until contact with the medical control physician can be reestablished.

The scope of practice defines a skill set for each team member. Periodic assessments of skill to determine competence should be performed and the results documented in personnel records. If the team is not able to provide an appropriate intervention owing to a need for specialty equipment, medications, or personnel, the team should divert to the closest receiving hospital. Transport team personnel should notify the receiving hospital of the diversion and the patient's status as soon as possible. No transport personnel should be placed in a position of monitoring, administering a drug, or performing a procedure outside their scope of practice or in an unstable environment.

As per the Emergency Medical Treatment and Active Labor Act (EMTALA), the transferring physician has the final responsibility for the appropriateness of the transferring team and personnel (along with mode of transport; see Chapter 7 on legal issues). Ideally this decision is accomplished in conjunction with the transport team and/or receiving personnel. These decisions must be made on the basis of the severity of the patient's illness, physical assessment findings, treatment requirements, and support requirements. To improve patient safety, knowledge of the transport environment and local options for transfer should be understood. At all times, the transport team should be well versed and trained in the care and support of critically ill neonatal and pediatric patients.

Transport in Support of Resident Education

Interfacility transport requires a unique set of skills, distinct from the traditional training of most hospital-based residency training programs. It is essential that personnel used to provide care during interfacility transport be properly trained, familiar with the unique demands of providing care during ground or air transport, and prepared to handle the variety of patient contingencies that might arise during transport. Providing an educational experience for residents in transport medicine is desirable but may present challenges in the service area. Because patient care must not be compromised, personnel in training who are not trained or capable of fully participating in the care of the patient should not replace experienced transport team members. Practically, space for inclusion of additional personnel in training during the transport process might be an issue with limited space vehicles. The Accreditation Council for Graduate Medical Education (ACGME) states that general pediatrics residency training programs must offer residents a minimum of two 1-month blocks of pediatric emergency and acute care medicine and exposure to emergency medical services. Given these requirements, it would seem that active participation of pediatric residents on transport teams is desirable, but this must be accomplished in a manner that ensures maximal quality and efficiency of the care provided. Furthermore, ACGME work-hour constraints might present programmatic challenges for programs interested in including a transport rotation or transport call to augment the emergency and acute care medicine requirements.

Residency and fellowship training programs that include transport medicine as a rotation should develop and require a specific curriculum for physicians in training. To be consistent with ACGME requirements, the syllabus should reflect specific educational goals, expectations, and measurable objectives. An assessment of the trainee's performance that measures the degree to which educational objectives were met is required at the completion of the rotation. Finally, adherence to resident work rules, which limit the number of continuous hours house staff may work and the cumulative hours of work in a given week, is mandatory.

Because traditional rotations in the pediatric residency are geared toward managing inpatients and ambulatory care patients, pediatric residents might not be specifically educated about the management of critically ill transport patients. If pediatric residents are to be part of a transport team, specific transport, critical care, and neonatal medicine education should be developed and presented before these physicians are included in the transport process. Studies are warranted to determine whether pediatric resident involvement in a transport medicine rotation improves the resident's level of skill and confidence and adds value to the service.

To ensure the quality of patient care, scopes of practice, policies, and educational guidelines must be developed to outline duties of all personnel, including physicians in training (residents and fellows) who serve on transport teams. A separate training curriculum should be developed that includes instruction in pretransport evaluation, triage, communication, transport safety, and medical management of critically ill patients who require transfer. Specific educational needs can be identified by a thorough practice analysis. These analyses will be required to identify knowledge gaps and steer the development of bridging curricula.

Insurance Needs and Options

Participants

Because transport team members are exposed to activities that might place them at greater risk of injuries or death, program administrators are often asked to provide additional insurance coverage for them while in the transport environment.

Team members must be adequately covered for the risks undertaken during transport on a daily basis. Unlike personnel who function solely in a hospital environment, transport team members are exposed to a higher risk of accidents during ground and air transports. Although it has been determined that collisions and crashes by pediatric and neonatal teams are uncommon, collective data suggest that 1 collision or crash occurs for every 1000 patient transports. Collisions or crashes involving injury or death are less common and occur at rate of approximately 0.546 per 1000 transports. Although death occurs most frequently as the result of aircraft crashes, ground collisions accounted for most transport-related injuries. Injuries sustained during ground collisions tend to be moderate to severe and in a category that can affect a victim's ability to work (see Chapter 10).

Patients

Hodge[8] states that the growth of managed care has provided health benefits to millions of children while attempting to control the increase in health care costs. Transport team administrators find that third-party payers frequently require preapproval for transport coverage. Many programs have found it important to proactively work and partner with third-party payers and define groups of patients who will meet criteria for transport. Medicaid rules and notification requirements are different in each state, and, as new programs are developed, Medicaid reimbursement can be adjusted or denied. It is, therefore, important for transport team administrators to remain aware of Medicaid reimbursement rules and trends in their respective states to ensure optimal Medicaid reimbursement. This is vital for programs that serve multiple states by virtue of location or specialty service. For those who currently, or foresee, transfer and care of patients with out-of-state government sources of reimbursement, anticipatory negotiations can reap significant dividends for patients, families, and transport and hospital services and can increase efficiency of the entire process.

Federal regulations protecting the right of patients to receive adequate emergency evaluation and care have been in effect for some time. It is important that transport personnel understand COBRA (Consolidated Omnibus Budget Reconciliation Act) and EMTALA regulations and requirements that must be met by referring and receiving facilities before a patient is transferred (see Chapter 7). Patients must be adequately evaluated in the facility from which they seek initial care, life-threatening conditions must be stabilized to the best of the providers' and facility's capabilities, and a facility that can provide an appropriate level of care for a patient's condition must be located and a receiving physician identified before transport to comply with EMTALA guidelines. Stabilizing medical care for critically ill children must be provided regardless of the family's ability to pay or the patient's insurance status.

Relationships With Referral Personnel

It is not uncommon for neonatal-pediatric transport teams to coordinate patient care and transfer. Referral personnel and organizations can benefit from development of a professional working relationship with the receiving facility. It is not uncommon for facilities to refer patients owing to managed care contracts. Transport teams can collaborate to facilitate transfer of patients to appropriate levels of care. It can be cost-effective for teams to work together when providing staff education opportunities and periodic tabletop transfer scenario drills.

Teams that perform only ground transports should develop a strong working relationship with services that provide rotor- and fixed-wing transports (and vice versa). This relationship will allow for optimal coordination of transport efforts when requests for critically ill children are time-sensitive or involve long distances. Patient transport care and options should not be limited to the services provided by a local or preferred vendor or service if that vendor or service has a limited array of transport staffing or transportation mode alternatives.

Patient Condition for Transfer

Stabilization of the patient before transfer should include adequate evaluation and initiation of treatment to ensure the transfer will not, within reasonable medical probability, result in death or loss or serious impairment of bodily functions, parts, or organs. It is recognized that there are times when complete stabilization is not possible because the referring facility does not have the personnel or equipment needed. In such cases, the patient should be stabilized to the best of the ability of the referring physician, staff, and facility and then promptly transferred by the most expert personnel. No transfer should be made without the consent of the patient and/or family and receiving physician and, if a standard in the local area, confirmation of acceptance from the receiving hospital's respective unit.

Transfers from patient care areas of an acute care hospital require that the patient (when applicable) and the family be informed of the reason(s) for transfer and the destination proposed by the transferring facility. The family's (and patient's when applicable) written consent for the transfer should be obtained, if possible. For patients who are wards of the state or cared for in areas where their guardian is not immediately accessible, anticipation of and potential for transfer and care in a local facility, as well as prospective transfer to a specialty facility, should be anticipated, authorized, and documented before a need arises. All patient records and copies of pertinent patient information, including diagnostic imaging and laboratory values, should be transferred with the patient. If not available at the time of transfer, test results may be faxed or telephoned as soon as possible to the receiving institution.

Communication Between Facilities

There must be clear communication between the sending and receiving personnel when a child needs to be transferred. The referring hospital must provide enough information about the child's condition for the receiving hospital to help determine the appropriate level and mode of transport, to advise on further care until the referral center is reached, and to arrange appropriate services at the definitive location. When a critical care transport team arrives at a referring facility, staff at the referring facility should be available and prepared to work with transport team members to the best of their ability, ensuring that the information flow, patient care, and handoff are complete, optimal, and seamless.

Once the patient has reached the receiving hospital, information about the patient's condition and care given during the transport should be sent back to the referring physician and staff in a timely manner. This information might be especially important when parents or other family members cannot accompany the child during the transfer or reach the receiving hospital promptly. Alternative methods and numbers for contacting family members about medical updates, changes in required therapies, and/or obtaining consents should be determined before the transport. It is important for all parties in the transfer process to communicate clearly to avoid misunderstandings that might adversely affect patient care. The receiving hospital should also inform the staff who cared for the child at the transferring hospital about the child's status during the hospital stay if permission has been granted by the patient and/or family and communications are within the scope of the regulations in the Health Information Portability and Accountability Act (also known as HIPAA).

The appropriateness of care given, timeliness of referral, and review of any problematic or exceptional issues that occurred should be provided to the referring personnel at a later time, in a constructive manner, to encourage thoughtful and joint evaluation of the care provided and the preparation for transport. Teams also should encourage and solicit feedback from referring personnel on their perceptions of the quality and delivery of the transport services.

References

1. Drohan WM. Writing a mission statement. *Assoc Manage.* 1999;51:117
2. Bart CK. Making mission statements count. *CA Magazine.* 1999;132:37–40
3. Bailey JA. Measuring your mission. *Manage Accounting.* 1996;78:44–46
4. Cohen S. Live your mission statement. *Nurs Manage.* 2001;32:13
5. Prowse MA, Lyne PA. Clinical effectiveness in the post-anesthesia care unit: how nursing knowledge contributes to achieving intended patient outcomes. *J Adv Nurs.* 2000;31:1115–1124
6. Aiken LH, Clarke SP, Cheung RB, Sloane DM, Silber JH. Educational levels of hospital nurses and surgical patient mortality. *JAMA.* 2003;290:1617–1623

7. White CL. Changing pain management practice and impacting on patient outcomes. *Clin Nurse Spec.* 1999;13:166–172
8. Hodge D. Managed care and the pediatric emergency department. *Pediatr Clin North Am.* 1999;46:1329–1340

Selected Readings

Bengo A. The outlook is bright for critical care nurses. *Crit Care Nurse Suppl.* February 2002:6

Buchnan J. Health sector reform and human resources: lessons from the United Kingdom. *Health Policy Plann.* 2000;15:319–325

Cunning SM. Avoid common management pitfalls. *Nurs Manage.* 2004;35:18

Hooker R, Berlin L. Trends in the supply of physician assistants and nurse practitioners in the United States. *Health Aff.* (Millwood) 2002;21:174–181

Jaques E. Managerial accountability. *J Qual Participation.* 1992;15:40–44

Jaques E, Cason K. *Human Capability.* Falls Church, VA: Cason Hall & Co; 1994

King B, Woodward G. Pediatric critical care transport: the safety of the journey: a five-year review of vehicular collisions involving pediatric and neonatal transport teams. *Prehosp Emerg Care.* 2002;6:449–454

Kraines GA. Essential organization. In: *Leadership for Physician Executives.* Boston, MA: The Levinson Institute; 1999

Moyers E. Principles of leadership: think and communicate. *Vital Speeches of the Day.* 2000;66:595–598

Regional news: South. *Mod Healthcare.* September 2000;30:34

Wright JN. Mission and reality and why not? *J Change Manage.* 2002;3:30–44

Questions

1. Which of the following conditions would *not* warrant a critical care pediatric transport referral?
   a. The patient requires a higher level of care.
   b. The patient's acute condition has been stabilized for the present, but further evaluation or management is needed.
   c. The patient's family (not the medical providers) is requesting a transfer for a patient in stable condition.
   d. The patient's health insurance supports the accepting facility.
2. Transport staff must be educationally prepared and competent to transport patients. It is the administrator's responsibility to ensure staff competencies. List 5 national course certifications available for transport team staff members.
3. Productive relationships with referral hospitals can be established by using all of the following methods *except:*
   a. providing staff education during outreach at the referral facility.
   b. completing annual drills involving referral staff and transport staff.
   c. providing immediate, corrective criticism at the bedside when the child's care is thought to have been mismanaged.
   d. encouraging coordination of multidisciplinary, professional referrals.

Answers

1. c
2. Advanced Cardiac Life Support (ACLS)
   Basic Life Support (BLS)
   Pediatric Advanced Life Support (PALS)
   Advanced Pediatric Life Support (APLS)
   Neonatal Resuscitation Program (NRP)
   Trauma Nursing Core Course (TNCC)
   Emergency Nurses Pediatric Course (ENPC)
   Critical Care Emergency Medical Transport Program (CCEMTP)
   S.T.A.B.L.E. (Sugar, Temperature, Artificial breathing, Blood pressure, Lab work, and Emotional support)
   Advanced Care of the Resuscitated Newborn (ACoRN)
   Critical Care Registered Nurse (CCRN)
   Neonatal/Pediatric Specialist Credential (NPS) (respiratory therapy)
   Pediatric Education for Prehospital Professionals (PEPP)
   Advanced Trauma Life Support (ATLS)
   Basic Trauma Life Support (BTLS)
3. c

■ Transport Team Clinicians, Health Care ■ Professionals, and Team Composition

Outline

■ Team composition
■ Personnel selection
■ Training

Team composition and educational processes vary considerably between transport programs. The choice of personnel usually depends on the availability of professionals in the base (sponsoring) facility, the anticipated patient population, financial support for the program, and other practical considerations. A transport program might choose a standard team composition or might vary the configuration depending on the nature of an individual transport request. Teams that transport a relatively similar population of patients (eg, neonates) are more likely to have a standardized team composition than teams that transport a more heterogeneous group, such as pediatric medical, surgical, and cardiac patients or patients with widely variable acuities. Training needs depend on the role of a specific professional group in the care of transported patients, their experience in neonatal-pediatric health care, and their familiarity with the transport environment. Guidelines for determining team composition, selecting personnel, and training are outlined in detail in this and the next chapters.

Team Composition

The patient population defined as *pediatric* is diverse and can range from premature newborns to adults receiving care for conditions developed during childhood. Transport locations can be limited to interfacility locations or might include prehospital medical and trauma locations. A variety of health care providers participate in

■■■■■■■■■■■■■■■■■■■■■■■■■■■■■■■■

the care of these patients and might be considered candidates for participating in the transport team (Table 3-1):

■ Specialty-trained attending physicians (eg, intensivists, emergency medicine physicians, neonatologists)
■ Transport physicians (eg, pediatricians with or without subspecialty training, hospitalists)
■ Physicians in training (eg, fellows, residents) (see chapters 2 and 4)
■ Advanced practitioners (eg, nurse practitioners, physician assistants)
■ Critical care, emergency, or neonatal nurses
■ Respiratory therapists
■ Paramedics
■ Emergency medical technicians

The choice of a particular type of professional might depend on the level of responsibility one is credentialed for or routinely assumes in the inpatient setting and on the availability of specific types of practitioners and other factors. The responsibilities of individual team members should take into consideration licensure, education, training, experience, and program policies. Many dedicated pediatric (nonneonatal) transport teams traditionally included a resident or attending physician, although there is little published evidence that this configuration results in improved outcome compared with nonphysician teams. Many neonatal teams are led by certified nurse practitioners or advanced practice nurses, a configuration that has been well accepted in the transport industry. Many programs that transport a significant volume of older pediatric patients have transitioned to the use of nonphysician transport team members while maintaining the option to include a physician on selected transports.

Consideration must be given to the allowable scope of practice of transport team members and established state, local, and program standards when determining team composition. The choice of personnel also might be strongly influenced by the need to fill other workforce needs within the primary facility. For example, these might include the following:

■ The need for care providers with advanced skills within intensive care units
■ Other care demands within the primary facility
■ The need of a particular service to use transport experience as an incentive for hiring personnel

Table 3-1: Potential Advantages and Disadvantages of Various Personnel for Neonatal-Pediatric Transport Teams

Transport Personnel	Advantages	Disadvantages
Specialty-trained attending physician	Expertise; public relations; critical care training and skills	High salary cost; limited availability for full-time coverage; care and supervision limited to 1 patient at a time
Non–intensive care-, nonneonatology-, or non–emergency medicine-trained attending physician	Expertise; public relations	High salary cost; limited availability for full-time coverage; care and supervision limited to 1 patient at a time; critical care skill acquisition as needed
Fellow	Expertise; valuable training experience	Transport demands might overburden training availability; availability might be limited by ACGME work rules
Resident	Valuable training experience; salary cost may be built into the training program	Demands of transport compete with other aspects of training and education; limited clinical experience; availability might be limited by ACGME work rules
Advanced practice neonatal or pediatric nurse practitioner	Expertise; consistent quality of care	High salary costs; usually limited to discipline for which they are trained (eg, neonatal nurse practitioner vs pediatric nurse practitioner); acceptance as specialized provider by referring care team can be an issue if community expectations are for physician-led team
Critical care nurse	Availability; expertise with appropriate training; uniform quality of care	Initial acceptance by referring care team can be an issue; requires intensive training to function independently in the transport environment
Respiratory therapist	Focused respiratory assessments; knowledge of respiratory equipment; advanced airway and ventilatory expertise	Focused airway training and experience; requires intensive training to expand to more global patient care
Paramedic or emergency medical technicians	Expertise in prehospital setting; availability; less costly than other team members	Lesser formal medical and pediatric training and perhaps experience; requires intensive training to assist with other areas of patient care

ACGME indicates Accreditation Council for Graduate Medical Education.

Some pediatric and emergency medicine residency programs require trainees to participate in transport medicine. Most residents report that transport experience is valuable and provides them with an important perspective on the differences in care resources and provision outside a specialty or tertiary facility. The intermittent incorporation of rotating trainees can be challenging for a busy critical care team, so it is important that there be discussions in advance about the roles and responsibilities of residents on the team. Limitations imposed by trainees' restricted schedules combined with the unpredictable nature of transport activities might make the residents less available for participation in transport. If residents are to work as members of the transport team, there should be a clear understanding and delineation of the educational goals of the rotation and the role of the trainee on the team (see Chapter 2).

Personnel Selection

The team member selection process is critical to the success of a program. A primary determinant of the type of team members to be selected is the specific staffing requirements of the transport program in terms of roles and responsibilities. Team members should be selected on the basis of their experience and competence in the care of children in the inpatient setting and on other personality traits required for success. Human resource colleagues can be invaluable in preparing the team managers and directors for the interviewing and decision-making processes. The team members should collectively have the ability to provide a level of care that is similar to that of the admitting unit. It is imperative for the team leader to have excellent assessment skills specific to the transport patient population. Beyond basic certification or licensure, some services require completion of one or more certification programs (see Chapter 2 and Appendix E). These certification programs can be provided as a component of the initial and/or recurrent training programs. The possession of personality traits that ensure a high level of performance in the variable and sometimes unpredictable transport environment is crucial. These include leadership, flexibility, independence, initiative, intelligence, inquisitiveness, and ability to solve problems and exercise good clinical judgment. Transport personnel must demonstrate excellent interpersonal and communication skills. Team members must have good crisis management skills, with the ability to negotiate, defuse stressful situations, and safely improvise as needed.

Training

Preparing a team of professionals, particularly a multidisciplinary team, to reach the level of expertise required to transport critically ill infants and children can be a daunting task. The guidelines in Chapter 4 include suggested content and format for training programs. By necessity, they are generic but are intended to be adaptable to the wide variety of professionals who participate in neonatal-pediatric transport. They have been developed under the assumption that trainees will have had considerable experience in the care of critically ill neonatal and/or pediatric patients in the inpatient setting, acute care setting, or both. Reaching proficiency in all areas may not be necessary for all team members, as long as at least 1 team member during each transport has achieved the requisite level of expertise. For example, programs that include intensivists on every transport need not train nonphysician personnel to be the primary providers of advanced airway intervention. However, it is preferable that all members understand the principles and typical process of every technique so that they are best able to offer assistance and comple-ment each other during the transport. The team should also have general medical and trauma stabilization and emergency response skills in case these are needed during a transport.

Although the specific requirements of initial training depend on the professional background of team members, their experience, and roles in patient care, the goals and general content of training are the same, regardless of the type of personnel. The team transport-ing a critically ill pediatric patient should include at least 1 member who is experienced in assessment, diagnosis, and treatment of life-threatening illnesses or injuries in neonates and children. This team member must understand pathophysiology, pharmacology, and the usual clinical course and complications of common neonatal and pediatric illnesses and the nuances of the transport environment. Ideally, all personnel have sufficient knowledge, training, skills, and ability to assume the team leader role as required. Cross-training of personnel in this regard will improve the ability to understand roles and should enhance a coordinated team approach. The team leader must also understand the use of appropriate laboratory and radiographic tests as diagnostic aids and have experience in managing neonates and children who require intensive pharmacologic intervention. Other team members must be familiar with pediatric and neonatal critical care so as to effectively provide apprpropriate support to the team leader.

The team should be capable of performing all standard emergency and stabilization interventions, management, and procedures required in the care of critically ill neonates and children. A high level of expertise in performance of and confidence in procedural decision making and implementation is necessary because those interventions are often performed under less than optimal conditions (eg, in a moving vehicle, with limited lighting and space, without redundant personnel). Even a low failure rate may be unacceptable if the procedure is potentially lifesaving.

All transport team members should be adept at communication during transport. A critical aspect of communication is an understanding of the milieu of the referring hospital and the sensitivity surrounding transport. Team members must have finely tuned public relations skills because they are the "ambassadors" of the receiving facility. Clear, thoughtful, and collegial communications with the referring personnel are essential and occasionally challenging during the stressful situations surrounding a critically ill child. Open and direct communication among team members also is important. It is essential for all team members to function together as a group to provide safe, competent care. Team members must be clear and precise when discussing actions and plans. They also must communicate well with families under stress. The team members are often the first representatives from the receiving (definitive) care location that the family will meet and might be first medical professionals encountered with specific pediatric or neonatal skills. The impressions made at this time will carry forward throughout the patient's hospitalization and beyond.

Selected Readings

Commission on Accreditation of Medical Transport Systems (CAMTS). *Accreditation Standards.* 5th ed. Sandy Springs, SC: 2002

Gomez M. Hiring, staffing, and team composition. In: McCloskey KA, Orr RA, eds. *Pediatric Transport Medicine.* St Louis, MO: Mosby; 1995:89–99

Lee SK, Zupnancic JA, Sale J, et al. Cost-effectiveness and choice of infant transport systems. *Med Care.* 2002;40:705–716

Leslie A, Stephenson T. Neonatal transfers by advanced neonatal nurse practitioners and paediatric registrars. *Arch Dis Child Fetal Neonatal Ed.* 2003:88:F509–F512

McCloskey KA, Johnson C. Critical care interhospital transports: predictability of the need for a pediatrician. *Pediatr Emerg Care.* 1990:6:89–92

Warren J, Fromm RE Jr, Orr RA, Rotello LC, Horst HM. Guidelines for the inter- and intrahospital transport of critically ill patients. *Crit Care Med.* 2004:32:256–262

Woodward GA, Insoft RM, Pearson-Shaver Al, et al. The state of pediatric interfacility transport: consensus of the second National Pediatric and Neonatal Interfacility Transport Medicine Leadership Conference. *Pediatr Emerg Care.* 2002:18:38–43

Questions

1. List 4 factors that may be considered in determining neonatal-pediatric transport team composition.
2. List 5 different types of health care personnel who might participate in transport.
3. List 4 factors that should be considered when making decisions about personnel selection.

Answers

1. • Availability of professionals in the base (sponsoring) facility
   • The anticipated patient population
   • Financial support for the program
   • The level of responsibility assumed by particular personnel in the inpatient setting
2. Attending physicians, physicians in training, nurses, respiratory therapists, paramedics
3. • Experience and competence in the care of children in the inpatient setting
   • Excellent communication skills
   • Personality traits that include flexibility and the ability to act independently and to reason and exercise good judgment
   • Ability to cope effectively in high-stress situations

Transport Program Personnel, Training, and Assessment

Outline

- Personnel and training
- Transport qualifications, performance expectations, and assessment
- Transport team training and program orientation
- Training strategies
- Skills development for neonatal-pediatric transport
- Continuing education and assessment

Personnel and Training

As noted in Chapter 3, many types of providers serve on neonatal-pediatric transport teams (Table 4-1). Although many teams include physicians, nurses, and respiratory therapists, prehospital (emergency medical technicians and paramedics) providers, nurse practitioners, and physicians' assistants are also commonly included. In addition, there may be differences in the level of training or experience among providers of the same general classification. For example, the term *physician* can refer to an attending or resident physician or to a fellow. Likewise, a *nurse* might be a nurse practitioner, a clinical nurse specialist, a nurse with specific advanced practice skills, or a staff nurse. No one team configuration is ideal for every situation, although there are minimum requirements that must be met for transport. The type of providers employed is best determined by the team's mission(s) and clinical needs. Teams that respond to out-of-hospital emergencies will need personnel with prehospital experience, and those whose mission is restricted to the transport of critically ill neonates will need providers with extensive experience in neonatal medicine. In some cases, team configuration might be influenced by local statutes that,

Table 4-1: Transport Program Personnel:
Potential Roles and Responsibilities
(see Appendix A1)

Program director
- Organization of the transport system
- Liaison between team and hospital administration
- Budget development
- Develop and implement quality improvement and safety programs
- Oversight of day-to-day transport team and supervisors
- In conjunction with transport team medical director, sets employment criteria and devises methods for continuing education to maintain and enhance skills

Transport team medical director
- Specialist in pediatric critical care, pediatric emergency medicine, or neonatology
- May function as program director and medical director
- May require codirector or other available expertise regarding specialty issues for combination neonatal-pediatric teams
- Partners with transport team coordinator regarding transport planning and operations
- Ensures consultation is available for pediatric trauma, surgical emergencies, and other required services
- Medical director or designee is available to transport team coordinator 24 hours a day, for online clinical expertise
- Participates in program fiscal planning and management
- Oversees and participates in design of the team training programs
- Oversees and participates in the selection and training of team members
- Develops and/or approves all transport policies and protocols
- Assists in development and implementation of outreach and follow-up programs
- Reviews transport cases, providing feedback to team personnel
- Conducts morbidity and mortality reviews with team members
- Reviews data and team statistics
- Designs research initiatives
- Serves as liaison with administration (base and referring facilities)
- Oversees and participates in quality reviews, and designs resulting education for staff

Transport team coordinator
- Health care professional (eg, nurse practitioner, registered nurse, respiratory therapist, paramedic)
- Coordinates day-to-day program activity
- Holds position equivalent to a manager for the transport team
- Partners with medical director regarding transport planning and operations
- Participates in design and implementation of the team training programs
- Develops and/or approves all transport policies and protocols, in conjunction with the medical director
- Oversees transport data collection
- Is responsible for equipment selection and maintenance
- Is responsible for budget management
- Is responsible for team scheduling and scheduling staff meetings and in-service offerings

Table 4-1: Transport Program Personnel: Potential Roles and Responsibilities, *continued*

- Participates in teaching and quality improvement reviews
- Assists the medical director in conducting morbidity and mortality reviews with team members

Medical control physician

- Designated medical control physician(s) (sometimes known as medical control officer) or designee available 24 hours a day
- Responds promptly to transport or consultation requests for medical management of individual patients
- Reports to the medical director or may hold both positions
- Is competent in acute and critical care, including pediatric critical care, pediatric emergency medicine, pediatric surgery, neonatology, cardiology, and other specialties as appropriate
- Has demonstrated experience with medical and logistical aspects of transport services
- Triages transport requests and activates backup system when necessary
- Assists in determining team composition and mode of transport
- Provides medical management suggestions before the arrival of the transport team
- Communicates with team via online (eg, telephone, radio) and off-line (eg, using written protocols) methods during transport
- Is kept informed of patient's clinical status
- Relays pertinent information to receiving unit for preparation for patient arrival
- Documents or ensures documentation of patient-related information and advice given
- Is knowledgeable of (or has immediate access to) available care resources (eg, area bed capacity, other transport team configuration, and therapy treatment options)
- Has the authority to accept transferred patients without further consultation
- Assists in admission to alternative receiving hospitals in region
- Has access to subspecialty consultation (eg, cardiology, nephrology, endocrinology, surgery)
- Is involved in quality improvement and safety programs (development and implementation)

Transport physician

- Licensed physician (attending, fellow, or resident status)
- Has the defined skill level for treatment of patient population
- Participates in the training program designed by the medical director and transport team coordinator using defined, established criteria
- Collaborates in stabilization and management of patient's condition during transport
- Documentation reflects assessment and required interventions during the transport
- Participates in teaching and quality improvement reviews

Transport nurse

- Licensed registered nurse
- Has the defined skill level for treatment of patient population
- Has specific experience and training in neonatal, pediatric, acute, intensive, and emergency care medicine
- Participates in training program designed by medical director and transport team coordinator using defined, established criteria

Table 4-1: Transport Program Personnel: Potential Roles and Responsibilities, *continued*

- Is responsible for coordinating stabilization and management of patient's condition; documenting assessments, communication, and care provided; and monitoring during transport
- Participates in teaching and quality improvement reviews

Transport respiratory therapist
- Licensed respiratory therapist
- Has additional specific training and experience of seriously ill patients
- Has specific experience and training in neonatal-pediatric patient management during interfacility transport
- Participates in training program designed by medical director and transport team coordinator using defined, established criteria
- Assists team leader with stabilization and management of the patient's airway, pulmonary care, ventilator management, and other care according to license and privileges during transport
- Participates in teaching and quality improvement reviews

Transport paramedic
- Licensed paramedic
- Has additional specific training and experience with seriously ill pediatric patients
- Has specific experience and training in neonatal-pediatric patient management during interfacility transport
- Participates in training program designed by medical director and transport team coordinator using defined, established criteria
- Assists team leader with stabilization and management of the patient's condition during transport within scope of licensure and practice
- Participates in teaching and quality improvement reviews

Transport emergency medical technician (EMT)
- Licensed EMT
- Has additional specific training and experience with pediatric patients
- Has specific understanding of and training in neonatal-pediatric patient management during interfacility transport
- Participates in training program designed by medical director and transport team coordinator using defined, established criteria
- Assists team leader with stabilization and management of the patient's condition during transport within scope of licensure and practice
- Participates in teaching and quality improvement reviews

for example, might restrict the performance of procedures to certain licensed personnel. As a guideline, transported infants and children should receive the same level of care en route as will be provided in the unit to which they will be admitted, within the constraints of a transport environment.

There is considerable debate about the role of physicians on the transport team. At one time, many, if not most, transport teams included a resident or attending physician. New regulations dictate resident work hours and place restrictions on independent practice by resident physicians. Furthermore, limited research (mostly from aeromedical teams) has demonstrated that well-trained nurses, respiratory therapists, and other professionals can function safely and effectively in the transport environment without the direct presence of a transport physician. Although this evidence suggests that the resident physician might not be a necessary member of the transport team, there is evidence that participating in transport medicine provides an important educational experience for the resident. Attending physicians and subspecialty (acute care) fellows can augment the skills of the transport team by providing additional expertise. Their technical and cognitive skills might be helpful in the care of certain critically ill infants and children. In addition, as members of the transport team, they can educate other team members and perform a quality assurance–quality improvement role.

Regardless of the type of practitioner, certain characteristics are vital for the effective practice of transport medicine. Team members must meet certain physical requirements (see Chapter 9 and Appendix A1). Transport personnel might be asked to perform procedures and tasks not usually associated with their roles. They must be able to function relatively independently and as part of a multidisciplinary team.

When team members have been selected, they must be trained thoroughly. The scope of training will be largely dictated by the experience and background of the candidates and the mission of the team. Some providers will require extensive initial cognitive and procedural training, but even highly experienced providers require significant orientation to the transport environment. Likewise, teams with a more restricted mission may need less extensive training than those with a broad mission. In many cases, transport personnel will be drawn from the ranks of experienced nurses and respiratory care practitioners. These staff members will need to undertake training designed to enhance their knowledge base and will need to learn and interpret certain assessments, techniques, studies, such as laboratory and radiographic analyses, and procedures not usually expected in their

███████████████████████████████████████

standard positions. Initial cognitive training of large groups of providers can be conducted in a classroom environment. However, this approach might not be practical when training the 1 or 2 people needed to fill a periodic vacancy. Therefore, teams should consider alternative teaching methods. Examples include videotaped lectures and self-learning modules. All candidates should be required to demonstrate that they have acquired the basic functional knowledge needed for the role (Table 4-2).

Most providers will need training to efficiently, expertly, and safely perform technical procedures in the transport environment. Suggested methods for acquiring these skills include actual practice with patients, use of manikins and simulators, and use of models.

Basic skill acquisition is only the first step. Continuing education is an essential component of team development for several reasons. First, advances in knowledge and changes in technology are likely to make some therapies less desirable or even obsolete. Second, certain vital technical skills are likely to be used only occasionally, if ever, in actual practice. Prudence dictates that teams should always be prepared to use these skills, making competency and proficiency assurance mandatory. Finally, some important disease entities are rare. Practice sessions and continuing education allow team members to rehearse the management of unusual conditions in advance of need.

In addition to initial training and continuing education, all teams should incorporate a program of quality improvement into their educational offerings (see Chapter 8). Such programs can take many forms, but most include several basic components. All sentinel, serious, and adverse events and near misses, as defined by the by the Joint Commission on Accreditation of Healthcare Organizations, and critical incidents, including death during transport, medical errors, compromised care, injury or death of personnel, and care conflicts should be carefully reviewed, as should all unexpected outcomes and procedural complications. In addition, most programs include mandatory review of certain types of transports, such as of patients with certain diagnoses or patients with a certain degree of illness as assessed by objective parameters.

███████████████████████████████

Table 4-2: Sample Diagnosis-Based Educational Checklist for Neonatal Transport*

Neonatal Diagnosis	Date learning module completed
Cardiac	
Cardiac arrhythmia	
Congenital heart disease (ductal-dependent defect)	
Congenital anomalies	
Ambiguous genitalia	
Bladder or cloacal exstrophy	
Choanal atresia	
Cleft lip and/or palate	
Down syndrome	
Genitourinary (renal, hydronephrosis, prune belly)	
Hygroma	
Multiple congenital anomalies	
Myelomeningocele	
Syndrome (enter specifics)	
Teratoma	
Metabolic, Medical	
Infant of diabetic mother	
Hydrops	
Hyperbilirubinemia	
Sepsis	
Neurologic	
Hematoma (epidural, subdural, subgaleal); skull fractures	
Intraventricular hemorrhage	
Neurologic defect other than meningomyelocele (encephalocele, hydrocephalus, anencephaly)	
Neuromuscular defect	
Seizures	
Respiratory	
Long-term ventilation or tracheostomy	
Prematurity, RDS	

Table 4-2: Sample Diagnosis-Based Educational Checklist for Neonatal Transport,* *continued*

Neonatal Diagnosis	Date learning module completed
Respiratory, *continued*	
Term RDS (TTN, pneumonia, PPHN, MAS, asphyxia)	
Surgical	
Bowel obstruction (abdominal distension, bilious emesis, malrotation, pyloric stenosis, volvulus)	
Diaphragmatic hernia	
Gastroschisis or omphalocele	
Esophageal atresia or tracheal-esophageal fistula	
Imperforate anus	
Intestinal perforation	
Masses (chest, abdominal)	
Necrotizing enterocolitis	
Skills used	
Arterial puncture, blood gas analysis	
Venous access, antibiotic administration	
Intraosseous access, fluid bolus, resuscitation medications	
Intubation, ventilator management, inhaled nitric oxide	
Needle aspiration, chest tube insertion and management	
Umbilical artery or vein cannulation	
Surfactant administration	

*RDS indicates respiratory distress syndrome; TTN, transient tachypnea of the newborn; PPHN, persistent pulmonary hypertension; and MAS, meconium aspiration syndrome.

Transport Qualifications, Performance Expectations, and Assessment

Assessment of the applicant's qualifications for team membership is based on but not limited to the following characteristics:

- Educational and experiential background
- Clinical and technical competence
- Leadership skills
- Critical thinking skills

- Communication and interpersonal skills (team approach, adaptability)
- Skill in public and community relations

The transport team member will successfully complete an orientation program. The program is based on a specific job description and set responsibilities and is of sufficient scope and duration to assure competency. It is based on a curriculum and identified individual learning needs of the transport team member. Successful completion is appropriately documented in the employee's record and personnel file and is required before performance of independent transport care activities.

Collectively, transport team members should demonstrate competency in at least the following transport and medical content areas, as indicated for their patient population (see Chapter 3):

- American Heart Association and American Academy of Pediatrics' pediatric and neonatal curricula
- Maternal physiologic and pharmacologic factors affecting the neonate
- Pediatric and neonatal assessment
  1. Physical examination
  2. Gestational age assessment
  3. Interpretation of clinical, laboratory, radiographic, and other diagnostic data
- Thermoregulation
- Oxygen monitoring
- Fluid and electrolyte therapy
- Pharmacology, including drug dose calculations
- Anatomy, pathophysiology, assessment, and treatment of
  - Acute and chronic respiratory diseases
  - Cardiovascular abnormalities
  - Surgical emergencies
  - Infectious diseases
  - Musculoskeletal abnormalities
  - Neurological and spinal cord injuries
  - Prematurity and postmaturity
  - Gastrointestinal emergencies
  - Hematologic disorders

- ❖ Metabolic and endocrine disorders
- ❖ Disorders of the head, eyes, nose, and throat
- ❖ Congenital and genetic disorders, congenital heart disease
- ❖ Injury (trauma, poisoning, child abuse)
- ❖ Aviation and transport physiology
- ❖ Psychosocial and bereavement support and crisis intervention
- ❖ Mechanical ventilation techniques during transport
- ■ Management of pain and agitation
- ■ Provision of developmentally supportive care
- ■ Transport relations and communication
  - ❖ With the referring hospital
  - ❖ With the receiving hospital
  - ❖ Within the hospital
  - ❖ Within the team
  - ❖ With parents, siblings, and significant others
- ■ Problem solving, crisis management, and priority setting
- ■ Medical-legal and ethical issues
  - ❖ Scope of practice of all team members
  - ❖ State and federal regulations regarding transport and advanced practice
  - ❖ Informed consent
  - ❖ Documentation guidelines and requirements
- ■ Continuous quality monitoring and improvement
- ■ Advanced practice protocols, if applicable
- ■ Transport safety issues
- ■ Orientation to the transport vehicles
- ■ Transport equipment, including troubleshooting and backup systems (Table 4-3)

Specific cognitive knowledge should include the ability to recognize and manage the following potentially life-threatening conditions, as appropriate for the transport population. A clear and direct path to obtain immediate medical knowledge and direction for unusual or medical issues that fall outside the team's usual scope is required.

- ■ Cardiopulmonary arrest
- ■ Upper airway obstruction
- ■ Respiratory failure
- ■ Air-leak syndromes

Table 4-3: Sample Transport Equipment Review and Competency Checklist*

By completion of the transport team orientation and yearly thereafter, the transport provider will satisfactorily have demonstrated proper equipment use and patient care skills as listed.

	Date Initial Demonstration	Date Return Demonstration
Ambulance		
Campus vehicle location; extra keys		
Hydraulic lift override		
Power inverter		
Incubator mounting options: single vs dual installation		
Infant seat policy		
Cell phone and contact numbers		
Use of priority status and seatbelt policy		
Oxygen, air, nitric oxide: cylinder storage; system 1 and 2 supply ports		
Suction, continuous vs low intermittent		
Patient care supplies: cupboard inventory; exam gloves; goggles; hand sanitizer		
Point-of-care meter supplies		
Specimen and breast milk coolers		
X-ray viewing board		
Medication refrigerator: inventory and daily log		
Pharmacy formulary		
Forms: cupboard inventory		
Policy manuals: transport procedures; infection control; point-of-care testing		
Transport incubator operation		
Power sources: A/C and battery		
Battery percentage of charge; battery operation meter		
Temperature control: digital panel; warmer; Mylar wrap		
Skin temperature probe		

Table 4-3: Sample Transport Equipment Review and Competency Checklist,* *continued*

	Date Initial Demonstration	Date Return Demonstration
Transport incubator operation, *continued*		
Incubator alarms		
Observation light		
Patient seatbelt restraint system		
IV pumps		
Power sources: A/C + detachable cord; battery		
Pump operation; syringe options, rate, bolus volume over time, volume limit		
Pump alarms		
Quick-release clamp vs screw release		
Cardiorespiratory–BP–Sao₂ monitor		
Power sources: A/C and battery		
Vital sign setup menus: ECG/respirations; lead options		
Respiration		
Pulse oximetry		
Thermometer		
Invasive BP: transducer calibration		
Noninvasive BP: transducer calibration		
$ETCO_2$		
Alarm limits		
Recorder: setting VS chart; record function; changing recorder paper		
Pulse oximeter		
Power sources: A/C and battery		
Backlight screen operation		
Alarms: preset limits; alarm reset		
Transport ventilator		
Power sources: A/C and battery		
Gas supply: minimum cylinder psi		
Specific adapters		

Table 4-3: Sample Transport Equipment Review and Competency Checklist,* *continued*

	Date Initial Demonstration	Date Return Demonstration
Transport ventilator, *continued*		
Low-flow blender: options with ventilator, nasal cannula, manual ventilation		
Hand ventilation: humidified vs nonhumidified gas, manometer		
Ventilation modes: CMV; SIMV; CPAP; PS; IAC		
Humidification system vs vent adapter		
Ventilation circuit assembly; system test		
Nitric oxide transport ventilator and delivery system		
Power sources: A/C and battery		
Rail mounting bracket		
Tubing; supply bag; spare cylinder		
Inhaled nitric oxide transport delivery regulator		
Portable suction		
Power sources; A/C and battery		
Mode of operation: low continuous		
Medication bag		
Controlled drug use policy: locking mechanism; medication sign-out form		
Inventory: medications; IV fluids; supplies		
Drip calculation charts		
Inventory sheet: patient charges		
Restocking responsibilities		
Refrigerated medications pouch		
Controlled drug use policy: locking mechanism; medication sign-out form		
Inventory sheet: patient charges		
Restocking responsibilities		

Table 4-3: Sample Transport Equipment Review and Competency Checklist,* *continued*

	Date Initial Demonstration	Date Return Demonstration
Supply box		
Inventory		
Restocking responsibilities		
Patient transport and admission records		
Forms: referring patient records; transport documentation; consent; X-rays; billing sheet		
Transport restocking policy		
Completion of restocking: equipment; medications; supplies		
Ambulance repairs; incidents		
Processing laboratory samples: specimens (including point-of-care testing materials)		
Trauma supplies		
Cervical spinal stabilization equipment		
Spinal immobilization equipment		
Splinting equipment		

*A/C indicates alternating current ventilation; IV, intravenous; BP, blood pressure; ECG, electrocardiogram; ETCO$_2$, end-tidal carbon dioxide; VS, vital signs; CMV, controlled mandatory ventilation; SIMV, synchronized intermittent mandatory ventilation; CPAP, continuous positive airway pressure; PS, pressure support ventilation; and IAC, interposed abdominal compression.

- Congenital malformations and associated diseases
- Anatomic abnormalities
- Metabolic disorders
- Birth injuries
- Prematurity
- Status asthmaticus
- Shock
- Congestive heart failure
- Cardiac arrhythmias
- Seizures and status epilepticus

- Altered mental status
- Intracranial hemorrhage
- Increased intracranial pressure
- Multiple trauma and burns
- Toxic ingestions
- Hematologic emergencies
- Metabolic disorders, including diabetic ketoacidosis
- Near-drowning and other global hypoxic-ischemic injuries
- Sepsis, meningitis, and other life-threatening infections

The transport team should have the combined expertise and legal scope of practice to perform at least the following procedures with respect to the anticipated patient population and established program guidelines and protocols, and organizational polices:

- Oxygen administration
- Bag and mask ventilation
- Application of nasal continuous positive airway pressure (CPAP), endotracheal intubation, laryngeal mask airway
- Surfactant administration
- Needle aspiration of pleural air or surgical placement of a chest tube
- Initiation and maintenance of mechanical ventilation, including high-frequency ventilation and inhaled nitric oxide if indicated
- Intravenous and intra-arterial access, which might include
  - Peripheral venous puncture and cannulation
  - Umbilical arterial and venous catheterization
  - Central venous access
  - Percutaneous arterial line and puncture
- Intraosseous access
- Venipuncture for laboratory specimen collection
- Cardiopulmonary resuscitation
- Medication preparation and administration
- Hemorrhage control
- Initiation and maintenance of cervical spine and general spinal precautions
- Initiation and maintenance of general immobilization and splinting techniques

At regularly scheduled intervals and on completion of orientation, knowledge and clinical competency will be evaluated and documented. Evaluation methods might include the following:
- Written examinations
- Simulated practice skills laboratories
- Transport faculty–supervised skills and transports
- Case presentations
- Oral examinations conducted by the course faculty, transport team coordinator, and transport team medical director
- Medical record review

Mechanisms to evaluate continued competency of transport team members might include periodic and recurring practice review sessions in the following.
- Cardiopulmonary resuscitation and stabilization
- Respiratory emergencies and ventilation
- Radiographic interpretation
- Management of suspected infection and infection control
- Fluid and electrolytes
- Monitoring equipment and techniques
- New equipment orientation and training
- Transport and client safety issues
- Public relations
- Advanced procedure laboratories for identified low-volume, high-risk proficiency
- Other topics based on annual learning needs survey or practice deficiencies
- Update on policies affecting functions of transport personnel
- Methods of communication with referring facilities, accepting facilities, and families

Transport Team Training and Program Orientation

The goal of transport team training is to develop a program that ensures that members will have the combined expertise to effectively assess and manage actual and potential problems, in addition to demonstrating their ability to plan, implement, and evaluate ongoing stabilization and interventions during transport. The depth and scope of an individual orientation program regarding initial interhospital or return transport and scene and prehospital response when applicable is determined based on job descriptions and specific transport responsibilities. An orientation period should include a training format such as outlined below. During this time, the trainee should participate in transport under the supervision of an experienced team member. This period should end when the training program director and the trainee are confident of the trainee's abilities. Formal evaluation regarding newly acquired and expected skills should be a standard part of the transport curriculum and provider assessment process.

Departmental Overview

- Department orientation plan and objectives
- Scope of service
- Mission and goals and objectives
- Department structure
- Patient flow and workflow
- Related departments
- Tour of facilities
- Department quality improvement activities

Job Responsibilities

- Work content description and responsibilities
- Performance standards and skills checklist
- Reporting and working relationships
- Patient and family relationships
- Customer service
- Information management

Safety Responsibilities

- Incident reporting
- Infection control
- OSHA (Occupational Safety and Health Administration) guidelines
- Latex precautions
- Material Safety Data Sheets
- Safety guidelines
- Utilities management
- Waste disposal

■ Disaster plan
■ Patient safety awareness

Departmental Policies and Procedures

■ Dress code
■ Identification badge
■ Locker assignments
■ Work schedules
■ Attendance and punctuality
■ Vacation and holiday requests
■ Policy and procedure manuals
■ Disciplinary process
■ Department meetings
■ Education in-service offerings
■ Competency review
■ Quality management review

Training Strategies

Each program should define the cognitive and technical skills required for each professional group and should include methods to document the acquisition and quality of these skills. Procedural capabilities of the providers should be sanctioned and approved by the base facility and, where appropriate, by the state regulatory agencies that govern the activities of each professional group. In addition, members of each professional group should become familiar with the care typically provided by members of other professional groups on the team so that they will be prepared to assist with procedures or provide care when necessary (see Chapter 23).

Instruction during training may be provided by persons knowledgeable and skilled in the required area of interest. Instructors in the pediatric critical care transport curriculum might include pediatric intensivists, anesthesiologists, emergency physicians, cardiologists, critical care registered nurses, critical care nurse practitioners, respiratory therapists, pediatric surgeons, traumatologists, clinical pharmacists, and other experienced transport personnel. Instructors in the neonatal critical care transport curriculum might include neonatologists, neonatal nurse practitioners, pediatric surgeons, respiratory therapists, clinical pharmacists, and other experienced transport personnel. For certification in some subspecialty transport services, instruction by a specifically credentialed professional might be required by the base facility or a governing agency.

Educational sessions designed to assist personnel to acquire, refresh, and update knowledge can be provided in several formats, including didactic lectures and audiovisual-assisted and computer-assisted interactive self-study programs.

Skills Development for Neonatal-Pediatric Transport

Considerable resourcefulness is required to create optimal procedural training opportunities for pediatric transport personnel. Potential sites of actual patient care training experiences include the pediatric and neonatal intensive care units, the emergency department, delivery rooms, and operating room. In addition, laboratory and facsimile simulations are available for some procedures. The use of electronic, computer-linked simulators is a promising training adjunct for transport and other health care personnel. This modality is currently limited by availability and the expense to purchase and maintain an educational program. Creative financing and management solutions, such as partnering with other departments, personnel, and institutions, could be considered when approaching how to make simulators cost-effective.

Examples of skills appropriate to specific resource locations might include the following:

1. *Anesthesia and operating room experience*
   - Airway assessments
   - Identification of airway complications
   - Bag-valve-mask ventilation (self-inflating and anesthesia bags)
   - Airway management and endotracheal intubation
   - Use of laryngeal mask airway
   - Vascular access, central line placement
   - Endotracheal intubation under pharmacologic control, including rapid-sequence intubation
   - Difficult airway management and rescue airway techniques
2. *Pediatric intensive care experience*
   - Critical care patient assessment

CHAPTER 4

- Airway management, endotracheal intubation, and tracheostomy management
- Aerosol treatment
- Oxygen therapy
- Ventilator and ventilation management
- Arterial puncture
- Needle thoracostomy
- Vasoactive infusions
- Central line placement
- Interpretation of laboratory test results and radiographs
- Thoracostomy tube placement
- Team approach to resuscitation

3. *Emergency department experience*
   - General patient assessment
   - Fluid resuscitation
   - Medication administration
   - Procedural opportunity (intravenous catheters, urinary catheters, nasogastric and orogastric tubes, airway/tracheostomy management, and oxygen therapy)
   - Aerosolized medications
   - Intravenous and intraosseous access
   - Spinal immobilization
   - Fracture splinting
   - Burn and wound care
   - Interpretation of laboratory results and radiographs
   - Team approach to resuscitation

4. *Neonatal intensive care and delivery room experience*
   - Neonatal patient assessment
   - Bag-valve-mask ventilation (self-inflating and anesthesia bags)
   - Nonintubated positive-pressure assistance and ventilation
   - Airway management and endotracheal/nasotracheal intubation
   - Delivery room resuscitation
   - Arterial puncture and peripheral arterial line placement
   - Needle thoracostomy
   - Vasopressor infusions
   - Umbilical venous and arterial line placement
   - Thoracostomy tube placement
   - Peripheral intravenous line placement

- Ventilator and ventilation management
- Surfactant administration
- Interpretation of laboratory test results and radiographs
5. *Laboratory experience (facsimile training)*
    - Endotracheal intubation
    - Intraosseous line placement
    - Central, including umbilical, line placement
    - Thoracostomy tube placement
    - Cricothyrotomy
    - Pericardiocentesis
    - Resuscitation management
    - Spinal immobilization

Competency testing of academic knowledge and clinical decision-making skill might include the following:
- Written examinations
- Transport and clinical case presentations and reviews
- Oral examinations
- Simulator assessment
- Medical record review
- Periodic performance appraisals
- Criterion-based performance evaluation
- Self-assessment instrument

Documentation of satisfactory performance of advanced practice skills as defined by the transport medical director or other supervisors and assessors might be based on the following:
- Simulated practice skills laboratories
- Transport faculty–supervised skill sessions
- Outsourced skills assessments (anesthesia staff supervising in the operating room)
- Documentation of the transport team member's review of practice guidelines
- Adherence to accepted standards of care, standards of practice, policies, procedures, job description, and certification requirements
- Quality improvement management findings
- New and updated policy dissemination

Continuing Education and Assessment

Continuing education for the transport team member will be based on:

- sufficient scope and duration to ensure continued competency,
- performance and findings from quality improvement activities and changes in technology and pharmacologic interventions,
- identified or stated education requirements of the transport team member,
- input and involvement of the transport team medical director, and
- the educational content identified by state or national organizations.

Continuing education will be appropriately documented in the employee's record and personnel file with regard to the content and scope of the program and the transport team member's successful completion of required annual competency.

All or a representative subset of transport cases should be reviewed routinely by the medical and program directors of the transport team. This review should also include presentations during team meetings with participation of all team members. A minimum number of neonatal-pediatric transports should be required to maintain skill levels. Periodic and recurrent experiences through instructional sites such as the delivery room, operating room, and simulator suite should be considered to maintain skills for use in the transport environment. Expectations for students and instructors regarding exposures and learning experiences should be elucidated before those experiences. Student and teacher should be aware of the specific purposes of the process and have an objective method to document experience, progress, and deficiencies and to enact required corrective training.

Transport team members should be encouraged to validate competency through local and national professional certifications.

Selected Readings

Accreditation Standards. 5th ed. Sandy Springs, SC: Commission on Accreditation of Medical Transport Systems; 2002

Adams K, Scott R, Perkin RM, Langga L. Comparison of intubation skills between interfacility transport team members. *Pediatr Emerg Care.* 2000;16:5–8

Davis PJ, Manktelow B, Bohin S, Field D. Pediatric trainees and the transportation of critically ill neonates: experience training and confidence. *Acta Paediatr.* 2001;90:1068–1072

Fazio RF, Wheeler DS, Poss WB. Resident training in pediatric critical care transport medicine: a survey of pediatric residency programs. *Pediatr Emerg Care.* 2000;16:166–169

King BR, Foster RL, Woodward GA, McCans K. Procedures performed by pediatric transport nurses: how "advanced" is the practice? *Pediatr Emerg Care.* 2001;17:410–413

King BR, Woodward GA. Procedural training for pediatric and neonatal transport nurses, part 1—training methods and airway training. *Pediatr Emerg Care.* 2001;17:461–464

King BR, Woodward GA. Procedural training for pediatric and neonatal transport nurses, part 2—procedures, skills, assessment, and retention. *Pediatr Emerg Care.* 2002;18: 438–441

MacDonald MG, Gomez MA, eds. *Guidelines for Air and Ground Transport of Neonatal and Pediatric Patients.* 2nd ed. Elk Grove Village, IL: American Academy of Pediatrics; 1999

McCloskey KA. Transport team training. In: McCloskey KA, Orr RA, eds. *Pediatric Transport Medicine.* St Louis, MO: Mosby; 1995:100–107

National Association of Neonatal Nurses. *Neonatal Nursing Transport Standards Guidelines for Practice.* DesPlaines, IL: National Association of Neonatal Nurses; 1998

Young T, Mangum B. *Neofax.* 17th ed. Raleigh, NC: Acorn Publishing, Inc; 2004

Questions

1. Consideration should be given to which of the following factors when determining transport team composition? Circle all that apply.
   a. The level of expertise and varied job responsibilities of the transport team
   b. The degree of supervision required by and available to the team members
   c. The complexity and seriousness of the patient's condition
   d. The type of technology to be used during the transport
   e. The legal scope of practice of transport team members
      1. a, b, and c
      2. b, c, and e
      3. a, d, and f
      4. All of the above

2. True or False: All critical care patient transports are to be conducted by a team whose members have the combined leadership and clinical competency specific to job responsibilities to safely transport critically ill patients.

3. At regularly scheduled intervals, theoretical and clinical competency needs to be evaluated and documented. Evaluation methods might include which of the following? Choose from the combinations listed.
   a. Written examination
   b. Simulated practice-skills laboratories
   c. Case presentations
   d. Oral examinations conducted by the medical director or coordinator of the transport team
   e. Medical record and quality improvement reviews
   f. Competency validation through professional certification
      1. a, b, and c
      2. b, c, and e
      3. a, d, and f
      4. All of the above

Answers

1. 4 (all of the above)
2. true
3. 4 (all of the above)

Communications and the Dispatch Center

Outline

- Emergency medical communications systems
- Online medical control
- Development of a communications center
- Communications specialists
- Integration of centralized communications systems into practice
- Follow-up communication with referring providers
- Role of the communications center during disasters and with EMS
- Information processing and documentation during transport

Effective communication is an essential component of an emergency transport service. By its very nature, interfacility transport presents the need for coordination among multiple parties: referring providers, medical control physicians, transport team staff, receiving facility staff, ground or flight crews, and public safety and administrative personnel. A system for communication should streamline the processes for access to services by referring providers: notification and mobilization of the transport team; response to the referring facility; and contact between and among the transport team, medical control physician, and receiving health care providers. Depending on the size and resources of the transport program, a communications system may be formally structured or may function as a component of a larger network. Even if a system is too small to support a more formal structure as outlined in this chapter, the principles of directed and efficient communications templates should be implemented. Ultimately, effective communication optimizes the utilization of the transport team, improves service to the referring providers, and, most important, ensures a safe and efficient transport process for critically ill neonates and children.

■ ■

Emergency Medical Communications Systems

There are multiple models for emergency medical communications systems: (1) 911 dispatch centers, responsible for public safety and emergency dispatch; (2) hospital-based communications centers (also known as dispatch centers), usually affiliated with an emergency department; (3) freestanding communications centers dedicated to one or more transport programs; and (4) unit-based communications sites within a hospital that use on-duty nursing or medical staff to coordinate transport services. Each model has advantages and disadvantages that should be considered when an individual transport program is designing a communications system. For example, 911 dispatch centers are usually governed by agencies such as law enforcement and fire services and, therefore, might not be as responsive to the needs of an interfacility transport program. Stand-alone communications centers are often desirable, but they are costly to equip, staff, and operate unless multiple programs or users are willing to pool resources. Unit-based communications centers use clinicians to coordinate the transport process, which could interfere with patient care responsibilities and delay the transport team's response.

There is no formula to determine the volume of calls necessary to justify the development of an independent communications center. Most costs are fixed, such as personnel salaries and equipment; therefore, use should be optimized to achieve the most favorable cost-benefit ratio. Justification for a centralized communications/dispatch center may be strengthened by identifying other areas in an institution that would benefit from coordination of communications, especially in emergency situations.

Establishment of a freestanding communications center has certain fixed expenses for hardware and software, in addition to necessary renovations. A list of equipment and representative estimate for equipping a communications center is shown in Table 5-1.

Online Medical Control

The medical control physician (MCP) is frequently involved in other patient care activities while directing an interfacility transport. Cellular phones, or low-power internal phone systems that do not

Table 5-1: Equipment Costs for a Communications Center	
Item	Estimated Cost, $
Dispatch software and database	30,000
Recording system	13,500
Radio system and console	21,500
Computers (hardware)	10,000
Fax machine, copier, printer	2,500
Telephone (multiline)	4,000
Telephones (wireless base)	1,500
Total	**83,000**

interfere with medical equipment, can facilitate communication with the MCP by enabling 2-way contact wherever the MCP is located.

Although all transport teams are likely to have written guidelines, policies, and procedures, nonphysician transport teams traditionally have written protocols to direct patient care under the authority of the transport team medical director. Nevertheless, it is essential that members of a nonphysician team have immediate access to the MCP if there is a significant deterioration in the patient's condition or patient care orders are needed that are beyond the scope of written protocols. The transport program should ensure that there is a contingency plan in case the MCP cannot be located or is temporarily inaccessible. Because the MCP might be a trainee (eg, critical care fellow) whose experience with interfacility transport is limited, it might be necessary to contact (or ensure involvement of) the responsible attending physician or transport team medical director for critical incidents or conflicts between the team and the referring providers.

Development of a Communications Center

A centralized communications center should coordinate all activities related to an interfacility transport request and should have the following essential features:
1. Operations 24 hours a day, 7 days a week
2. Trained communications specialists
3. Administrative transport policies and procedures

■■■■■■■■■■■■■■■■■■■■■■■■■■■■■■■■■■■■

4. Information about local and regional emergency care resources
5. Communications technology and equipment, including the ability
    to record all transport-related contacts

Space for the dispatch center should be chosen to permit operation 24 hours per day. Secure access and proximity to cafeteria and
restroom facilities are important because the center might be staffed
by only 1 communications specialist at times. The location of the dispatch center should take into account the need to monitor ambulance
and helipad activity, directly or indirectly. If indirect observation is
favored, video monitoring of the remote areas should be available in
the dispatch center. Furniture should be chosen with the understanding that the communications specialist will be seated for the majority
of a shift and needs ready access to manuals and reference materials.

A phone system is a critical component of any communications
system. Most hospital-based programs can link to existing digital
phone services. Multiline units are a necessity, as is the ability to
conference 3 or more parties at a time. A unit that is capable of
programming frequently dialed numbers improves efficiency. A
toll-free number can be established for in-state or multiple-state
calls. If possible, request a phone number that will be easy for the
referring providers to remember (eg, the last 4 digits represented by
"KIDS" or "HELP"). The communications center should be included
in the institution's emergency plan for phone system outages.

Many emergency medical services (EMS) systems use 2-way radios
in addition to cellular phones. Radios permit instantaneous contact
without dialing and can serve as a backup in case there are problems
with the phone system. Many bands are available, including UHF
(ultra high frequency) and VHF (very high frequency). Many hospital
services (eg, engineering) already might be using 2-way radios; the
hospital's vendor will likely offer the use of another rented frequency
to suit the transport system's needs. Alternatively, the transport program can apply to the Federal Communications Commission for a
license to operate its own frequency. Applications are available at
http://www.fcc.gov. Radios are linked to the dispatch center by use
of a console, which can also monitor other frequencies such as local
EMS providers, fire and police agencies, and the local C-MED (central
medical emergency dispatch) system. The console will usually permit
the radio operator and the phone user to be patched into the same

call. Many hospitals are equipped with a radio system that is part of the nationwide Hospital Emergency and Administrative Radio, or HEAR, system. This could be monitored in the communications center as well.

It is strongly recommended that all communications pertaining to an interfacility transport be recorded. The advantages of recording are multiple and include the opportunity to review intake conversations for educational and quality improvement purposes, the ability to review conversations when there are questions or concerns related to the transport process or patient management, and the availability of recorded information in case there is a regulatory or legal inquiry about an emergency transport. A digital recording device is preferred. Most recording devices need to be kept within a certain range of the main phone system, although some can be remote. The advantage of having recording hardware located within the communications center is that tapes or digital video disks (DVDs) from previous periods can be easily accessed for review. A disadvantage is the need for physical space for recording equipment. Computer-based digital recording alleviates the need to have equipment other than a personal computer in the communications area and eases distribution of recorded conversation for quality review. A variety of media are available for recording and storing conversations and sources of communication, including cassette tapes, VHS (video home system) tapes, and DVDs. The DVDs have the advantage of holding the most data per disk and are easy to store. All stored copies should be remotely located from the originals in case of fire, flood, or other catastrophe. Although the time for retaining recorded materials is not mandated, it is important to have a policy that is similar to the institution's policy for storage of medical records and images. The hospital's legal counsel should be consulted to develop a clear policy. Software to operate the recording system can be loaded directly onto the communications center's computers, and most systems will allow for supervisor or manager access from the desktop. Separate software can be purchased to permit last message or last time interval playback for use by the communications specialist during a call.

Federal regulations permit the recording of telephone conversations as long as at least 1 party consents; in other words, recording conversations by third parties is illegal. The Federal Communications Commission has more specific requirements for interstate and foreign calls, during which recording can be done only under one of the following circumstances:

- Preceded by verbal or written consent of all parties to the telephone conversation
- Preceded by verbal notification that is recorded at the beginning and as part of the call by the recording party
- Accompanied by an automatic tone warning device, sometimes called a beep tone, which automatically produces a distinct signal that is repeated at regular intervals during the telephone conversation when the recording device is in use

For in-state calls, regulations vary by state and might require 1-party or 2-party consent. A list of state-by-state regulations can be found at http://www.callcorder.com/phone-recording-law.htm.

Communications Specialists

Communications specialists are often the first persons with whom the referring provider has contact, so a professional and service-oriented demeanor is essential. They must be skilled at managing multiple tasks under stressful circumstances. They should not have concomitant duties that might delay the transport process. They must be familiar with institutional resources and procedures. Communications specialists are trained to follow guidelines or protocols established by the transport program's leadership.

It is recommended that the communications specialist have experience in EMS or in a hospital setting. Familiarity with dispatch procedures, radio communications, and computer data entry are desirable. Excellent verbal skills and hearing are required. A working knowledge of medical terminology is helpful. The specialist must be able to function independently and make decisions and recognize when additional resources are needed. Attention to detail is extremely important given the nature of neonatal-pediatric transport and the importance of accurate medical records and logs. A sample job description and performance evaluation for an emergency communications specialist are included in Figure 5-1 and Figure 5-2.

Figure 5-1: Job Description: Transport Team Dispatcher

JOB TITLE: Transport Services Dispatcher

DEPARTMENT: Critical Care Transport

SUPERVISOR:

SALARY GRADE/JOB CODE:

EXEMPT/NONEXEMPT: Nonexempt

General Summary
As an integral part of the emergency transport system, ensures and participates in coordinating the timely and efficient management of patient transports. Enters information into department databases as necessary.

The incumbent works alone and must possess and demonstrate, at all times, ability to make sound judgment with life-support alarms, ability to be versatile to handle multiple crises at once, and ability to maintain composure, and must possess good communication skills.

Principal Duties and Responsibilities
1. Receives and triages calls as a member of a 24-hour transport communications center. Obtains information from caller required to assess urgency of request and initiate appropriate response.
2. Enters all appropriate information into department databases as necessary.
3. Coordinates community outreach.
4. Assists in orienting and training new staff.
5. Keeps work area neat and orderly and free of fire and safety hazards.
6. Furthers knowledge and skills through attendance and participation at conferences, seminars, and in-service and continuing education programs.
7. Performs other related duties as assigned or requested.

Minimum Knowledge and Skills Required by the Job
1. Work requires a high school level of educational development and at least 1 to 2 years of previous experience, preferably in dispatch operations. Work requires some understanding of medical terminology through training or experience. EMT preferred.
2. Work requires the analytical skills to gather and interpret data in situations in which the information or problems are relatively routine.

Certification, Registration, or Licensure Required by the Job
No certification, registration, or licensure required.

Figure 5-1: Job Description: Transport Team Dispatcher, *continued*

Physical Requirements of the Job
1. Work requires frequently lifting and carrying patients, children, and/or objects weighing up to 10 pounds and occasionally lifting and carrying patients, children, and/or objects weighing 11 to 20 pounds.
2. Work requires occasionally stooping and bending.
3. Work requires regularly reaching and grasping objects below shoulder level, frequently reaching and grasping objects at shoulder level, and regularly grasping and fine manipulation with hands.
4. Work requires regularly proofreading and checking documents for accuracy and inputting/retrieving words or data into or from an automated/computer system.

Bloodborne Pathogen Category
No Potential Exposure: Job requires performance of duties that involve no potential for exposure to blood, body fluids, or tissues. Tasks that do involve exposure are not an expectation of employment.

Job Document Attributes

Human Resources Approval	[Click **here** and type name] [Click **here** and type job title] Human Resources Department	Last Modified Date	05/09/2006
Manager Approval		Dates Reviewed Revised	

Revision Notes
Document actions taken when reviewed or revised.

Date	Review/Revision Action	Reviewer

Figure 5-2: Transport Team Dispatcher Performance Evaluation

Employee Performance Evaluation Form

EMPLOYEE NAME:

DEPARTMENT: Critical Care Transport

JOB TITLE: Transport Services Dispatcher

PERFORMANCE PERIOD:

Policy, Procedure, and Work Rule Compliance
Please mark each statement where the employee has complied with hospital and departmental policies, procedures, and standards of conduct. Mark nonapplicable standards N/A. Please comment on items not in compliance.

☐ Always conforms to hospital's standard of conduct as detailed in the hospital's personnel policy manual. Adheres to ethical and legal standards of practice.

☐ Complies with position-specific work schedule, arrives at work on time, starts promptly, works scheduled hours.

☐ Uses earned time per departmental and hospital policy; requests time off in advance; calls supervisor to explain unscheduled absence in a timely manner as defined in the departmental policies.

☐ Always complies with all job-specific safety and infection control standards. Follows departmental/hospital universal precaution and infection control policies and procedures.

☐ Displays hospital ID badge at all times while on hospital premises. Dresses appropriately for work assigned.

☐ Always treats patients, coworkers, and staff with dignity, courtesy, and respect.

☐ Follows departmental/hospital policies and practices to protect patient and employee confidentiality.

☐ Complies with and enforces hospital's visitation policy.

☐ Complies with hospital procedures for responding to and reporting incidents involving patient or personal injury. Reports work-related injuries immediately to supervisor.

☐ Attends safety training sessions and/or reviews manuals for fire and disaster procedures provided by the hospital annually. Knows fire and emergency procedures for the area. Follows departmental/hospital procedures regarding handling and disposal of infectious and/or hazardous materials. Completes mandatory annual review documentation.

☐ Completes TB screening within 3 months prior to performance review date.

☐ Completes CPR training as required by policy. CPR certification expiration date:_____

☐ Maintains up-to-date licensure/certification/registration/visa in departmental file.

Comments

Figure 5-2: Transport Team Dispatcher Performance Evaluation, *continued*

Employee Performance Evaluation Form, *continued*

Employee Self-evaluation
If applicable, please attach the employee's self-evaluation and make any comments about this self-evaluation here.

Goals, Objectives, and/or Accomplishments
If applicable, please attach the employee's goals, objectives, and/or accomplishments for the past and upcoming year and make any comments about these goals here.

Principal Duty and Responsibility
Receives and triages calls as a member of a 24-hour transport communications center. Obtains information from caller required to assess urgency of request and initiate appropriate response.

Performance Standards
1. Receives incoming calls, and arranges for immediate and scheduled transfers.
2. Receives calls from an outlying institution requesting patient transport, and triages the call to the appointed medical control physician and transport nurses.
3. Coordinates patient placement with bed control nurse.
4. Obtains patient demographics (name, diagnosis, and name of hospital, location within hospital).
5. Notifies ambulance company and/or drivers.
6. Calls referring hospitals with ETA, and updates if known deviation is greater than 5 minutes.
7. Maintains immediate contact capability with team, referring or receiving hospital.
8. Contacts consultants if requested.
9. Monitors other radio frequencies (helicopter, fire rescue, 911).
10. Participates in in-services for patient transports.
11. Acts as trouble-shooter for the transport communication system equipment.
12. Coordinates information among ambulance, helicopters, fixed-wing service, referring hospitals, and receiving hospital personnel for expedient and efficient transports.
13. Maintains up-to-date information on bed availability, physician and team member's coverage, and contact numbers.

Rating
[ ] Exceeds job performance standards
[ ] Meets job performance standards
[ ] Does not meet job performance standards

Comments

Figure 5-2: Transport Team Dispatcher Performance Evaluation, *continued*

Employee Performance Evaluation Form, *continued*

Principal Duty and Responsibility
Enters all appropriate information into department databases as necessary.

Performance Standards
1. Able to use spreadsheets and databases for data entry.
2. Generates statistical reports from computer programs.

Rating
[ ] Exceeds job performance standards
[ ] Meets job performance standards
[ ] Does not meet job performance standards

Comments

Principal Duty and Responsibility
Coordinates community outreach.

Performance Standards
1. Ensures that form letter to referring physician is sent within 2 days.

Rating
[ ] Exceeds job performance standards
[ ] Meets job performance standards
[ ] Does not meet job performance standards

Comments
Not a responsibility at this time

Principal Duty and Responsibility
Assists in orienting and training new staff.

Performance Standards
1. Effectively assists in the training of new staff, following departmental policies and procedures.
2. Maintains accurate and thorough documentation of skill levels and makes appropriate suggestions for progression.

Rating
[ ] Exceeds job performance standards
[ ] Meets job performance standards
[ ] Does not meet job performance standards

Comments

Figure 5-2: Transport Team Dispatcher Performance Evaluation, *continued*

Employee Performance Evaluation Form, *continued*

Principal Duty and Responsibility
Keeps work area neat and orderly and free of fire and safety hazards.

Performance Standards
1. Work area is left clean, neat, and orderly at end of shift.
2. Doorways are not blocked, and fire and safety hazards are reported to the appropriate person.

Rating
[ ] Exceeds job performance standards
[ ] Meets job performance standards
[ ] Does not meet job performance standards

Comments

Principal Duty and Responsibility
Furthers knowledge and skills through attendance and participation at conferences, seminars, and in-service and continuing education programs.

Performance Standards
1. Pursues opportunities to advance knowledge of materials management through attendance at relevant programs, seminars, or academic course work.
2. Regularly attends department-specific in-service programs as offered.
3. Identifies when help or instruction is required, and seeks it appropriately.

Rating
[ ] Exceeds job performance standards
[ ] Meets job performance standards
[ ] Does not meet job performance standards

Comments

Principal Duty and Responsibility
Performs other related duties as assigned or requested.

Performance Standards
1. Demonstrates ability to complete additional tasks in a timely manner.
2. Responds quickly to situational or assignment changes.
3. Demonstrates flexibility and adaptability in work assignment.
4. Identifies and suggests areas of opportunity for quality improvement.

Figure 5-2: Transport Team Dispatcher Performance Evaluation, *continued*

Employee Performance Evaluation Form, *continued*

Rating
[ ]   Exceeds job performance standards
[ ]   Meets job performance standards
[ ]   Does not meet job performance standards

Comments

Employee Development
(In completing this section, the evaluator should review information from the department's continuous improvement activities.)

In what ways would you suggest the employee could improve and/or enhance his/her performance?

Agreed-upon action for improving and/or enhancing performance:

What job knowledge/skills might you suggest the employee acquire or further develop to improve his/her performance and/or prepare for changes in the patient population and/or other career opportunities?

Agreed-upon action plan for acquiring and/or further developing job knowledge and/or skills:

Performance Summary
Overall Performance Summary
[ ]   **Exceeds job performance standards.** Performance that exceeds performance standards for assigned job duties or responsibilities. This is a level infrequently achieved even by very experienced incumbents.
[ ]   **Meets job performance standards.** Performance that is consistently strong in all job duties. The incumbent makes a contribution to the hospital that demonstrates a commitment to patient care, support services, or research.
[ ]   **Does not meet job performance standards.** Performance that does not meet standards for one or more job duties. A performance improvement agreement is necessary, or if performance is significantly below standard, disruptive, or inhibiting the unit's productivity, immediate disciplinary action may be necessary.
[ ]   **Deferred Overall Rating/Merit Increase.** Performance that needs improvement in some responsibility areas. No merit increase will be given at this time. Areas that do not meet standards are documented in this review, as well as expectations and plans for performance improvement. Performance will be reviewed again on _____ (date within the next 6 months), and merit increase may be given at that time if performance has improved and meets standards. The merit increase will not be retroactive.

■■■■■■■■■■■■■■■■■■■■■■■■■■■■■■■■■■■■■■

Figure 5-2: Transport Team Dispatcher Performance Evaluation, *continued*

Employee Performance Evaluation Form, *continued*

Employee Comments and Signature
Do you feel your job description is still current?   Yes _____   No _____

If no, indicate below what changes you feel need to be made.
Have your questions about career opportunities been answered?   Yes _____   No _____

If no, indicate below what opportunities you would like to know more about.

Use the following space to comment on your job or evaluation (optional):

Confidentiality Statement
In signing your employee evaluation form, you are indicating that you have received and understand your evaluation. In addition, your signature indicates that you understand and agree with the following statement:

I understand that in the performance of my duties as an employee of the Hospital, I may have access to and work with confidential information such as
a. *Patient medical, social, financial, and demographic information.*
b. *Sensitive and personal information of or about employees, including medical and personnel information, private correspondence, etc.*
c. *Hospital business information, such as financial and payer information, strategic planning, fundraising and reporting information, and internal memoranda.*
d. *Research information, including information describing or relating to inventions and discoveries.*
e. *Information concerning outside companies with which the Hospital does business, including data the Hospital is contractually obligated to keep confidential.*

I understand that I must maintain the confidentiality of these data at all times, both at work and off duty. I will access, use, and disclose such information only in accordance with Hospital policies related to privacy and the scope of my job and recognize my responsibility to become familiar with those policies. I understand that a violation of these confidentiality considerations may result in disciplinary action, including termination. I further understand that I could be subject to legal action.

In addition I acknowledge that the Hospital policy states that Hospital computer resources may be used only for clinical, research, and other legitimate Hospital purposes and only in a responsible, ethical, professional, and courteous manner. I have read and agree to comply with the Guidelines for Ethical Use of Computers and Computer Information. These guidelines describe requirements and obligations of accessing and using Hospital computer resources, accessing sensitive or confidential information stored on Hospital computer resources, and the copying and use of software.

■■■■■■■■■■■■■■■■■■■■■■■■■■■■■■■

Figure 5-2: Transport Team Dispatcher Performance Evaluation, *continued*

Employee Performance Evaluation Form, *continued*

I certify by my signature below that I have read and understood the above statements concerning privacy, confidentiality, and information access at the Hospital. My supervisor has discussed the contents of my evaluation with me. I understand that this form will be filed in my personnel file and that I may have a copy of it.

Employee's signature   **Date:**

Supervisor and Manager Signature and Comments
The contents of this form have been discussed with the employee. I will follow up with Human Resources on any changes the employee and I agree need to be made to the employee's job description.

Supervisor's signature   **Date:**

Manager's signature   **Date:**

In general, the communications specialist is responsible for coordination of all aspects of the emergency transport process. Specific duties of communications specialists include the following:

- Initial point of contact with referring providers and facilitation of prompt access to the MCP
- Appropriate documentation of all interactions (Figure 5-3)
- Team notification; ground or flight service dispatch; updates on team status for the referring and receiving facilities; facilitation of the acceptance and admission process; contact with security or public safety personnel; and, for some programs, coordination with discharge planners and/or third-party payers
- For flight services, coordination of landing zones, flight position monitoring, weather reports and advisories, and communication with law enforcement, air traffic control, and other aeromedical programs

Figure 5-3: Dispatch Documentation*

Children's Hospital Boston
Transport Call Report

Date: / /   Time: :   Referring MD:

Referring Facility: Location of Child:

Callback Phone: ( ) -

Are you looking: ☐ To use our Transport Team   ☐ Consult

Patient Information:

Name: Sex: Age:

Gestation Age: Weight: DOB: / /

Diagnosis:

Medical Control:

Transport Fellow:

PMH:

HPI:

Labs:

Is any special equipment being used?

IV access:

Given any meds:

Vitals   HR: RR: BP: /

Do you need our transport team? ☐ Yes   ☐ No

What kind of bed is needed?

☐ NICU   ☐ PIC   ☐ CICU (P6)   ☐ Floor   ☐ ED

Run Times:

Transport Team Informed	Time: :	**Who was paged:**	
COPP notified	Time: :	**Name of COPP:**	
Referring Hospital advised of ETA	Time: :		
Team left TCH	Time: :		
Team reached referring facility	Time: :		
Team departs referring facility	Time: :		
Team arrives at accepting facility	Time: :		
Call Logged in Access			

Notes:

Figure 5-3: Dispatch Documentation,* *continued*
Children's Hospital Boston
Transport Team: Special Circumstances

No Beds at Children's Boston:

Accepting Physician: Call back number: ( ) -

☐ Confirmed our team's ETA at their facility.   Time: :

Air Transport:

Call back phone: ( ) -   Time: :

Type: ☐ Fixed Wing   ☐ Rotor Wing

Fixed Wing:

☐ Insurance Approval Obtained   Call Back phone: ( ) -

Time: :

Insurance Company: Policy #:

☐ Children's Security Contacted   Time: :

☐ Brigham's Security Contacted   Time: :

☐ Contacted Floor with 5-min ETA   Time: :

Alternative Transport Team:

Arrangements by: ☐ TCH Dispatch   ☐ Referring Facility   Time: :

Alternative mode of transport:
☐ Air   ☐ ALS   ☐ BLS   ☐ Another TT   ☐ Other

Company: Contact:

Call back number: ( ) -

Notes:

Used with permission: Monica Kleinman, MD, FAAP, Children's Hospital Boston

*DOB indicates date of birth; PMH, past medical history; HPI, history of present illness; IV, intravenous; HR, heart rate; RR, respiratory rate; BP, blood pressure; NICU, neonatal intensive care unit; PICU, pediatric intensive care unit; CICU, cardiac intensive care unit; COPP, coordinator of patient placement (bed control); ED, emergency department; TCH, The Children's Hospital; ETA, expected time of arrival; ALS, advanced life support; BLS, basic life support; and TT, transport team.

▪ Maintenance of logs for all transport requests, referrals, and missed or cancelled transports
▪ Input of demographic and transport-related data into the program's database
▪ Monitoring and maintenance of communications center equipment
▪ Attendance at safety and staff meetings
▪ Maintenance of on-call schedules and contact information for clinical services, MCPs, and transport team staff
▪ Monitoring of neonatal and pediatric intensive care bed availability and trauma center status internally and for other area institutions
▪ Consultation with transport program leadership for unusual circumstances or critical incidents

Integration of Centralized Communications Systems Into Practice

Establishment of an emergency communications center might represent a significant change in procedure for referring providers and MCPs. Educating the principal parties involved will hasten acceptance and promote cooperation among services. For example, a referring provider might believe that directly contacting the potential accepting physician will result in the most expedient transport, when in fact the dispatch center might be able to simultaneously facilitate mobilization and contact with the appropriate physician so the transport team can be en route before the intake conversation is completed. For referring providers not familiar with the institution, a "one call does it all" approach can prevent the caller from being routed to multiple people when making an emergency referral. Ideally, a transport program will have a policy in which the transport team can be dispatched before formal physician acceptance. Because there invariably is some time during travel to the referring institution, bed assignment and notification of the receiving clinical team can be accomplished while the transport team is responding. A unit-based program may be concerned about yielding control of its communications with referring providers. Demonstration of the decrease in administrative time spent by busy clinical personnel involved with a transport is usually a persuasive argument in favor of a centralized dispatch center.

An emergency dispatch center should perform self-evaluation by surveying its "customers" to ensure that referring providers and receiving staff are satisfied with the system. Because the dispatch center represents an institutional expense and is not a direct source of revenue, hospital leaders must be given data that show the unmeasured value of well-coordinated communications and improved satisfaction of referring physicians.

Follow-up Communication With Referring Providers

The communications center can also support the transport program by serving as a source for follow-up information for referring providers. Consideration should be given to sending a written or electronic communication at the completion of each transport to inform the referring physician of the patient's safe arrival and subsequent disposition. Although Health Information Portability and Accountability Act, or HIPAA, regulations might prevent sharing of certain medical information without the explicit written consent of the patient or parent, the practice of providing follow-up for referring physicians is important to education, quality improvement, and, perhaps, financial aspects of patient transports. When communicating in writing with referring physicians, the receiving facility must take appropriate safeguards to ensure that a patient's personal health information is protected. An alternative is to provide the referring physician with contact information for the receiving unit and/or attending physician for follow-up. The Air Medical Physician Association has published a position statement on the issue of patient follow-up letters and HIPPA. A sample of correspondence for a referring physician is shown in Figure 5-4.

Role of the Communications Center During Disasters and With EMS

For the same reasons that prehospital EMS dispatch systems might not be ideally suited for coordination of interfacility transports, a transport dispatch center is often not designed to manage EMS communications. Inbound ambulance staff might request medical control from an authorized emergency physician or nurse; this requires familiarity with state and regional prehospital care protocols and the capabilities of individual systems or services. Nevertheless,

---

Figure 5-4: Sample Follow-up Correspondence

Date: 00/00/00

Dear Dr. _____:

Thank you for referring your patient, **Johnny Doe,** for transport to Children's Hospital on **00/00/00. Johnny** was admitted to **the pediatric intensive care unit** with a preliminary diagnosis of **bronchiolitis.**

For further information, you may contact the **PICU** attending physician through the hospital's page operator at **(555) 555-5555.** If you have difficulty contacting the appropriate physician, please contact Dr Ambulance, medical director for the neonatal-pediatric transport team, at (555) 444-4444.

Thank you for the opportunity to serve you and your patients. If you have questions or comments about our transport services, please contact us at the following numbers or e-mail addresses:

> **Emergency Communications Center:** (800) 888-KIDS (5537)
>
> **Medical Director:** Dr Ambulance (555) 444-4444
> **E-mail address:** dr.ambulance@childrens.transport.edu
>
> **Transport Team Coordinator:** Tom Transport, RN/EMT (555) 333-3333
> **E-mail address:** tom.transport@childrens.transport.edu
>
> **Communications Center Supervisor:** Terry Telephone, EMT (555) 222-2222
> **E-mail address:** terry.telephone@childrens.transport.edu

We would appreciate your completion of the enclosed brief survey about our service and return in the enclosed self-addressed envelope.

Sincerely,

Children's Hospital Neonatal-Pediatric Transport Team

enclosure

---

the transport dispatch center can be used to coordinate communications and to notify receiving providers of a patient's imminent arrival. See Chapter 23 for further discussion.

In a disaster, hospitals are frequently overwhelmed by phone calls and inquiries from families, friends, employees, and the media. Incorporation of the dispatch center into the institution's disaster response system can provide additional resources for fielding phone calls. In addition, the dispatch center can notify other hospitals and ambulance services that "routine" emergency patients should be diverted to other institutions during the time standard resources are limited. The dispatch center often has valuable information about other facilities, including bed capacity and contact persons and phone numbers.

Information Processing and Documentation During Transport

Administrative Protocols

Each transport system differs in the policies and procedures used to guide operations and decision making. Examples of topics that should be covered in a comprehensive set of administrative protocols for the dispatch center include the following:

- Identification of the MCP
- Notification tree for specific types of patients (eg, trauma, surgical emergencies)
- Criteria for ground vs air transport
- Procedures to follow when the primary or preferred transport team is unavailable
- Weather-related policies and procedures
- Patient triage and disposition

Several sample flow diagrams for communication and decision making are included in Figure 5-5 and Figure 5-6.

The Intake Process

Essential information that should be obtained by the communications specialist at the time of a transport request is as follows:

- Name of caller and referring provider
- Patient's name, age, date of birth, and weight
- Call-back phone numbers, including the unit where patient is located and the referring provider's pager, if indicated
- Name of referring facility and location of the patient within the referring facility
- Landing zone information, if indicated
- Name of receiving facility and destination within the receiving facility, if known

Figure 5-5: Communications Center Flow Sheet, Emergency Department Referral*

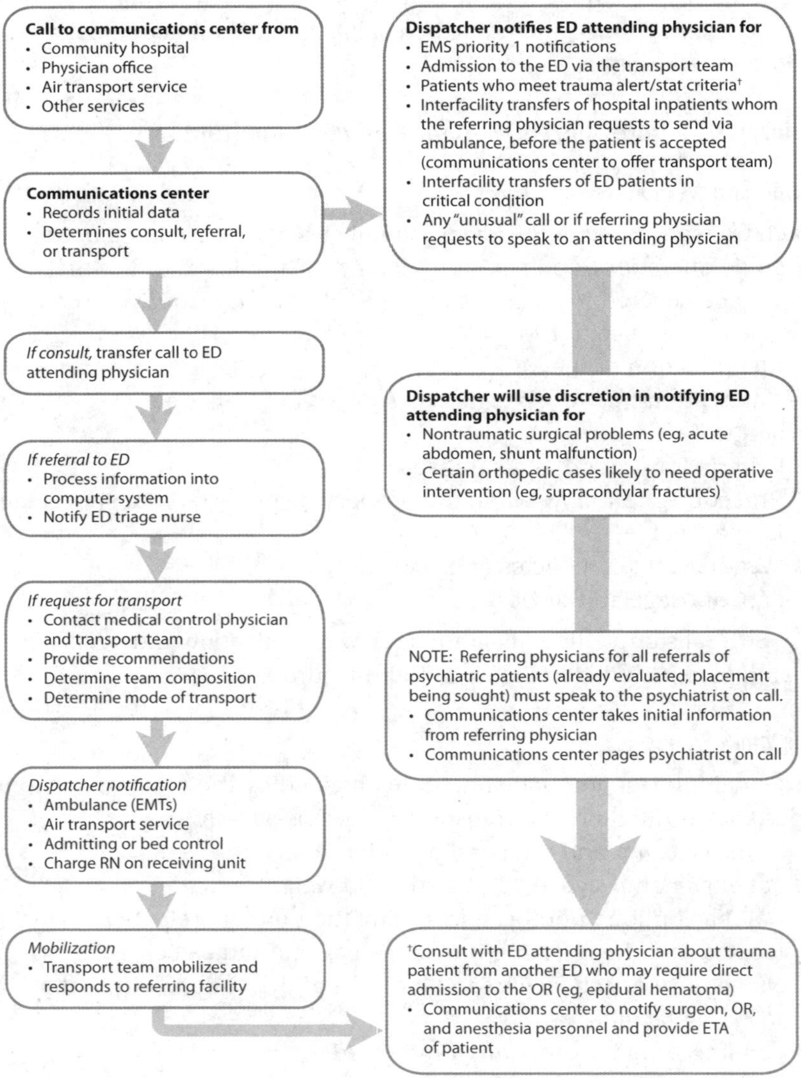

Call to communications center from
- Community hospital
- Physician office
- Air transport service
- Other services

Communications center
- Records initial data
- Determines consult, referral, or transport

If consult, transfer call to ED attending physician

If referral to ED
- Process information into computer system
- Notify ED triage nurse

If request for transport
- Contact medical control physician and transport team
- Provide recommendations
- Determine team composition
- Determine mode of transport

Dispatcher notification
- Ambulance (EMTs)
- Air transport service
- Admitting or bed control
- Charge RN on receiving unit

Mobilization
- Transport team mobilizes and responds to referring facility

Dispatcher notifies ED attending physician for
- EMS priority 1 notifications
- Admission to the ED via the transport team
- Patients who meet trauma alert/stat criteria†
- Interfacility transfers of hospital inpatients whom the referring physician requests to send via ambulance, before the patient is accepted (communications center to offer transport team)
- Interfacility transfers of ED patients in critical condition
- Any "unusual" call or if referring physician requests to speak to an attending physician

Dispatcher will use discretion in notifying ED attending physician for
- Nontraumatic surgical problems (eg, acute abdomen, shunt malfunction)
- Certain orthopedic cases likely to need operative intervention (eg, supracondylar fractures)

NOTE: Referring physicians for all referrals of psychiatric patients (already evaluated, placement being sought) must speak to the psychiatrist on call.
- Communications center takes initial information from referring physician
- Communications center pages psychiatrist on call

†Consult with ED attending physician about trauma patient from another ED who may require direct admission to the OR (eg, epidural hematoma)
- Communications center to notify surgeon, OR, and anesthesia personnel and provide ETA of patient

*ED indicates emergency department; EMTs, emergency medical technicians; RN, registered nurse; EMS, emergency medical services; OR, operating room; and ETA, expected time of arrival.

Figure 5-6: Communications Center Flow Sheet, Intensive Care Unit Referrals*

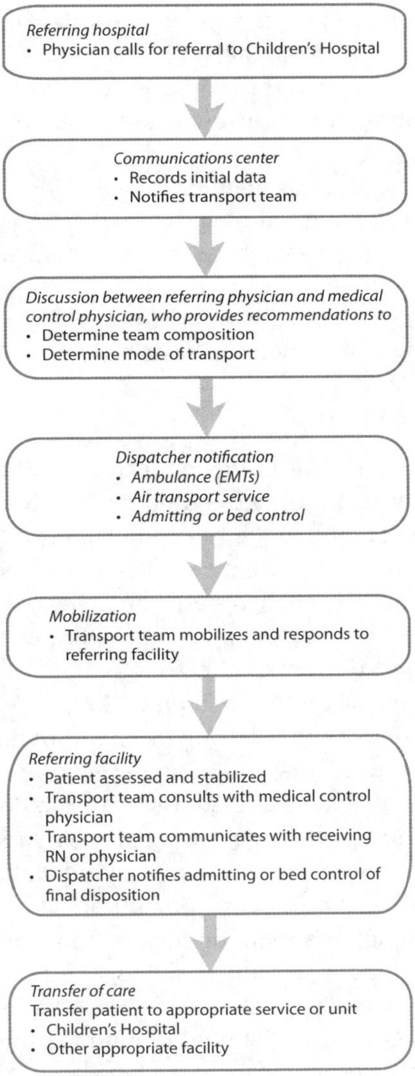

Referring hospital
- Physician calls for referral to Children's Hospital

Communications center
- Records initial data
- Notifies transport team

Discussion between referring physician and medical control physician, who provides recommendations to
- Determine team composition
- Determine mode of transport

Dispatcher notification
- Ambulance (EMTs)
- Air transport service
- Admitting or bed control

Mobilization
- Transport team mobilizes and responds to referring facility

Referring facility
- Patient assessed and stabilized
- Transport team consults with medical control physician
- Transport team communicates with receiving RN or physician
- Dispatcher notifies admitting or bed control of final disposition

Transfer of care
Transfer patient to appropriate service or unit
- Children's Hospital
- Other appropriate facility

*EMTs, emergency medical technicians; and RN, registered nurse.

- Name of accepting physician, if known
- Patient's preliminary diagnosis
- Time sensitivity (eg, emergency, urgent, nonemergency, elective)

Additional information that should be exchanged during contact between the MCP (or medical intake provider if a registered nurse or other professional) and the referring provider is as follows:

- Concise description of the current problem and pertinent medical history
- Patient's physiologic status, including vital signs
- Pertinent laboratory and radiologic data
- Current treatment (eg, vascular access, mechanical ventilation, medications)
- Interventions and response to interventions
- Special equipment or personnel requested (eg, isolette, inhaled nitric oxide)
- Infection control issues

It is essential that the MCP provide recommendations for evaluation and management during the time that the transport team is mobilizing and responding to the referring facility. The transport team should be advised of these recommendations so as to anticipate a possible change in the patient's status on arrival. If the referring provider indicates that he or she plans *not* to follow such recommendations, the transport team should be notified.

After the transport team has been mobilized, the communications specialist should contact the referring facility to obtain additional demographic information that might be necessary to process the admission. In general, access to insurance information is not necessary when ground or rotor-wing transport is being requested under emergency circumstances. For elective or scheduled transports or for long-distance fixed-wing transports, preauthorization of payment by third-party payers might be required for the transport program and/or the receiving facility to be reimbursed for their services.

To facilitate an expeditious departure from the referring facility, the communications specialist should remind the referring personnel of the need for copies of medical charts, laboratory results, and imaging studies (eg, radiographs, computed tomography, magnetic resonance imaging, ultrasound) to accompany the patient.

The Call-back Process

Once the transport team has had the opportunity to assess the patient and stabilize the patient's condition, there should be contact with the MCP. This contact updates the receiving institution about the patient's status and provides an opportunity to discuss management issues and patient disposition with the responsible physician. Essential data points are as follows:

- Patient's current condition
- Interventions and results of interventions performed by the transport team
- Special needs on arrival to the receiving facility (eg, high-frequency oscillatory ventilation, vasopressors, blood products, an isolation room) or immediate availability of the operating room, surgeons, diagnostic imaging (eg, computed tomography scan), or the resuscitation or trauma team
- Estimated time of arrival

Documentation

A standardized transport form can be used to distinguish care provided during interfacility transport from subsequent inpatient care. The form should concisely summarize the events during transport and provide a place to document information that the transport team might be in a unique position to obtain (eg, primary care physician, parent, or guardian contact numbers). Examples of EMTALA (Emergency Medical Treatment and Active Labor Act) forms for transport permission and documentation are included in Appendix A4.

Selected Readings

Fultz JF, Coyle CB, Reynolds PW. Air medical referring customer satisfaction: a valuable insight. *Air Med J.* 1998;17:51–56

Position statement of the Air Medical Physician Association: Patient Follow-up Letters and HIPPA. Available at: www.ampa.org/component/option,com_docman/task, cat_view/gid,23/. Accessed January 13, 2006.

Stanhope K, Falcone RE, Werman H. Helicopter dispatch: a time study. *Air Med J.* 1997;16:70–72

Thomson DP, Thomas SH. Guidelines for air medical dispatch. *Prehosp Emerg Care.* 2003;7:265–271

Questions

1. Emergency transport dispatch centers:
   a. have different priorities than prehospital emergency communications.
   b. should record all conversations regarding the transport.
   c. may be located in the intensive care unit, emergency department, or a remote location.
   d. have all of the above the characteristics.
2. Initial intake information should include:
   a. the patient's insurance information.
   b. call-back numbers for the referring provider and patient's unit.
   c. results of all laboratory and diagnostic tests.
   d. differential diagnosis.
3. Responsibilities of the dispatch center include:
   a. coordination of communications between the referring and receiving physicians.
   b. contact with air and ground ambulance service providers.
   c. communication with staff in the receiving unit.
   d. all of the above.

Answers

1. d
2. b
3. d

■ Equipment and Medications ■

Outline

- ■ Overview
- ■ Equipment
- ■ Medications

Overview

The interfacility transport of critically ill neonates and children requires basic and specialized equipment and medications geared toward the needs of pediatric patients (see appendices C1 and C2). Transport teams should be self-sufficient, with dedicated, organized supplies for quick, efficient access. Storage packs especially designed for neonatal-pediatric transports are commercially available and can be manufactured to be resistant to water and bloodborne pathogens. These packs and equipment containers should be organized, maintained, and verified by members of the transport team on a routine and documented basis. If any equipment needs to be shared among transport programs, local hospitals, or emergency medical services teams, plans and checklists should be developed to ensure that equipment is available and properly maintained. It is not advisable to rely on or plan to borrow equipment or medications from a referring hospital on a routine basis to serve a transport team's needs.

Transport equipment needs to be lightweight, portable, rugged, and easy to clean; to meet or exceed all hospital, local, state, federal and Federal Aviation Administration (FAA) requirements; and to have been tested in the transport environment. Use of a single universal equipment pack to treat patients ranging from premature neonates to adults is not recommended. There are too many age-specific tools, medications, delivery devices, and techniques to enable efficient use of this type of equipment organization. The weight of stocked packs should be documented for air transports. All medical packs should be checked before and after each transport, as well as daily. All electrical equipment must have independent, rechargeable power sources that can easily connect to power outlets in ground and air transport vehicles. These issues can be especially troublesome in the international transport arena. Compatibility of all mechanical equipment is critical (eg, the oxygen and air connectors must be compatible with all such connectors on all vehicles to be used) to avoid potentially disastrous interruption of therapy. Routine, scheduled equipment maintenance should be done by competent, well-trained biomedical technicians.

The safety of all equipment used in transport is mandatory. Approved methods must be used to secure all equipment inside all transport vehicles and aircraft, whether equipment is portable or a permanent part of the vehicle. Techniques for securing patients, incubators, ventilators, stretchers, and equipment and drug packs need to be reviewed rigorously, and all personnel should be trained in these vital aspects of transport safety (see Chapter 9, 10).

Changes in weather and environmental conditions encountered during transport may affect performance of equipment. The real effects of vehicle vibration, temperature swings, and barometric pressure changes with altitude or sudden decompression must be determined before equipment is used. If this has not been accomplished by the manufacturer or by another organization, local biomedical testing services may be helpful in simulating transport conditions while testing proposed equipment.

Proper storage and dispensing of medications is essential for providing safe, effective care. Medications such as prostaglandins and surfactant require special procedures for refrigerated storage, shelf-life adjustment when not refrigerated, and additional training regarding their use on transport. A clinical pharmacist can be a valuable resource for identifying specific issues related to medication use during transport. Most transport teams carry controlled substances; institutional, state, and federal regulations should be consulted for security and documentation requirements. The Joint Commission on Accreditation of Healthcare Organizations (JCAHO) has mandated the use of standardized medication concentrations in hospitals and intensive care units (ICUs) but has not specifically required this change for interfacility transport. It is recommended that each transport program, however, consult its compliance experts to determine how to interpret JCAHO standards within the transport environment.

Equipment

The essential features of equipment used in neonatal-pediatric transport are listed in Table 6-1, and a specific equipment list is shown in Table 6-2. Packs may need to be tailored to the needs of the individual transport service, and all team members should be facile in locating all supplies. Specialized teams (eg, neonatal, cardiac, extracorporeal membrane oxygenation, nitric oxide, and trauma) need additional equipment and medications to support these particular services.

Various transport incubators (isolettes) are available commercially. The type selected must provide regulated temperature, oxygen, and humidity and allow visibility and easy emergency access to the infant during transport. Review and approval of the FAA are required if the incubator is to be used on rotor- or fixed-wing aircraft.

Table 6-1: Essential Features of Equipment Used in Neonatal-Pediatric Transport

- Lightweight and portable
- Durable, able to withstand 4g acceleration and deceleration forces
- Easily maintained and cleaned
- Portable power (twice the expected mission time as minimum)
- AC/DC capable (use vehicle or hospital power source when possible)
- Production of no electromagnetic interference
- Resistant to electromagnetic interference
- Well-labeled (including return address of transport team)
- Audible and visible alarms
- Completely securable
- Compatible with all other equipment
- Able to meet all local, federal, state, and Federal Aviation Administration codes, including hazardous material regulations
- Able to tolerate altitude and temperature changes, sudden decompression, and vibration without performance change
- Able to fit easily through standard hospital doors
- Loadable in vehicles by 2 transport personnel

■ ■

Table 6-2: Specific Equipment Used in Neonatal-Pediatric Transport*

- Transport incubator (patients <5 kg) or stretcher
- Ventilator, humidification and oxygen delivery equipment
- Cardiovascular, blood pressure (invasive and noninvasive), and pulse oximetry monitors
- Portable transilluminator, chest tubes, and Heimlich valves
- Portable glucometer (essential)
- Point-of-care testing equipment, including blood gas analyzer (optional)
- Temperature monitoring probes and devices
- Airway equipment (endotracheal tubes, laryngoscopes, resuscitation bag and mask, and laryngeal mask airways)
- Portable suction
- Air-oxygen blender capable of delivering F_{IO_2} 0.21 to 1.0 with flow meter up to 15 L/min
- Infusion pumps with low (0.1 mL/h) to high (1000 mL/h) capability
- Intravenous, central venous, intraosseous, and umbilical lines
- Defibrillator-cardioverter/pacer (see text)
- Intracranial pressure monitor (for certain pediatric patients)
- Nitric oxide administration equipment
- Trauma packs (for selected pediatric teams) including bandages, splints, chest tube kits, large bore venous access, and cervical spine immobilization equipment

*All electrical equipment must have an independent (battery) power source. The batteries should have power for at least twice the anticipated mission time when vehicles to be used have no power source. F_{IO_2} indicates fraction of inspired oxygen.

The choice of ventilators is not easy and should be based on projected use, cost, team skill-level, and team configuration to ensure proper operation. The availability of a respiratory therapist may influence the range of ventilator options during transport. Modes of ventilation for infants and children range from pressure-limited, time-cycled to volume-cycled or flow-triggered pressure support. Most ventilators are capable of delivering positive end-expiratory pressure. Some ventilators can perform multiple functions and can be adjusted for use with patients ranging from neonates to adults; other ventilators are ideally suited to a more limited patient population. Most neonates are ventilated using a pressure-limited, time-cycled mode. However, there are data to support the use of continuous positive airway pressure, assist-control, or high-frequency oscillatory or jet ventilation modes on transport. It is important to note that the equipment providing these newer ventilation modes in a mobile environment may be in the development phase, and most data are team-specific and have not been thoroughly reviewed. The use of untested or uncertified custom-built ventilators is not recommended unless approved by local institutional review boards for research purposes. If transporting a patient using a home ventilator that has not been tested in the transport environment, special considerations should be made, such as transfer to a transport ventilator before transport to ensure adequate transition and support or ensuring availability of a backup transport ventilator in case problems are encountered with the home ventilator.

The use of inhaled nitric oxide to treat severe, persistent pulmonary hypertension in term and near-term neonates is standard of care. Teams transporting neonates receiving inhaled nitric oxide require specialized personnel and delivery devices to provide the correct mixture of gases through transport ventilators. The use of inhaled nitric oxide during transport is not recommended until transport personnel are well trained with the equipment in the intensive care setting (see Chapter 17).

It is standard for infants and children to have end-tidal carbon dioxide monitored during assisted ventilation via an endotracheal tube during transport. Disposable end-tidal carbon dioxide detectors are available commercially in several sizes for use in patients ranging from infants (> 2 kg) to adults. These colorimetric detectors are light- and moisture-sensitive and are most commonly used to confirm tracheal tube placement at the time of intubation rather than to monitor tracheal tube position during transport. Capnography during transport is available with a portable device or as a built-in component of a transport monitor. The advantage of end-tidal carbon dioxide monitoring, as opposed to detection, is the continuous graphic display of each respiratory cycle. In addition to the ongoing confirmation of endotracheal tube position, capnography can provide valuable information about ventilation and circulation when interpreted by knowledgeable providers. It should be noted that the efficacy of these monitors and detectors has not been tested as thoroughly with neonates, especially those who are preterm, compared with children and adults.

Oxygen and air cylinders must be labeled and checked regularly. A desirable supply estimate is based on at least double the anticipated needs for the transport. A portable supply must be available for the transfer of the patient to and from the transport vehicle, with appropriate tubing lengths for maneuvering equipment in and out of ambulances and aircraft. It is essential to be able to provide oxygen concentrations between 21% and 100% during interfacility transport, especially for infants with congenital heart disease who are at risk for pulmonary overcirculation in the presence of high concentrations of oxygen. Certain air-oxygen blenders are less wasteful of gases than others, and the most efficient gas-conserving model should be selected. Monitoring of the delivered oxygen concentration also is required.

Suction capability in all aspects of transport is essential. Whether it is for airway clearance or for thoracostomy tube drains, a stand-alone, battery-powered unit is required. The ability to regulate vacuum pressure is essential for the neonatal population.

Many cardiovascular and vital sign monitors are available commercially. Multifunction monitors that include oximetry and invasive and noninvasive blood pressure monitoring are desirable but can be costly. For noninvasive blood pressure monitoring, appropriate cuff sizes for a variety of patients must be available.

Pulse oximeters used in aircraft must pass electromagnetic interference testing. Pulse synchronization is essential to avoid erroneous readings during transport, when patient movements and vibration may interfere with optimal operations.

Monitoring of patients' temperature is mandatory. Hypothermia and hyperthermia are common findings in pediatric patients (eg, prematurity, sepsis, cold-water drowning, and febrile seizures). Hypothermia may result from the exposure involved in stabilization and transport, especially in preterm neonates. Personnel should be familiar with the myriad of skin and tympanic membrane probes available for transport.

Intravenous infusion pumps must have stand-alone capability and be capable of accurate, controlled, and even delivery of infusion fluids and medications through various intravenous and umbilical line apparatus. Battery-operated pumps that can deliver rates as low as 0.1 mL per hour and high-flow rates may be required and are readily available commercially. Transport teams should use pumps that can be secured safely on intravenous poles attached to transport stretchers or isolettes so that they do not have to be carried separately.

■■■■■■■■■■■■■■■■■■■■■■■■■■■■■■■■

Blood glucose monitoring strips or portable glucometers are essential during transport. Many teams now use point-of-care portable testing equipment, which allows for accurate electrolyte and/or blood gas measurements. Portable blood gas analyzers are also commercially available. When considering whether to provide point-of-care testing, a transport program should be aware that there are considerable requirements for quality control and documentation in conjunction with the sponsoring institution's laboratory services.

A separate, designated pediatric defibrillator-cardioverter/pacer is highly recommended, but it might not be used during most transports owing to the low incidence of arrhythmias in the neonatal and pediatric age groups. Each team must consider the weight and cost of such equipment vs the realistic needs based on patient population, thereby potentially making the routine inclusion of this equipment less practical for some exclusively neonatal transport teams. If teams take defibrillators-cardioverters/pacers on transport, they should ascertain that pediatric-sized pads or paddles are included. Although it is uncommon, transport teams may be asked to provide transthoracic pacing for pediatric patients with conditions such as toxic ingestions, myocarditis, and implanted pacemaker failure.

The use of intracranial pressure monitoring during neonatal-pediatric transport may also be encountered. Specific training and equipment are needed to optimally manage the care of patients who need such monitoring.

Medications

Table 6-3 lists the basic groups of medications and intravenous fluids used by neonatal-pediatric transport teams. Important indications, contraindications, and special considerations for administering neonatal-pediatric transport drugs are accessible via local, published, and online formularies. A sample transport team drug dosage card is included in Appendix B.

Medications need to be checked and restocked routinely before and after every transport and their use logged appropriately. A routine and scheduled inspection for expired medications and a rotation plan for near-expired medications are recommended. Transport medications should be stored in a safe, dedicated place between transports

---

Table 6-3: Basic Groups of Medications and Intravenous Fluids Used by Neonatal-Pediatric Transport Teams

- Intravenous fluids
  - $D_{10}W$, D_5W, D_5W 0.2 NS, D_5W 0.45 NS, lactated ringer's, NS (normal saline), albumin 5%
- Inotropic agents
  - Dopamine, dobutamine, epinephrine, norepinephrine, milrinone
- Code medications
  - Epinephrine, sodium bicarbonate (infant and adult preparations), naloxone, lidocaine, amiodarone, atropine, adenosine, calcium chloride, calcium gluconate, magnesium sulfate
- Rapid-sequence intubation medications
  - Fentanyl, midazolam, ketamine, etomidate, thiopental, rocuronium, vecuronium, succinylcholine, atropine
- Diuretics: furosemide
- Antibiotics
  - Ampicillin, gentamicin, cefotaxime, ceftriaxone, cefazolin, acyclovir
- Prostaglandins
- Surfactant preparations
- Asthma and croup medications
  - Methylprednisolone, racemic epinephrine, albuterol, terbutaline
- Anticonvulsants
  - Lorazepam, phenobarbital, fosphenytoin
- Intracranial pressure medications
  - Mannitol, dexamethasone, hypertonic saline

---

so they are not depleted inadvertently by use in another clinical area. Transport teams should always assume that community hospitals will not have the medications or specialized fluids needed to treat most neonatal and pediatric conditions. Any incorrect dose or unexpected adverse drug reaction should be documented and reviewed with the team's medical director and the pharmacist immediately following the transport.

Most analgesics, sedatives, and induction agents are considered controlled substances by state and federal agencies. All controlled substances must be prescribed by a physician with a valid US Drug Enforcement Agency license and state controlled substance certificate. For a nonphysician transport team, orders for controlled substances

■ ■

must be signed by the medical control physician or appropriate designee. For hospital-based transport teams, institutional policies govern the documentation requirements for controlled substances and the process for replenishing supplies after use. For freestanding transport teams, an arrangement with one or more medical control facilities should be made to provide replacement of controlled substances through a hospital pharmacy.

The use of endotracheally administered surfactant for neonates with respiratory distress syndrome is standard of care in the neonatal ICU. Many transport teams or referring medical teams administer surfactant to appropriate patients at referring nurseries before transport to the tertiary center. It is highly recommended that each team standardize its surfactant protocol and be well trained in its administration to minimize confusion and potential adverse effects, such as accidental extubation, pneumothorax, and pulmonary hemorrhage. Lung compliance changes should be anticipated during the first 30 minutes following surfactant administration. Some transport teams wait a specified time after administering surfactant to initiate the return transport.

Drug packs optimally should be constituted according to the needs of an individual team. Because most drugs used in pediatrics are given on a dose-per-kilogram basis and the weight of some critically ill pediatric patients may not be available at the time of transport, it is recommended that a length-based tape or length-weight or weight-for-age chart be used to approximate the child's weight. This chart can be used for emergency drug and fluid calculations until a definitive weight can be obtained. Teams that use length-based tapes on which doses are provided in *milliliters* should ascertain that the concentration of the drug preparation used matches that used on the tape.

Weight-drug-dose tables should be attached to drug packs and intake sheets to facilitate efficient mixing and administration of drugs (eg, vasopressors, antibiotics, and medications used during cardiopulmonary resuscitation). Drug cards, developed by each team, may be laminated and pocket-sized and should include important telephone numbers.

Questions

1. Do neonatal-pediatric transport teams need specialized equipment and medications?
2. Is one ventilator suitable for all pediatric transport patients?
3. Should transport teams consider separate medication and equipment packs for neonates and older pediatric patients?

Answers

1. Yes. Neonatal-pediatric transport is a specialized aspect of transport medicine. Neonatal-pediatric teams must have equipment and medications geared to the specific illnesses and conditions of the neonatal-pediatric population.
2. Modes of ventilation range considerably from premature neonates to older pediatric patients. Each team needs to assess its patient population and purchase a transport ventilator that is easy to use and most applicable to the anticipated needs of patients. No single ventilator is optimal for use with all neonatal and pediatric patients and conditions.
3. Yes, the drug doses and needs of neonates, especially preterm neonates, are different from those of pediatric patients. Personnel should be trained in the storage, dosing, and administration of drugs specific to their patient populations.

Legal Issues

Outline

- Legal concepts and issues
- Sources of the law
- Court concepts
  - Venue
  - Case law
  - Role of the trial judge
  - Role of the jury
  - Standard of care
- Basic concepts of health care law
- Medical liability
  - Criminal
  - Licensure
  - Civil liability
- Emergency Medical Treatment and Active Labor Act
  - Presents to the dedicated ED
  - Ambulances and helicopters
  - Designated hospitals
  - Disaster status exception
  - Patient transfers: stable vs unstable
  - Outpatient vs inpatient transfers
  - Administration of the law
- Health Insurance Portability and Accountability Act
  - HIPAA disclosure to law enforcement
  - Public health reporting
  - Communicable diseases
  - Abuse or neglect

- When medical responsibility attaches to the transport team
  - Dispatch
  - Diversion en route
  - On-scene responses
  - In the hospital
  - Delivery at the receiving facility
  - When civil legal liability attaches
- Transfer agreement issues
  - Liability issues with transfer agreements
- Role of risk management
  - Credentialing
  - Policies, procedures, and protocols
  - Quality measures
  - Incident management
  - Litigation support
- Documentation
  - What should be in the record
- Quality of care issues at the sending facility
  - Duty to intervene
- Quality of care issues during transport
- Transporting nonpatients

Legal Concepts and Issues

By offering care to a patient, the provider takes on a duty. This duty results in medical and civil legal liability, forming a contract, actual or implied, for services. A *tort* occurs when there is negligence that results in an injury or harm to the patient. A *criminal liability* occurs when there is a breech of criminal statute. Some acts may be a tort and a crime (eg, battery).

As medical transport services take an increasingly important role in the provision of health care, it is important to recognize that the laws that govern the legal liability of these services are not new. In fact, the laws and rules come from a progressive development of case law, statutes, and regulations over time. The rules of law that apply to medical transport, therefore, are a composite of general rules, transportation rules, and ambulance rules flavored with recent aircraft and emergency medical services (EMS) regulation.

Understanding the source of the rules and the applications that have arisen are essential to consideration of legal liability and distinctions for transport application.

Sources of the Law

The Constitution, statutes, and case law (laws established by court decision) are the foundation of our judicial system. During the last half of the 20th century, a new source of laws has emerged in the form of administrative regulations. These regulations, developed by various agencies and bureaus, have blurred the distinction between the legislative and executive branches of government and now represent the vast majority of the written law in the United States. The Warsaw Convention and associated agreements and protocols generally cover cases involving international commercial air transport.

In the malpractice liability context, however, constitutional issues are seldom involved beyond whether a jury trial must be provided to determine a malpractice claim. The dominant sources of law in the medical field have been the court system with its decisions on interpersonal rights and responsibilities and the jury system driving the price of liability. To a limited degree, legislatures have attempted to reform the court system and limit liability in malpractice cases, but at the same time, increasing volumes of regulations have created new standards that may become the basis for claims of malpractice liability.

Court Concepts

The courts of the United States function on a number of basic principles that are essential to an understanding of legal liability for health care providers in general and transport providers specifically. These principles include venue, case law, roles of the trial judge and jury, and the standard of care.

Venue

Most medical malpractice cases are based on state standards and tried in state courts, unless the case involves "diversity of citizenship" (residents or services of different states involved). The state laws determine the rights of all parties to the case, the procedures they must follow, and the damages (money) or limits to damages that plaintiffs may recover.

State courts are typically organized by counties, and juries are usually obtained from the community where the case is filed (venue). Where a case is filed, depending on the state's rules, can vary from where the transport of the patient originated or terminated to where the company is headquartered. The likely verdict or size of award may also affect the venue. In situations such as air medical transport, the location of the care might involve multiple states or countries and further expand the options of where the case may be tried. In some cases involving multiple locations, a judicial panel on multi-district litigation may decide the case venue.

Case Law

Courts are expected to follow established precedent to the extent that it fits the case. This expectation is called *stare decisis*. The process of following prior decisions is often referred to as *common law* or *case law*. It is essentially following legal tradition and abiding by the existing information that people have available to guide their actions.

Role of the Trial Judge

The role of the trial judge is to rule on the law, the process, and the evidence in a case. The trial judge controls the issues allowed to be presented by ruling on the legal sufficiency of various elements of court documents and the items of information the parties can have access to through the process of *discovery.* In medical malpractice cases, the trial judge often must rule on what items of information are confidential and exempt from disclosure, such as certain peer-review documents.

During the trial, the trial judge serves as the referee to ensure that both sides follow the rules of courtroom decorum and rules on motions and objections that determine what evidence is presented and how it is presented. The rulings on the evidence often have a profound influence on the ultimate outcome of a case.

At the conclusion of the evidence and following the arguments of the attorneys for both sides, the judge gives a verbal *charge* to the jury.

This charge involves a reading of the written instructions the jury members will take with them into deliberations on their verdict.

Following the verdict, the trial judge may rule on motions for a new trial or to overturn the verdict of the jury. These posttrial motions are usually in preparation for an appeal to a higher court. Once an appeal is filed, the trial judge loses jurisdiction over the case until the higher court returns the case with instructions or rulings. The reality of trial courts, however, is that most cases end with the jury verdict at the trial level and are not appealed.

Role of the Jury

Most state and all federal courts allow either side of a medical malpractice case to request a jury trial. The number of jurors varies by locality or jurisdiction. Procedures differ between jurisdictions for selecting jury members from the pool of potential jurors. The jury must reach its decision in a medical malpractice case based on the facts it finds to be true by a preponderance of the evidence. This means that the jury must be convinced that a given fact is more likely true than untrue, or just beyond 50% probability. The number or percentage of jurors necessary to reach a verdict varies by jurisdiction.

The jury is considered the conscience of the court system. It is charged with the duty to make its decision based on the facts, evidence, and law presented to it, without allowing sympathy or prejudice to interfere in the process. The jury members may rely on their common understanding and experience in life to judge the reasonableness of the evidence and testimony and to decide what is true and not true.

Standard of Care

Often, the most significant fact that the jury must determine is whether the health care provider's care in the case was within the *standard of care*. This essentially is a determination whether the health care provider "negligently injured" the patient in some way as claimed in the lawsuit.

Simply, the standard of care is based on how competent practitioners with similar qualifications would have managed the patient's care under the same or similar circumstances. The standard is generally based on usual practices that exist in a community. In current legal terms, *community* may mean a region or the entire nation, depending on the jurisdiction. The standard may also be based on the *respectable minority* rule. This rule lets the jury decide whether the practitioner, using best judgment, followed an alternative treatment recognized by a respectable minority of those in the profession. There is no current legal definition of what constitutes a respectable minority. Generally, a medical expert of the same provider specialty will testify that the care provided did or did not meet the standard of care expected in similar circumstances.

Although the court often makes legal rulings on issues that may affect what goes to the jury for its decision on facts, we will consider the concept of liability for medical malpractice claims as made up of 4 basic factual elements that the jury generally determines:

1. Duty: Did the health care provider establish a relationship with the patient that created a duty to provide care?
2. Breach: Did the health care provider fail to provide the care or provide it in a manner that fell below the standard of care of the specialty or profession?
3. Injury: Did the action or inaction of the health care provider that failed to meet the standard of care cause a legally recognized injury (physical, psychological, property damage, or damage to another legal right), worsen the injury, cause or increase expense, or (in some states) reduce the chances for a favorable outcome? Was there a logical connection between the failure to meet the standard of care and the resulting injury?
4. Damages: What award of money will compensate the victim for the injury or losses suffered and reasonably likely to be suffered in the future? This award typically includes medical expenses, hospitalization, home care, loss of wages, and pain and suffering.

Basic Concepts of Health Care Law

First and foremost in health care law consideration is the concept of patient choice as a fundamental right. The competent, unimpaired, adult (a person who has reached the age of majority) has the right to choose whatever health care treatment he or she will receive, even if that choice might otherwise seem illogical or result in death. The right of *informed consent* may be involved in the malpractice liability issues that will confront a transport service and is especially important when considering pediatric transport (see Chapter 18).

Informed consent shows the patient's agreement to a course of treatment and must be obtained before any treatment of a patient. Lack of informed consent may be grounds for medical malpractice claims and potential (but rare) criminal prosecutions. For example, touching a person (such as providing medical care) without consent is considered *battery* under the law—illegal touching that causes some legal or physical harm to the patient. In addition, an allegation of insufficient informed consent can be added to an allegation of malpractice to imply that the physician is careless.

Consent may be legally obtained from competent, unimpaired adults for their own care. However, there may be issues about who may consent for a minor, such as in the case of a pediatric transfer. Generally, a parent may consent for health care to his or her minor child. Other adults may consent for care of a minor based on state statutes that establish *health care surrogate* or *in loco parentis* (someone standing in for the parent) laws. The legal order in which decision-making power is conferred on relatives or significant others varies significantly from state to state. Some states allow minors to consent for care related to reproductive and sexually transmitted disease concerns.

Another area of concern is the issue of minors who are pregnant or who are parents, whether married or unmarried. Some states clearly establish by law that minors who are parents may consent for the care of their children and for themselves. Other state laws allow minor parents to consent to the care of their child but not to their own care unless they are married. In some states, a pregnant minor female may consent to her own care and that of her unborn child, whereas in others, she may not do so, and the mother's parents retain legal power of consent over the pregnant minor and the unborn child.

In some states, minors may gain limited adult rights when they are emancipated. Depending on the state, a child may be considered emancipated by demonstrating freedom from parental control or support or by court declaration. Emancipated minors may give their own informed consent and enter into contracts.

There is also the principle of *implied* or *emergent consent*. This form of consent exists when the surrounding circumstances lead a reasonable person to believe that consent would have been granted even though the patient or legal surrogate did not directly express agreement. For example, one would expect lifesaving measures to be taken in the sudden, unforeseen circumstance that required action to protect a life. Common and statutory laws generally have supported physicians and health care professionals providing emergency care for children without the consent of a parent or guardian.

Providers must be familiar with the laws and regulations dealing with consent in their state of operation. With advice from legal counsel who have expertise in health care law, transport services should develop written policies and guidelines that conform to federal and state laws regarding consent for the treatment of minors, including specific guidelines on parental notification and patient confidentiality for unaccompanied minors.

For consent to be valid, the patient must be properly informed. The *informed* requirement means that the responsible, consenting party was provided information on the benefits, risks, and alternatives of the proposed treatment before consent. Some states require that the disclosure of risks must be all things a reasonably prudent person would want to know when making a decision on care (reasonable patient standard). Other states limit the necessary disclosure to things a reasonable physician would consider important to disclose (reasonable physician standard).

Ideally, informed consent is documented on a specific form that details the service to be provided (such as helicopter transfer with medical care en route) and a simple, clear statement of the risks associated with the transfer. A statement that "risks and benefits were discussed with the patient" is not sufficient. Hospitals should use a standardized form that includes the reason for transfer, medical benefits and risks, mode and level of transport, care to be provided during the transport, and the name of the receiving facility and authorized accepting person or physician (Appendix A4).

Where possible, the consent should be signed by the patient. If written signature is not possible, verbal authorization or phone consent should be obtained from the legal surrogate and noted and signed by the person obtaining the consent (and witness if required) when possible. Patients who are unable to consent owing to injury or medical condition, intoxication, mental illness, or legal incompetency (eg, a minor) who do not have a legal surrogate available are presumed to have given implied consent for reasonably necessary care. The law generally requires that a reasonable effort must be made to contact the parent(s) or legal guardian or responsible party (such as a state agency guardian for children or developmentally disabled patients or prison warden for incarcerated patients) for consent unless physicians have determined that the delay would endanger the patient. The American Academy of Pediatrics, the American College of Surgeons, the Society of Pediatric Nurses, the Society of Critical Care Medicine, the American College of Emergency Physicians, the Emergency Nurses Association, and the National Association of EMS Physicians have endorsed the statement that "Appropriate medical care for the pediatric patient with an urgent or emergent condition should never be withheld or delayed because of problems with obtaining consent."

It is of import to note that under the Emergency Medical Treatment and Active Labor Act (EMTALA; see the "Emergency Medical Treatment and Active Labor Act" section), a minor can request an examination or treatment for an emergency medical condition. A hospital is not to delay care while waiting for parental consent. If no emergency is found to exist, further care may be deferred while awaiting consent.

Medical Liability

Legal liability concerns for neonatal-pediatric transport providers involve malpractice liability, in addition to regulatory actions, licensure concerns, and the possibility of criminal charges in the most extreme cases. Transport providers may primarily be concerned with malpractice risk issues in legal discussions of liability, but the interactions of all types must be considered. In fact, violations of regulatory or licensure standards may be the basis for a malpractice allegation.

Criminal

Unlicensed or substandard operations are the most likely to result in criminal charges. Issues of unlicensed operation may occur when transport units cross state lines to pick up or deliver patients.

It is essential that transport teams have a clear understanding of neighboring state laws and licensure clearance before responding across a state line. Reciprocal agreements or multistate licensure may be required to ensure that medical care may be legally performed in a neighboring jurisdiction. In the case of rotor- and fixed-wing services, the issue may extend to an even greater radius of potential service. Responses into some states, whether by fixed-wing or rotary aircraft, may be prohibited by state or local law except in cases of disaster. It is the responsibility of the transport service's legal counsel to determine the types of clearance needed in each potential destination state and to obtain the appropriate permissions, licenses, and/or waivers needed and educate the teams on the requirements. In addition, the service should ensure that its malpractice and liability policies are in effect when traveling to other states.

Licensure

Failure to meet or maintain the standards and requirements for licensure can result in actions against the service and individual personnel. These actions can result in fines, probationary status, suspension, or revocation of licenses.

Civil Liability

In most states, a basic case of liability can be made by showing that the regulations were violated and that the regulations were in place to protect the safety of the public. In some cases, the law explicitly creates a new statutory cause of action for liability. These new causes of action, however, are legislative changes and typically are not created by regulation.

The rules that apply to regulatory violations and their effect on liability vary from state to state. In some states, when that standard is violated and harm results, "normal" medical malpractice may be established without resort to experts to establish the standard of care. One such approach is called *negligence per se*. A violation of the law or regulations is proof of failing to meet the appropriate standard of care. In a negligence per se claim, the plaintiff has to show that a law intended to prevent the type of injury that occurred was violated. A negligence per se claim may be made even if the defendant has not been convicted or administratively sanctioned under the law in question. In such cases, the plaintiff must prove that the defendant violated the law. Other states use a *prima facie rule*. In prima facie cases, it is presumed that the evidence is sufficient to establish the fact in question unless rebutted. The burden shifts to the defendant to prove that the violation of the regulation was not negligence. In either case, however, there must be resulting harm to the patient for liability to exist.

Not every violation of the regulations, however, would result in liability. If vehicle maintenance regulations were violated, for example, it would not be grounds for a medical malpractice claim, but it might be grounds for liability for patient injuries incurred in a crash that resulted from improper maintenance. On the other hand, a violation that involved failure to restock mandated equipment and the lack of equipment made it impossible to properly care for the patient would likely support a malpractice claim by a patient who was harmed by the lack of equipment. In the absence of explicit intent of the legislature or agency to create a safety standard or prior court rulings on the issue, it is up to the injured party to prove to a judge that the regulation is a safety standard that should be applied to create liability.

Emergency Medical Treatment and Active Labor Act

For years, many indigent patients were turned away from hospital emergency departments (EDs). Patients in unstable condition were transferred or denied care simply because they did not have the financial means to make or guarantee hospital payment. Congress passed an amendment to the Social Security Act, EMTALA, as part of the Consolidated Omnibus Budget Reconciliation Act of 1986. Intended as an "anti–patient dumping" law, it required Medicare-participating hospitals to provide necessary emergency care for patients. Hospitals had to provide a medical screening examination (MSE) and stabilization of any emergency medical condition (EMC) regardless of the patient's ability to pay. Subsequent revisions of EMTALA have expanded its scope and better defined its role, especially with respect to EMS. Laws that contradict or conflict with EMTALA are considered preempted by it. The Centers for Medicare and Medicaid Services (CMS) issue and enforce regulations under the act.

Congress did not intend for the statute to be used as a federal malpractice statute. A number of court decisions have supported this (*Bryan v Rectors and Visitors of University of Virginia*, 95 F3d 349, 351 [4th Cir 1996]; *Lopez-Soto v Hawayek*, 175 F3d 170, 177 [1st Cir 1999]; and *Baker v Adventist Health, Inc*, 260 F3d 987, 994 (3rd Cir 2001).

EMTALA provides that any patient who "presents" to the hospital's "dedicated" ED requesting evaluation or treatment must receive an MSE to determine the presence of an EMC. If an EMC is present, the patient's condition must be stabilized within the capacity of the treating hospital. Patients requiring care beyond the hospital's capacity may be transferred to an appropriate facility. The obligations related to the transfer depend on whether the patient's condition is stable. Protection under EMTALA also covers psychiatric patients and the unborn children of women in labor.

Presents to the Dedicated ED

The latest revision of EMTALA clarifies the old "comes to the hospital" standard. Any person who comes to the hospital's dedicated ED requesting an evaluation or a treatment must have an MSE. The request can be made on the patient's behalf (eg, a minor). A request is considered to have been made if a prudent layperson observer would believe, based on the person's appearance or behavior, that the person needed an evaluation or treatment. A *dedicated* ED is any department of the hospital (1) licensed by the state as an ED, (2) held out to the public as a place for emergency or unscheduled care, or (3) in which at least one third of the outpatient visits were for emergency care during the previous calendar year. The ED does not have to be located on the main hospital campus. The CMS considers labor and delivery and psychiatric units to fall under the dedicated ED definition. However, EMTALA does not apply to a person who comes to a hospital outpatient department and an EMC unexpectedly develops during a scheduled visit.

The "250-yard" rule has also been modified. The request for care, using the aforementioned criteria, may still occur anywhere on the hospital property (including driveways and sidewalks). However, CMS uses other Medicare rules (42 CFR §413.65) to define the hospital campus. Areas such as physician offices, skilled nursing facilities (and similar separate Medicare-participating units), and nonmedical facilities are not included in the hospital's zone of responsibility. Non-EDs off the main hospital campus no longer fall under EMTALA. They still must have written policies for dealing with emergencies.

Ambulances and Helicopters

The new rules have clarified a number of issues for hospital and non–hospital-owned and -operated ambulances and helicopters. Hospital-owned and operated ambulances and helicopters are not considered part of the hospital's dedicated ED if they are

1. operated under community-wide EMS protocols that direct where to transport the patient (eg, to the closest appropriate facility) or
2. given online medical directions to where to transport the patient by a physician who is independent of the hospital that owns the ambulance.

Telephone or telemetry contact with ED personnel by non–hospital-owned and -operated ambulances and helicopters does not trigger that hospital's EMTALA obligation. The hospital may divert the ambulance to another facility if the hospital is on "diversionary status" (insufficient staff or facilities to accept additional emergency patients). However, if the ambulance drives on to the hospital property despite being told to divert, the hospital has an EMTALA obligation.

In *Arrington v Wong,* the US 9th Circuit Court of Appeals ruled that diverting an ambulance requesting access may result in EMTALA liability. In this case, it was alleged that a patient with severe breathing difficulties was diverted en route from an ED to a military hospital. The patient died on arrival at the military facility, and the family sued the hospital that did not accept the patient. The hospital was not on diversion status. The court ruled that the allegations were enough to force the matter to trial on potential EMTALA liability. The CMS partially addressed this issue in the revised rules. Hospital and non–hospital-owned and -operated ambulances may be diverted

■■■■■■■■■■■■■■■■■■■■■■■■■■■■■■■■■

when the diversion is part of a community-wide EMS protocol. Should a hospital that is not on diversionary status fail to accept a telephone or radio request for transfer or admission, the refusal could represent a violation of other federal or state requirements.

Under the *helipad exemption,* ambulances may bring patients onto the hospital grounds without triggering the hospital's EMTALA obligation under certain circumstances:

■ The use of a hospital's helipad by local ambulance services or other hospitals for the transport of patients to tertiary hospitals located throughout the state does not trigger an EMTALA obligation as long as the sending hospital conducted the MSE before transporting the patient to the helipad. The sending hospital is responsible for conducting the MSE before transfer to determine whether an EMC exists and implementing stabilizing treatment or conducting an appropriate transfer. Therefore, if the helipad serves simply as a point of transit for patients who have received an MSE before transfer to the helipad, the hospital with the helipad is not obligated to perform another MSE before the patient's continued travel to the recipient hospital. If, however, while at the helipad, the patient's condition deteriorates, the hospital at which the helipad is located must provide another MSE and stabilizing treatment within its capacity if requested by medical personnel accompanying the patient.

■ If as part of the EMS protocol, EMS activates helicopter evacuation of a patient with a potential EMC, the hospital that has the helipad does not have an EMTALA obligation if it is not the recipient hospital unless a request is made for the examination or treatment of an EMC by EMS personnel, the patient, or a legally responsible person acting on the behalf of the patient.

So the patient who had an MSE at Hospital A could be taken by ambulance to the helipad located on the grounds of Hospital B for transfer to Hospital C without triggering Hospital B's EMTALA obligation unless the patient's condition deteriorated before loading on the helicopter. In addition, a patient picked up in the field who is brought to the helipad at Hospital X for transfer to Hospital Z under local EMS protocol would not launch Hospital X's EMTALA obligation unless the EMS personnel (or patient) requested care before loading on the helicopter.

Designated Hospitals

Although community-based EMS protocols may determine the appropriate facility for a patient from the field, once a patient has arrived in the ED, he or she must be provided with an MSE and appropriate stabilizing care. Hospitals are not relieved of their EMTALA obligation to screen or provide stabilizing treatment or an appropriate transfer because of prearranged community or state plans that have designated specific facilities to care for selected patients (eg, Medicaid patients, psychiatric patients, pregnant women, and trauma patients). Hospitals located in states with laws that require certain patients (eg, psychiatric) to be evaluated and treated at designated facilities may violate EMTALA if the hospital disregards the EMTALA requirements and does not conduct an MSE and provide stabilizing treatment or conduct an appropriate examination before referring or transferring the patient to the designated facility. If, after conducting the MSE and ruling out an EMC (or after stabilizing the EMC) the sending hospital needs to transfer a patient to another hospital for treatment, it may elect to transfer the individual to the hospital so designated by the state or local laws (these patients are not considered in unstable condition under EMTALA). The existence of a state law requiring transfer of certain patients to certain facilities does not preempt the requirement to meet federal EMTALA requirements.

Disaster Status Exception

For a national emergency or crisis (eg, bioterrorism), state or local governments may develop community response plans that designate specific entities (eg, hospitals and public health facilities) with the responsibility of handling certain categories of patients during these catastrophic events. Although CMS added a section to the rules eliminating sanctions for inappropriate transfers in these circumstances, hospitals could still be held responsible for providing an MSE to any patients who presented to the ED. For example, a patient potentially exposed to a toxin arrived at a hospital not designated, pursuant to a state or local EMS plan, as a hospital where patients exposed to toxins should go. After interviewing the patient and determining that the patient falls into the category for which the community has a specified screening site, the patient may be referred to the designated community facility without risking sanctions under EMTALA. It is important to note that this exemption applies only to declared national—not state or local—emergencies.

Patient Transfers: Stable vs Unstable

Not all transfers between hospitals are subject to EMTALA. In fact, only patients who have an unstable EMC fall under the rules. Although the CMS interpretive guidelines and court decisions have confirmed that EMTALA does not apply to a patient in stable condition, surveyors of an EMTALA complaint may not understand the differences. In addition, a professional review organization may be asked by the survey agency to determine whether the patient was in stable condition at the time of the transfer. Some states may have rules applicable to the transfer of patients in stable condition. For good patient care and medicolegal purposes, it is reasonable to follow the same guidelines for all transfer patients.

For EMTALA purposes, a patient is considered in stable condition when the EMC that resulted in ED admission has resolved; however, the underlying medical condition may persist. The determination of the stability of a patient's condition is based on the reasonable clinical confidence of the treating physician or practitioner that the EMC no longer exists and there is no material risk of deterioration in the condition. The example for this given by CMS is a patient with an asthma exacerbation. Although the patient's acute attack is controlled (stabilized EMC), the underlying asthma still exists.

In psychiatric emergencies, CMS interpretive guidelines state that any patient expressing suicidal or homicidal thoughts or gestures or determined dangerous to self or others would be considered to have an EMC. Psychiatric patients would be considered in stable condition when they are protected and prevented from injuring or harming themselves or others. The use of chemical or physical restraints to effect a transfer may stabilize the psychiatric patient for a time and remove the immediate EMC, even though the underlying medical condition may persist.

Patients in unstable condition may be transferred because of medical need or the patient's (or surrogate's) request. A transfer for medical need is indicated when the hospital no longer has the capacity to perform the MSE (additional specialized equipment is needed) or stabilize an EMC (provide a higher level of care). *Capacity* includes staff, resources, and physician expertise. *Higher level of care* includes facilities with specialized units, staff, and equipment (eg, pediatric intensive care unit, cardiac bypass, and neurosurgeon). A patient may request a transfer for any reason. Patients in unstable condition who request a transfer for economic reasons (eg, managed care plan) do so at their own risk.

The referring hospital is responsible for coordinating the transfer. EMTALA requires the transferring physician to certify in writing that at the time of the transfer:

1. the benefits of the transfer outweigh the risks;
2. the patient (or surrogate) has given informed consent for the transfer; and
3. an appropriate transfer has been arranged.

If a physician is not physically present in the ED at the time of the transfer, the certification may be signed by hospital-designated qualified medical personnel after consultation with the physician. The physician then will need to countersign the certification.

In documenting the benefits and risks, the physician should be as thorough as possible. Terms such as "Needs level I trauma care," "No orthopedic services available," or "High-risk L&D [labor and delivery] services required" clearly show specific medical needs. Description of risk should also be straightforward (eg, "Risk of deterioration or death") but more detailed than simply "Risk of ambulance ride."

Informed consent should be obtained from the patient. If the patient is not capable of providing consent and no surrogate is available, the transfer may proceed under implied consent. Refusal to an appropriate transfer by the patient (or surrogate) should clearly be documented in the medical record. Documentation should include details about the risks and benefits of the transfer that were explained to the patient (or surrogate) and an assessment of the patient's competency to make the decision. In this situation, the hospital's EMTALA obligation is complete.

EMTALA does not require the transporting service to obtain a separate consent. Services should discuss with their legal counsel the advisability of having a separate transfer consent form. A separate form may be particularly useful for air transport services to affirmatively document that the patient or family is aware of the specific risks associated with air transport.

A separate certification form should be used. The form should include the following:

1. Description of the patient's diagnosis and condition
   - No EMC
   - Stable EMC (no material risk of deterioration during transfer)
   - Unstable EMC (material risk of deterioration during transfer)
2. Reason for transfer (medical need, patient request, refusal or failure of on-call consultant to respond within a reasonable time)
3. Mode and method of and care during transport
4. Name, time, and date that accepting physician and/or authorized receiving hospital personnel agreed to the transfer
5. List of documentation being sent with patient
6. Vital signs before transfer
7. Signed informed consent for transfer

An appropriate transfer occurs when the:

1. transferring hospital has provided medical care within its capacity to minimize risk to the patient's health (or to the unborn child of a woman in labor),
2. receiving hospital has agreed to accept the patient and has the space and resources available for treatment,
3. transferring hospital sends available medical records with the patient, and
4. transfer is effected by qualified personnel and transportation equipment.

Care within capacity (see the definition earlier in this section) is different for each patient. Performing an MSE that determines that other services are needed may be the only service within a hospital's capacity for certain conditions. Other care to minimize the risk to the patient's health can range from stabilizing airway, breathing, and circulation to the administration of medications and fluids.

The transferring hospital must determine whether the potential receiving hospital has the resources available to care for the patient. For example, it would not be appropriate to transfer a patient with a severe head injury from a rural hospital ED without a computed tomography (CT) scanner or neurosurgeon to another hospital similarly situated. Hospitals with specialized services are required to accept transfers for patient's requiring those services if they have the capacity. Having the capacity has come to mean that if the hospital could care for a similar patient in its ED, it would have to accept the transfer.

A patient in unstable condition cannot be transferred to a particular hospital simply for economic reasons, whether insured or not. A health care plan cannot require a patient be transferred to a contracted or in-network facility during the MSE or if the treating facility is capable of stabilizing the EMC. Neither can the plan require the patient be transferred to a facility with less capability than medically needed by the patient. If there are two hospitals of equal capabilities and transport time and one is a plan in-network facility, the patient may choose based on the insurance. Lack of or delay in obtaining health care plan authorization cannot defer a transfer to an appropriate receiving hospital.

EMTALA does not require a physician to be the accepting party for the receiving hospital. In fact, it is up to the hospital to determine who can accept patients on its behalf (eg, physician, nurse, or admission clerk). For good patient care and other medicolegal reasons, it is prudent for the transferring physician to discuss the patient's condition with the receiving physician or health care team member.

At a minimum, a copy of the medical record including triage note, physician record, patient care staff notes; records of treatments, test results, and radiographs; and transfer certification and consent must be sent with the patient. In situations in which the physician was not present at the time of the transfer, the record must include the name and address of the on-call physician who authorized the transfer. Some states may have additional requirements. A patient's transfer should never be delayed because of paperwork. Paper or electronic records may be faxed or sent by e-mail and hard copy items (eg, radiographs) may be sent by courier. However, a record of the patient's most recent vital signs and status at the time of the transfer should be available to go with the patient.

Transport teams should check that they have the appropriate documentation before loading the patient or be able to inform the receiving hospital about how the records will be delivered. Delivery of the records should be documented by written receipt from the receiving staff or at least by notation in the transport record. Specific transport documentation is not required by EMTALA, but a copy of the transport record should be given to the receiving hospital.

The term *qualified personnel and transportation equipment* is not defined by EMTALA. The level of training and mode of transport should be consistent with the needs of the patient. The referring physician and hospital may be held liable for using inappropriate transport services. Although transferring a patient by private vehicle per se is not an EMTALA violation, it would be difficult to defend as an appropriate mode of transport for a patient in unstable condition.

It is important to remember that it ultimately is the referring physician's responsibility to determine the scope of the MSE, the existence and/or stabilization of an EMC, and the appropriate receiving facility and level and mode of transport for the patient.

Outpatient vs Inpatient Transfers

The revised rules distinguish between outpatients and inpatients. EMTALA no longer applies to inpatients. CMS applies the Medicare Conditions of Participation (42 CFR §482) to monitor the hospital's continued responsibility to meet the inpatient emergency needs.

EMTALA defines an *inpatient* as a patient who has been admitted to the hospital with the reasonable expectation that he or she will occupy a bed at least overnight. It does not matter if the patient is directly admitted to the ward, stops in the ED to get a room assignment, or is boarded in the ED pending bed placement. Patients placed in temporary observation status or admitted for stabilizing care with the expectation of transfer without staying at the first hospital overnight are not "inpatients" under EMTALA. Patients admitted with the intent of avoiding EMTALA are not legally considered inpatients. The fact that a patient was admitted with the expectation he or she would occupy a bed overnight but whose condition deteriorated, requiring transfer, does not invalidate inpatient status.

Administration of the Law

Complaints of potential EMTALA violations are investigated by CMS through its regional offices or state oversight agencies. Complaints related to physician issues are reviewed by peer physician reviewers from the state's professional review organization. Review guidelines and policies are published and available on the CMS Web site (http://www.cms.hhs.gov/providers/emtala/default.asp).

If a hospital is found in violation of EMTALA and CMS determines that the violation poses immediate jeopardy to the health or safety of people who come to the ED, it is given a 23-day notice of termination from participation in federal insurance programs (Medicare, Medicaid, CHAMPUS [The Civilian Health and Medical Program of the Uniformed Services]). During that time, the hospital is to develop, present, and have approved a program to ensure compliance.

The Health and Human Services Office of Inspector General reviews all cases and may levy civil monetary penalties for violations and prosecute cases that are disputed. Hospitals with fewer than 100 licensed beds can be fined up to $25 000 per violation incident. Larger hospitals face fines of up to $50 000 per violation. Physicians found in violation can be fined up to $50 000 per patient violation incident in addition to termination from participation in federal insurance programs. The law also grants patients and aggrieved medical facilities the right to sue for damages for injuries sustained as a result of an EMTALA violation.

Health Insurance Portability and Accountability Act

An issue in medical communication is Health Information Portability and Accountability Act (HIPAA) privacy regulation compliance. HIPAA legislation, passed in 1996, includes a privacy rule that created national standards to protect personal health information (see Chapter 16). Although HIPAA greatly affects the flow of medical information, it does not prevent or require specific authorization for sharing of information among health care providers involved in the care of the patient. Each provider, however, is obligated to comply with HIPAA, and most attorneys favor separate disclosure of privacy practices and consents whenever possible. When an interstate transfer is involved, conflicting state laws may become an issue, and the "higher" or more restrictive standard applies.

Privacy notice forms are complex documents that must reflect many detailed elements of federal and state laws. These documents should be prepared by counsel and standardized for use by the transport service. All personnel should be trained regarding the content and use of the forms and in the privacy practices applicable in their jurisdiction. Emergency services such as transport teams are required to provide notice of privacy practices to patients "as soon as reasonably practicable after the emergency treatment situation." This determination of practicability will probably be somewhat lenient in scene response situations, and provision of the information at the destination hospital will likely be acceptable. In transfer situations, however, it is more likely that the privacy notice will be expected before transfer.

It is generally advisable to obtain a signature evidencing receipt of the notice of privacy practices, but when the patient or family refuses signature or it is not practical to obtain a signature, it should be documented that the notice form was given to the patient or family. If the situation is too involved for providers, patients, or family to rationally cope with legal notices, the situation should be documented, and notice may be provided later when circumstances permit.

Violation of HIPAA regulations may result in fines to a provider and federal criminal charges against individuals for certain intentional violations. State requirements may impose additional penalties, including criminal charges against individuals, for privacy violations. Although HIPAA creates a new civil liability, privacy violations can be used as grounds for medical malpractice suits in all jurisdictions. HIPAA also has the effect of standardizing privacy practices, which in turn has the effect of creating a new standard of care over time.

HIPAA Disclosure to Law Enforcement

Law enforcement personnel are frequently involved in ED or acute medical cases and may come into contact with transport teams. Transport teams will be appropriately knowledgeable about the information they may disclose and when they might be stepping across the line into a HIPAA violation. Investigators, on the other hand, might not be as familiar with HIPAA and its restrictions.

In many cases, there may be a conflict between the HIPAA regulations and existing state laws. HIPAA supersedes the state law in some cases, unless the state law is more restrictive, in which case the state law controls. It is neither feasible nor desirable to attempt to resolve these fine legal points in the acute care setting when these conflicts will impair the ability of the transport team and law enforcement to perform their respective functions. ED, transport, and police administration (and perhaps legal counsel) need to address these issues proactively to reduce the stress on officers and transport personnel.

HIPAA addresses several types of situations in which information might be requested or required from health care providers by law enforcement or public officials.

Public Health Reporting

Teams may report public health conditions *required by law* to a properly designated public health agency without permission or notice to the patient or representatives [45 CFR 164.512(b)(i)].

Communicable Diseases

Under HIPAA, health care personnel may report a person who may have been exposed to a communicable disease or may be a carrier of a communicable disease if the health agency has the power under the law to receive that information and track or notify the disease or condition [45 CFR 164.512(b)(iv)].

Abuse or Neglect

Transport team personnel may report suspected issues of child abuse without permission or notice to the patient, parents, or legal representative [45 CFR 164.512(b)(ii)]. As mandated reporters, transport team personnel may report cases of abuse or neglect to an authorized agency to the extent that it is *required by law*. They may report only the portion of information that is required by the law, *with the patient's consent to the extent required by state law.*

If the patient is not competent to consent, the disclosure can be made if the health care provider believes that:
1. it is necessary to prevent serious harm to the patient or other potential victims,

2. it is not intended to be used against the patient, and
3. an immediate investigation would be compromised by waiting until the patient was competent to consent.

In these circumstances, transport team personnel must inform the patient promptly that a report was or is going to be made, unless the health care professional reasonably believes that informing the patient or legal representative would place the patient or representative at risk of serious harm or that the representative is responsible for the abuse, neglect, or injury of the patient [45 CFR164.512 (c)].

When Medical Responsibility Attaches to the Transport Team

Acceptance of a call for response places the transport service under a duty to the patient, but when do the team members become individually responsible to the patient in a medical sense?

One of the first important concepts is that many people can have medical responsibility for a single patient at one time. The fact that one person has acquired medical responsibility does not automatically release someone else.

Dispatch

Once a team is dispatched to a particular response, the first medical responsibility attaches, that is to not unreasonably abandon the patient. To the extent that completion of the response remains within the control of the transport team members, they have a duty to continue with a response. If control is lost owing to weather, safety, mechanical issues, dispatch orders, or pilot decisions, the transport team members are not responsible for more than they can actually do. It may be reasonable to notify dispatch, but there is no requirement that team members place themselves at unreasonable risk, disobey orders, or violate flight rules to complete a response.

Diversion En Route

The implications of transport mission diversion are significant. The limited resources of transport teams in many areas makes triage, mission prioritization, and potential diversion not infrequent issues. The legal issues, however, may be more complex, and the exposure to a lawsuit is definitely increased if mission diversion occurs. Mission diversions must be firmly supported by written policies and procedures that clearly establish the service's position on whether mission diversion may ever occur, what priorities will be applied, who will make priority decisions, notification procedures for transport teams and hospitals, use of mutual aid, and documentation processes.

By and large, general liability law does not create a duty for a transport operation to provide service to any given patient or hospital. That duty, however, may arise in other ways. When a transfer contract exists with a hospital or EMS system, the contract may create a duty to respond and possibly also provide exceptions. Transfer contracts will be discussed in more detail later in this chapter. If a service or a team breaches the terms of a transfer contract, it may be possible for a patient to file a malpractice lawsuit for any harm caused by a delay or failure to respond.

Except for hospital-owned and -operated EMS units that are not operating under a community-wide protocol, ambulances are not subject to EMTALA. Mission diversion may have EMTALA ramifications for hospitals attempting an appropriate transfer. If a transport team intended for such a transfer is diverted, the transferring physician may have to seek alternative transportation to prevent a delay in the transfer.

Transport services should standardize all procedures to provide appropriate response and service to all patients regardless of which area of the hospital the patient occupies or the formal designation of patient status. Although some payment status issues may depend on these details, appropriate care standards do not. From a medical malpractice liability perspective, levels of patient care that depend on reimbursement status, rather than patient safety, are extremely difficult to defend in court.

The second source for a legal duty to respond to the patient is acceptance of the obligation to respond. Mission diversion after accepting a patient may be viewed as "abandonment" similar to other forms of medical abandonment. In this circumstance, once accepted, a rescuer has a duty to respond if the patient relies on the acceptance and, therefore, gives up the chance to find an alternative rescuer. Typically this would translate into whether the on-scene/referral team had sufficient time to make alternative arrangements for the safety of the patient (paramedic response, basic or nonmedical transport). The issue will then boil down to whether the mission diversion was reasonable, whether it was consistent with system policy, and whether adequate notice was provided to the transferring physician or on-scene rescue personnel.

One form of mission diversion is "stacking." In this circumstance, multiple calls are accepted for a transport team and "stacked" in order of priority or order of calls received. In these circumstances, a clear obligation exists to tell callers that a backlog of calls exists and the anticipated time of arrival. Most effective services have a policy for periodically reporting priority and response schedules. If a priority change occurs, any resulting delay should be reported expeditiously to all hospitals that will be affected.

The initial indications and subsequent notifications should be carefully documented regarding what the hospital or physician knew—and when. This information will be invaluable if review or investigation into care or delays is undertaken. The same process of documentation and notification would be expected in cases of weather delays or grounding.

The more problematic form of mission diversion occurs when an emergency response has been acknowledged and a subsequent request is deemed more urgent. This is clearly a case in which the reasonableness of the change in mission and practicality of alternative resources for the first patient may be questioned. Clearly, weather or other safety hazards may justify delay or even cancellation of critical rescue responses, but discretionary priority diversions can place credibility of the service at risk and expose the service to potential malpractice claims for abandonment. Unlike most malpractice cases, the primary source of the claim against the provider may be the physician who was left to care for a patient and felt abandoned along with the patient.

It is impossible to state that mission diversion of this type cannot legally occur under any circumstances. It seems prudent, however, to limit the types of cases and relative acuity deemed sufficient to allow mission diversion. This should be done with carefully drawn policies, protocols, standards, and notification procedures that have been thoroughly reviewed by legal counsel and the service's medical malpractice insurance company.

■ ■

On-scene Responses

Once the transport team arrives to a patient location, it shares medical responsibility with the other providers. The medical obligation as the most highly trained medical personnel on scene usually extends to direct medical care for the patient within a reasonably prompt time, allowing for assessing the scene, protecting the scene, and donning protective gear. That obligation extends to entering a hazardous environment to access the patient, but only if the team members are trained and equipped for that environment. If the transport team lacks appropriate protective gear or members are not trained for the type of environment involved, they are not required to place themselves at unreasonable risk to support the rescue. It may be appropriate to leave the extrication and patient care to the rescue crew until the patient can be brought to safety and accessed by the transport team.

This raises the question of when the duty to the patient exactly starts. If an EMS team did not initiate patient care, it may be considered to have no duty to the patient. In *Zepeda v City of Los Angeles,* the patient died after city paramedics who were summoned to the scene of a shooting allegedly refused to provide medical aid until the police arrived. The appellate court held that because the paramedics had not initiated care, they did not have a duty to the patient (223 CalApp3d 232). Two other cases found that once the paramedic made contact with the patient, even if it was a "one-minute look over," a duty had been established (*Wright v City of Los Angeles* [219 CalApp3d 318], *Hackman v American Medical Response* [2004 WL 823206 (Cal App 4th Dist) (unpublished opinion)]).

In the Hospital

One of the most complex interactions of medical responsibility is when the transport team is at a transferring hospital and is preparing the patient for transport. Hospital staff may step back and allow the transport team complete control of the patient with an understanding that the transport team has "assumed care." Often transport policies specifically state that the patient is deemed to be under the care of the service owner and the medical director of the transport service. These policies and assumptions may serve to make the alignment of tasks more convenient among the transport team and the hospital staff, but they fail to properly reflect the overlapping responsibility issues this setting produces.

There are definite reasons that a medical transport team that specializes in the care of pediatric patients should lead the process of preparing their fragile patient for transport. However, leading the effort does not translate into "command" or sole medical responsibility for the patient. The physician and other qualified medical personnel remain responsible for the patient until the patient physically leaves the hospital.

While the patient is still in the hospital, the physician cannot hand off the patient to the transport team and proceed as if the patient has left the hospital and his or her care. The issues include privileges (and, thus, hospital regulations) and EMTALA. If there are physicians or midlevel providers on the transport team, they are not usually privileged to function within the referring hospital. As such, they technically have no rights of practice within the facility, except as adjuncts to the attending physician. Even this concept stretches the bounds of most medical staff bylaws. The idea that care has been surrendered to the receiving facility or transport service on arrival of the transport team is erroneous. It is reasonable, however, for the transferring hospital to allow specialty or specifically trained providers to provide care under its authority and supervision. The transferring physician must retain involvement and ultimate responsibility and sign the transfer certificate at the *time of actual transfer*. At any time the transferring physician deems it in the best interests of the patient to intervene or cancel the transfer, it is that physician's right and duty to do so. At the same time, however, the transport team has a medical responsibility to the patient as well—it is concurrent, and it must be coordinated. A team approach to care is ideal and should be strived for by all participants in the process.

When there is unresolved disagreement between the transferring physician and the transport team in a plan of care for the patient, the team should suggest a phone conference with medical director of their service or the medical control physician. If the transferring physician still disagrees with the plan of the transport team, the team must defer to the transferring physician while the patient is still in the hospital. Refusal by the team to complete the transport could put them at medicolegal risk.

Delivery at the Receiving Facility

The issue of privileges may also have a role in the delivery of a patient to a hospital, especially when transport teams are delayed from removing the patient from their gurney. When a hospital-owned and -operated service delivers patients to its home hospital, the issue may be one of scope of practice or credentialed privileges within the hospital environment compared with the transport environment.

In a busy department, a new patient may be left in the hands of the transport team until it is optimal for the ED or inpatient staff to assume care of the patient. This obviously leaves the transport team with a patient for an extended time, when their services might be needed elsewhere. It also leaves the patient in transport "packaging" when other equipment and personnel should be available to provide the patient with optimal and definitive care.

Although the transport team might want to transfer the patient to a hospital bed and proceed with other duties, the medical responsibility to the patient requires that the transport team not abandon the patient. This, in turn, means that a detailed report and orderly turnover of responsibility be accomplished before leaving the patient at the destination. The transport team retains medical responsibility until proper hand off has occurred, even though the receiving facility shares responsibility.

Much like the idea that the sending facility can hand off responsibility when the transport team arrives, receiving facilities often assume that they do not acquire responsibility until they accept the patient from the transport team. Both concepts are erroneous in their literal application. The sending facility and staff surrender primary medical responsibility when the patient leaves their direction and control, which can mean when the patient leaves the physical premises or when the patient leaves the zone of their online medical control and enters the medical control of another off-hospital system. The receiving facility and staff begin to acquire medical responsibility for a patient when the patient arrives on their premises and staff becomes aware of the patient's presence, even if the patient is being attended to by the transport team.

■■■■■■■■■■■■■■■■■■■■■■■■■■■■■■■

When Civil Legal Liability Attaches

A question that frequently follows a description of this concurrent and overlapping medical responsibility is: "So when does *legal* liability attach—or detach?"

The answer to that question is that legal liability flows from medical responsibility—medical duty. As described, liability is a function of duty and violation of that duty in a manner that violates the standard of care and produces harm.

In any case in which a patient is harmed as a result of medical negligence (malpractice), any health care provider who had medical responsibility or duty to the patient has the potential for legal liability to the patient. Actual liability, however, depends on which health care provider violated his or her duty to the patient in a negligent manner and produced harm. It is possible that more than one provider meets the criteria or that no provider was liable. As with shared medical responsibility, often there is shared legal liability.

Shared legal liability has two factors that influence the financial impact in most states: proportion of fault and joint or several damages. In most states, a provider can be held liable only if the proportion of fault is 50% or more on the part of the provider. If more than one provider is found to be at fault by the jury, the verdict typically assigns the relative portion of fault so that the responsibility is apportioned among the negligent parties.

If there is sufficient coverage for all negligent parties, each pays his or her own proportion of the verdict. This is *several liability*, as the sum total verdict is recovered from the several negligent parties and each pays his or her own share. Under *joint liability*, the injured patient can collect 100% of the verdict from any one or more of the negligent parties. Joint liability typically becomes an issue if one or more of the negligent parties has insufficient insurance or settles before trial and another has a greater financial coverage. In effect, a health care provider who was only minimally negligent could be required to pay the entire judgment for those who were much more at fault. Some states have completely eliminated joint liability in favor of several liability, and others have required that a party must be at least "X %" at fault to be held jointly liable.

Two other mechanisms exist to balance legal liability with the medical responsibility. The first is *contribution*. In this case, health care providers cross-sue one another in the case to ensure that each provider pays his or her fair share to the others if a disproportionate recovery is taken against one party. Problems with this approach are that it can potentially set in opposition one health care provider against the others in a suit and potentially increases the risks of a perhaps unjustified finding of negligence.

The other mechanism is *indemnity,* which is based on the concept of active and passive negligence. A hospital, for example, might be negligent by failing to have proper policies and procedures that allowed negligent performance by a physician. The hospital would have passive liability and would ask that the physician indemnify or repay it for any liability caused by the physician's actions. The problem with this approach is that it sets one health care provider against another, with the same potential risks.

One may see actions for contribution or indemnity when several insurance companies are involved in a high-value case or when active hostility exists between providers.

Transfer Agreement Issues

Transfer agreements are written plans that exist between hospitals or between hospitals and transport services that define the roles, understandings, and procedures for moving patients from one facility to another. A sample transport agreement is included in Appendix A5. They do not have to be lengthy but should accurately reflect the understandings of the parties. These agreements often define how payment will be made and how nonreimbursed services will be handled. Transfer agreements are recommended for hospitals and transport services for business reasons, ease of interaction, and to meet legal requirements in some states.

One of the main reasons for transfer agreements is to create a smooth-working transfer system that serves the needs of all participants and helps set the expectations and standards of all parties. For patients, transfer agreements attempt to make care more efficient with the least risk of adverse outcome. For hospitals and transfer services, agreements allow participants to understand how the system is to work, what responses to expect, and how payment is to be addressed before actual need. Legal counsel is recommended to ensure the agreements meet state requirements and do not contain clauses with unintended risks. If state-mandated agreement forms are used, legal counsel should review them for compliance.

Liability Issues With Transfer Agreements

Transfer agreements seldom produce liability, except for issues pertaining to payment. If a transfer agreement provides that payment for transfers will be guaranteed by the hospital if insurance, Medicaid, or Medicare fails to pay or pays less than a specific percentage of the transport service bill and the hospital refuses to pay when properly billed, one can expect that liability might result from the contract.

If the transport service promises a specific response time or specific response personnel under given circumstances for a given price, it is likely that financial liability issues would be involved if the transport service failed to meet the conditions of the contract. If that failure resulted in harm to a patient, the hospital might cross-claim against the transport service if a medical malpractice case arose because of the lack of an appropriate and expected response. Patients can also sue directly for the breach, maintaining that patients were the parties intended to be served or protected (third-party beneficiary) by the contract terms.

The liability exposure of the transfer agreement seldom creates new liability, however, because the contract terms are usually carefully drawn to make the service conditional on availability, capacity, and other provisions to make the agreement a more nonbinding understanding than a document on which liability would rest.

Role of Risk Management

Transport services are well aware of the value of the preventive maintenance and flight checklists that must be used to keep their aircraft in safe operation. Similar attention to the services of the medical component through risk management activities likewise prevents quality, compliance, and legal issues from imperiling the operation.

The risk management role has many aspects that might be assigned to different members of the team and administration, rather than to a single risk manager, but the elements still need to be covered to ensure the long-term survival of the service as a viable business entity so that critical public safety needs can be met.

Credentialing

A critical factor in managing risk is attention to the credentialing of members of the transport team. Aggressive and well-documented follow-up is necessary on all applications to ensure that the team members are properly licensed, functionally competent, and free of significant loss histories that warn of possible future issues. It is not sufficient to rely solely on the fact that a hospital has granted privileges to a provider to enable privileges in an independent transport system. On the other hand, hospital owned and operated services might reasonably use the hospital credentialing office because they are part of the same entity.

Direct contact with previous employers, instructors, and team members is recommended to help identify personnel who might not be ideal for a transport team position. Assessment of personal proficiencies should be documented before placing a person on a team, and ongoing assessment of competencies of all team members should be documented in their personnel files. Ongoing tracking of certification renewals, continuing education, and performance reviews is necessary to document that the system has not allowed an unqualified or noncompetent provider on the transport team.

Policies, Procedures, and Protocols

Transport services should have detailed job descriptions, policies, and procedures, which may be modeled after those of an ED or critical care unit. As a risk-management objective, it is important to realize it is difficult to defend a practice if people do not approach events in a similar manner. Policies and procedures are useful and necessary to help create a systematic (ideally evidence-based) and defensible process.

The policies and procedures can be "care paths," protocols, guidelines, or other treatment algorithms. These may be legally necessary to allow hospital-based flight nurses, physician assistants, paramedics, or other nonphysicians to provide critical care outside the hospital.

Continuing education, training, competency, and quality review need to be documented to ensure that the team members remain qualified to perform necessary services and procedures. Deviation from protocols eases a plaintiff's burden of showing that transport team personnel were negligent and shifts the burden to the team to justify the variance from protocol.

Risk managers, in conjunction with clinical and legal leadership, are typically involved in the creation and drafting of policies, procedures, and protocols. They help clarify language for regulations or standard of clinical care, focus on potential risks in the process, and review documentation to ensure that it supports the care provided.

Quality Measures

One of the most important risk management tools is ongoing quality reviews of the records of transports. These reviews set specific standards for measurement and audit and track compliance. The information provided by this process helps identify the potential vulnerabilities or inadequacies of individual team members and of the system as a whole, thereby allowing the risk manager to focus training, compliance efforts, and counseling to close the vulnerable spots in the medical-legal operations of the team. Quality reviews may or may not have nondiscovery protection depending on state law.

All team members should be aware of exactly which quality indicators are being monitored, and they should be made aware of team performance and be made privately aware of their own marks to help motivate improvement or identify competency.

Incident Management

An incident can include unplanned deviations from protocol, complaints, internal concerns, adverse outcomes, a medical records request from a lawyer, or any other circumstance that triggers a review of the facts, potential legal issues, and potential ways to prevent the issue from arising again in the future. The actual management of the incident may include factual investigation, communication with the parties to contain the situation, preparation of information and notification of the insurance company, or recommendations for systems or performance improvement by the staff or team.

Ongoing issues in a system may not receive a primary focus for a variety of reasons. Competition among systems, problems with client hospitals, issues with getting paid by insurance companies, and lawsuits typically receive priority attention because they must be addressed at that time. On the other hand, many of these situations may have had warning signs for a period before the event and could have been managed with favorable outcomes at these early stages. Risk management responsibilities include identifying warning signs and ensuring corrective action early in the process, ideally before harm has ensued.

Litigation Support

If a transport service is involved in a litigated case, a great deal of effort will be expended in responding. The insurance company and defense lawyers will require the service and team members to be sources of information, documents, and records. A risk manager can provide oversight to the defense team and help keep team management informed on the progress of the case.

Documentation

The main purposes of medical record documentation are to ensure optimal patient care and to communicate appropriate and important information about the patient with other care providers. For transport services, continuity and communication are vital to the safety and well-being of patients as they transition from one system and/or group of providers to another. The documentation provides an ongoing history of the patient's course through the presentation, hospital treatment, and transfer to the next medical providers and location.

Additional functions of the record are proof of regulatory compliance and that the standard of care has been met. A complete record provides factual information for quality review and a basis to refresh one's memory for future testimony. Lawsuits, external inquiries, and, ultimately, trials typically occur several years after the events that form the basis of a claim or review. The medical record is permanent and reflects the information available and care provided at the time of the event. It generally proves to be a touchstone for the credibility of all aspects of the case or issue.

The number of people who will be looking at the record can be large and can include the following: subsequent treating physicians, nurses, coders, reviewers, compliance officers, risk managers, quality and other departmental committees, utilization review personnel, medical records personnel, peer review committees, third-party payers, professional boards, government reviewers, patients and their families under HIPAA, patients' lawyers, insurance company representatives, defense attorneys, outside experts, judges, and juries. Although not all records will receive this scope of exposure, each report must be written as if it will; often providers do not know in advance which records will receive intense review.

Documentation should be complete, legible, and signed. The use of care maps, template documentation styles, and documenting by exception is gaining popularity in the field and in billing enhancement circles, but the medical narrative report remains a solid and reliable method to document the facts, sequence, and details necessary to justify quality of care on review or defend a lawsuit. Documenting by exception and template-only documentation may lack sequence (time) entries, details, and observations that are the heart of the care. The subsequent treating physicians and the reviewers and juries are unable to get a clear view of the patient and the care provided, which, in turn, can lead to an assumption of less than optimal care (or caring) by the treating physicians and negative verdicts from juries.

What Should Be in the Record

It is perfectly acceptable to use blocks and checkboxes for routine administrative entries, such as verification of contacts, completion of chart segments, one-time entries such as gender and religion, and inclusion or completion of routine tasks. Beyond those types of entries, a clearly written and legible narrative entry should be made for all conversations, orders, observations, interventions, and rechecks. These entries should be timed, and each individual transport team member should sign the record. The documentation should also clearly indicate which team member performed which function.

The record should include a summary of the referral information and become more detailed from the point of initial contact with the receiving facility by radio or on arrival. Details should include patient evaluation, interventions and treatment before arrival, treatment at the referring facility by the transport team, preparation for transport, vital signs on an ongoing basis, care provided during transport, changes in patient condition during transport, and patient condition on arrival at the destination. Any issues encountered at any point should be detailed carefully and objectively. A wrap-up narrative should include details of any changes in patient condition after arrival at the receiving facility, to whom the patient was delivered, to whom report was given, and any issues arising at the receiving facility. Information should be documented factually and objectively. All entries should be timed as closely as possible.

Details and *narrative* imply that the record will contain specific vital signs, observations, and other specific items of information. Some generalization may be necessary, such as referring to a patient's general condition as "unchanged," but specific measurable items such as vital signs should be reported each time with numeric value. Comments such as "normal" or "within normal limits" are not generally useful for documenting or recognizing changes in patient condition unless those terms are clearly defined in the transport-documentation standards.

Quality of Care Issues at the Sending Facility

Transport teams may arrive and find that care the patient is receiving is different from that the transport team or receiving center recommended or would like to have provided. This may lead to a temptation to be critical in the medical record. It is important to simply document the facts of patient care, without opinion, criticism, or editorial comment. Initial entries should always state what was first observed about the patient and the ongoing treatment on arrival. Commenting on what drugs had been given, current monitoring, what procedures were conducted, and whether intravenous lines were in place and functional are among items that would typically be documented. Following the same procedure on all documentation will adequately record information without value judgments appearing in the record.

For concerns about the adequacy of care, an internal quality process should exist for review. A risk management specialist and/or qualified attorney can assist the service to develop a process that meets the requirements for confidentiality in the state involved. Incident or quality reports should recite the facts but not include editorial comments or opinions. In most cases, the rule for incident reports is that if the facts are reported sufficiently, the issues should be evident without the need to point them out. The only exception to this approach would be for circumstances that require reporting under state law, in which case, the team should follow mandated reporting procedures.

Duty to Intervene

Except in Vermont and Minnesota, individual EMS personnel do not have a duty to intervene. For example, an off-duty paramedic may not be not required to stop at a car wreck while driving to the store. An in-service EMS unit may have a duty to stop at the same accident if not on a higher priority call based on local rules, laws, and community protocols.

In transfer situations, the transport team may receive total deference when it arrives and care is ceded to them, sometimes to the point of almost literally stopping midprocedure to hand the patient over to the transport team. Occasionally, when the transport team arrives at the sending hospital, transport personnel may believe that the ongoing or planned care is not optimal or in the best interest of the patient. This situation can create an extremely challenging decision point for the team regarding how and when to intervene to help provide optimal care to the patient, which risks alienating the providers and hospital versus standing back and not participating in the care being provided.

It is important to keep in mind that the transport team is usually not privileged to treat patients in the sending hospital and has no inherent right to assume care of the patient. At the same time, failure to draw attention of the hospital staff to an issue raises a concern of moral duty and a possibility that the patient may receive less than optimal care. It is important to remember there is a chain of command and a physician-patient relationship while the patient is still in the transferring hospital. When there is unresolved disagreement, the transport team should contact its medical director or the medical control physician to discuss the patient's care with the referring physician. The team should document any significant issues in a matter-of-fact, nonaccusatory manner. Nonprivileged personnel may feel an ethical duty to intervene but may be on somewhat shaky legal ground. Consultation with the medical director or the medical control physician may be helpful to discuss alternatives and potential plans of action.

Quality of Care Issues During Transport

On occasion, quality of care issues or disputes between team members occur during transport. It is generally the responsibility of the senior medical team member to direct care (with input from online medical control as needed). Any team member has a duty to the team and to the patient to raise questions or issues of care during the transport, if there is a concern. Respect and trust are essential for all team members to function in the high-stress environment of a neonatal-pediatric transport. Team members need to be able to remind, recommend, and disagree in a manner that is supportive and not divisive. The team approach, however, does not mean that quality improvement is ignored.

In neonatal and pediatric care, it may be particularly difficult to deal with perceived errors or shortcomings that injure a child. Great care must be exercised to avoid team conflict about a care incident that places the focus on guilt or responsibility rather than quality improvement. In these cases, extreme caution must be used to avoid accusations or judgments in the medical record or other documents. Only factual medical details should appear. Verbal comments that are critical should likewise be limited entirely to the quality review process because they otherwise may result in additional performance and legal issues. Investigation may show that a perceived error had little or nothing to do with the adverse outcome, but premature comments or emotional criticism in the record can lead to a different conclusion. Unfortunately, misperceptions may expand into controversies and litigation that persist long after they could have been avoided or resolved. Careful handling of the issues in a systematic quality improvement process tends to prevent the unnecessary controversies and identify and resolve the justified concerns.

Transporting Nonpatients

One area that has potential legal exposure is the practice of transporting nonpatients. The potential risks include additional weight and space factors and that the nonpatient is physically present to witness events that later might be claimed to involve malpractice. In practice and the transport literature, however, the latter concern has not been shown to be a significant risk; indeed, parental presence may decrease risk of malpractice claims because the nonpatient passenger directly observed the care and concern demonstrated by the transport team members.

The noise, vibration, turbulence, enclosed space, and unfamiliarity with a helicopter or ambulance transport, coupled with the emotional aspects of a family medical emergency, can result in the nonpatient passenger becoming an additional patient who requires medical attention that could interfere with the team's ability to care for the primary patient. This disruption endangers the team in a legal sense and could endanger the original patient and the nonpatient-turned-new-patient with resulting medical and legal risk. There should always be a transport team member assigned to be the primary contact for the nonpatient passenger. If the team is unable to provide that support, it may not be ideal to include a nonpatient passenger on the transport. Children who are not patients should be transported in an alternative passenger vehicle, whenever possible.

For teams that allow or encourage nonpatient passengers or observers, insurance carriers should be consulted to ensure that there is appropriate liability coverage. Documentation and consent procedures suggested by the insurance company and/or attorney should be considered.

Examples of transport-related forms are provided in Appendices A4 and A5. The examples are supplied to provide drafting ideas and are not for direct incorporation into a program without local legal review. Examples of these forms are also provided in the text, *Providing Emergency Care Under Federal Law: EMTALA,* by the American College of Emergency Physicians and R.A. Bitterman and its 2004 Supplement (see Selected Readings).

Selected Readings

American Academy of Pediatrics Committee on Pediatric Emergency Medicine. Consent for emergency medical services for children and adolescents. *Pediatrics.* 2003;111:703–706

American College of Emergency Physicians. Fraud, compliance, and emergency medicine. 2004. Available at: http://www.acep.org/NR/rdonlyres/2BDCC528-8396-4090-A7FD-8943731AAFE4/0/fraud_compliance.pdf. Accessed January 19, 2006

American Medical Association. Pertinent changes to the EMTALA regulation. 2003. Available at: http://www.ama-assn.org/ama1/pub/upload/mm/395/finalrule2.doc. Accessed January 19, 2006

Andrews SS. Hospital helipads and the Emergency Medical Treatment and Active Labor Act. *Air Med J.* 2005;24:105

Bitterman RA. *Providing Emergency Care Under Federal Law: EMTALA.* Dallas, TX: American College of Emergency Physicians; 2000

Bitterman RA. Supplement to Providing Emergency Care Under Federal Law: EMTALA. American College of Emergency Physicians; 2004. Available at: http://www2.acep.org/library/pdf/emtalaSupplement.pdf. Accessed January 19, 2006

Centers for Medicare and Medicaid Services. Special responsibilities of Medicare hospitals in emergency cases. 42 CFR §489.24. Available at: http://a257.g.akamaitech.net/7/257/2422/12feb20041500/edocket.access.gpo.gov/cfr_2004/octqtr/pdf/42cfr489.24.pdf. Accessed January 19, 2006

Centers for Medicare and Medicaid Services. State Operations Manual Appendix V: Interpretive Guidelines: Responsibilities of Medicare Participating Hospitals in Emergency Cases (Rev. 1, 05-21-04). Available at: http://new.cms.hhs.gov/manuals/downloads/som107ap_v_emerg.pdf. Accessed January 19, 2006

Fosmire MS. Frequently Asked Questions About the Emergency Medical Treatment and Active Labor Act (EMTALA), 2003. Available at: http://www.emtala.com/faq.htm. Accessed January 19, 2006.

Frew SA. New Ambulance Regs Affect EMTALA Choices. 2005. Available at: http://www.medlaw.com/healthlaw/EMS/ambulance-regulations-aff.shtml. Accessed January 19, 2006

Keeton P, Prosser WL. *Prosser and Keeton on the Law of Torts.* 5th ed. St Paul, MN: West Publishing Co; 1984

Linzer JF. EMTALA: a clearer road in the future? *Clin Pediatr Emerg Med.* 2003;4:249–255

Maggiore WA. What's your duty? when your legal obligation starts and where it ends. *JEMS.* 2004;29:86–93

Section 1837 of the Social Security Act: examination and treatment for emergency medical conditions and women in labor. 42 USC §1395dd. Available at: http://frwebgate.access.gpo.gov/cgi-bin/getdoc.cgi?dbname=browse_usc&docid=Cite:+42USC1395dd. Accessed January 19, 2006.

Williams A. Diversion: air medical liability issue? *Air Med J.* 2001;20:11–12

Williams A: *Outpatient Department EMTALA Handbook.* 2004 edition. Gaithersburg, MD: Aspen Publishers; 2004

Woodward GA. Legal issues in pediatric interfacility transport. *Clin Pediatr Emerg Med.* 2003;4:256–264

Questions

True or False

1. A helicopter that lands at a hospital helipad to pick up a patient from an ambulance as part of a prearranged transfer puts the hospital that owns the helipad at risk of an Emergency Medical Treatment and Active Labor Act (EMTALA) violation if the emergency department physician does not do a medical screening examination.
2. EMTALA forbids transfer of any patient for economic reasons.
3. EMTALA supersedes local or state regulations for transfer.

Answers

1. False, unless the ambulance or air crew requests medical assistance from the hospital staff.
2. False. It requires a medical screening examination and does not allow patients in unstable condition to be transferred until their conditions have been appropriately stabilized. Once a patient's condition is stable, transfer for economic reasons is not prohibited by EMTALA.
3. True. EMTALA preempts local and state legislation requiring transfer to specific centers for specific issues. The condition of a patient who presents to an emergency department (as defined by EMTALA) must be stabilized to the best of the provider's ability before transfer.

Quality Improvement

Outline

- Basic terminology
- The QI process
- PDSA and the QI plan
- Essential elements of the QI plan
- Objectives of the QI plan
  - Table 8-1: QI coordinator job description
  - Table 8-2: Sample categories for process improvement opportunities in transport
  - Table 8-3: Samples of area-specific indicators
- Role of the medical director(s) in the QI process
- Accreditation and the QI process

Construction of a well-functioning transport program begins with building a strong foundation, including personnel, training, equipment, communication, and vehicles (ambulance, helicopter, or fixed-wing aircraft). How each of these cornerstones is designed and structured determines the caliber of service. Continual monitoring and evaluation of the transport program are critical to providing quality patient care and ensuring that the program can stand the test of time.

Basic Terminology

Many terms have been used in the pursuit of quality and excellence. This chapter provides a basic understanding of these terms and how a neonatal-pediatric transport program can incorporate the quality process into the fabric of the team. *Quality improvement* (QI) is a process that seeks to systematically, objectively, and continuously monitor, assess, and improve quality and the appropriateness of patient care provided based on predetermined standards.

Quality management involves all parties in the sphere of the transport program. It determines the leadership that will direct the people responsible for monitoring activities, reviewing events, and providing recommendations for individual and team improvement. *Scope of care* refers to types of patients transported by the program and identifies the basic clinical activities. *Key aspects* are the assessment and treatment modalities that are most important to quality care and that require ongoing evaluation. *Benchmarking* is the process of comparing one's performance with that of others and begins with standardized, comparative measurements and then examines performance differences between similar processes.[1]

As it applies to transport, benchmarking is the practice of setting operating goals by selecting the top performers within the transport industry and identifying best practices for the performance of the transport service. *Indicators* are objective, measurable criteria based on current knowledge and clinical experience. They outline the data to be obtained for analysis. *Thresholds* are statistical measures of compliance on a specific indicator based on preestablished, attainable levels of performance. *Data* and *review* outline the method used to direct the monitoring activity. *Evidence-based guidelines* and *critical pathways* analytically outline the development of outcome and performance measures that can be used in process improvement.[2] General knowledge of these terms will facilitate understanding the QI process as it applies to neonatal-pediatric transport.

The QI Process

Consumers and the health care industry mandate adherence to particular standards during the provision of patient care. Transport programs should analyze every component of the services provided to ensure effective, consistent, safe, and state-of-the-art care. *Quality Improvement in Emergency Medical Services for Children*[3] describes the commitment of the Emergency Medical Services for Children to the QI process in the transport of children, with goals to establish the following:

- Strong leadership at all levels
- A focus on the customer (children, families, and communities)
- Collaborative efforts that can improve processes and outcomes of emergency care for children

- Links to strategic planning goals, education, training, and program development
- Data and information that are reliable, rapidly accessible, standardized, and timely; pediatric clinical guidelines and performance measures that assist in guiding, evaluating, and improving emergency medical services for children
- Commitment to research that contributes evidence for changes in practice

The QI process should be integrated into every level of the transport program. One model to satisfy this requirement is Plan, Do, Study (or Check), Act (PDSA or PDCA).

PDSA and the QI Plan

PDSA is a basic method to implement the QI process. *Plan* is when the problem is identified and an action plan for change is developed. Table 8-1 lists process improvement categories applicable in the transport setting. Although the list is not all-inclusive, the categories of education, safety, communications, and overall aspects of transport operations represent the typical areas that should be addressed in the QI planning process.

Do is when the action plan is implemented with clearly defined roles and the change is monitored. Implementation of the QI plan requires thorough evaluation of clinical guidelines and algorithms that outline the process of clinical decision making and, thereby, direct the design of clinical practice. Data collection methods and tools used in health care may include simple check sheets, focus groups, interviews, process-related problems lists, flow charts, surveys, and voting. By using these methods, processes can be changed with the intent to improve patient care or services. For example, a flowchart depicts a process as a chronological sequence, breaking down the performance measure into parts that can be measured and improved. A focus group or interview may identify possible indicators important to the group.

Study (or Check) is the phase when process changes are reviewed, data are analyzed, and results of the change are compared with previous results or characteristics. Numerous methods exist to review data. Some data display techniques include bar charts, histograms, line graphs, and scatter diagrams. Data are plotted in such formats to

Table 8-1: Sample Categories for Process Improvement Opportunities in Transport*

Education and training
Hiring process: clinical performance, experience
Orientation
Ongoing continuing education
Skills competency training and procedural evaluation
Certifications: NRP, PALS, ACLS, ATLS or trauma equivalent
Annual performance appraisal

Safety
Personnel: annual physical and testing (eg, PPD)
Institutional and program mandatory yearly review
■ Environmental safety: fire, electrical, hazardous materials
■ Patient safety: infection control, sedation, pain management
■ Transport safety: helipad/helicopter, ambulance, fixed-wing aircraft, survival training

Administration
Budget: resource allocation and expenditures
Compliance with regulatory agencies
Health Insurance Portability and Accountability Act (HIPAA) compliance
Marketing and public relations

Communications
Internal: dispatch, triaging, meetings, logs, memos, committee minutes
External: referral institutions, vendors

Equipment standards
Reliability
Maintenance
Alarm parameters
Safety features
Technologically meets standards of the transport environment

Vehicles (ambulance, helicopter, fixed-wing aircraft)
Design
Configuration
Maintenance
Federal and state specifications and regulations
CAMTS standards

Patient care guidelines, protocols, procedures, policies, and documentation
Reviewed and updated regularly
Chart review
Documentation: meeting critical elements
Morbidity and mortality

Table 8-1: Sample Categories for Process Improvement Opportunities in Transport,* *continued*

Sample transport review triggers
Sentinel, serious, adverse, and near-miss events
Death during transport
Death within 24 h of admission
Cardiopulmonary resuscitation
Intubation or extubation
Transported without vascular access
Deviation from protocols
Use of vasopressors
Discharged patients directly from emergency department or within 24 h
Time at the referring institution exceeded acceptable limits
Change from floor to ICU within specified number of hours
Technical interventions completed (eg, CT, central lines, needle thoracotomy)
Mode of transport decisions questionable for particular patient or specific mode

Operational data (including quantity indicators)
Number of completed transports
Number of canceled transports owing to weather
Number of canceled transports owing to maintenance
Number of canceled or aborted transports
Response time
Team composition

*NRP indicates Neonatal Resuscitation Program; PALS, Pediatric Advanced Life Support; ACLS, Advanced Cardiac Life Support; ATLS, Advanced Trauma Life Support; PPD, purified protein derivative (tuberculin); CAMTS, Commission on Accreditation of Medical Transport Systems; ICU, intensive care unit; and CT, computed tomography.

assist in noting trends or problems areas and in making comparisons. Cause-effect analysis seeks to understand the process as a system of causal factors. Collaborative methods such as brainstorming, nominal group technique, and conflict resolution are also helpful. Another method is using collaborative efforts whereby organizations (other transport programs) can pool data and information resources when a common improvement goal exists. Sharing information can help groups learn from variation in practice and support problem solving during difficult phases of change.[1] Details of these methods are beyond the scope of this chapter and are reviewed further in other references and sources.

Act is the summary phase in which action is taken based on what has been learned. If standards are not met, the problem is identified and a new corrective action is taken with plans for follow-up outcome measures. Actions may include needs for education or training to meet the skill or certification criteria.

Essential Elements of the QI Plan

The Joint Commission on Accreditation of Healthcare Organizations (JCAHO), under its initiative Agenda for Change, outlined its integration of performance measurement data into the accreditation process. The JCAHO generic model for monitoring and evaluation lists the elements of the QI plan. It notes the cyclical nature and the requirement for continual reassessment to ensure that the practice criteria establish and maintain a quality service based on performance. The QI plan should:

- assign individual responsibility and accountability;
- define the scope of care;
- determine the important aspects of care, including clinical outcomes;
- characterize the important aspects of care and identify indicators;
- establish thresholds for evaluation that are appropriate to the individual service;
- obtain data for indicators using QI tools;
- evaluate the data in a multidisciplinary manner, and identify concerns about quality of service;
- recommend corrective action, and monitor its implementation;
- reassess, stressing the continuum, to develop new strategies for improving; and
- report the findings, and evaluate the improvement process.

A QI program should establish criteria to ensure that the standards of care are practiced by individuals and groups, linking the transport team with the medical director, administrative team, risk management personnel, and pertinent disciplines to identify opportunities to improve care.

Objectives of the QI Plan

The objectives of the QI plan should be defined and include the following:

- Identify important characteristics of neonatal-pediatric transport.
- Develop and maintain multidisciplinary communication links through the QI process, and provide a forum to present needs and areas for improvement via regularly scheduled meetings.
- Establish regular review of patient care guidelines and how they are applied to predetermined indicators and other criteria to permit objective monitoring of the key aspects of care.
- Respond in a systematic manner to sentinel, serious, adverse, and near-miss events. Expectations under JCAHO standards for an organization's response to a sentinel event include a root cause analysis and an action plan. Definitions and further explanations are available at http://www.jointcommission.org.

Accountability for oversight of various tasks should be assigned. Accountability rests with the QI coordinator, the QI committee, and the members of the transport team. The QI coordinator should be a person with expertise in neonatal-pediatric medicine and transport and quality monitoring. The QI coordinator is responsible for organization and direction of the QI program (Table 8-2). Crucial to the support of such a role is the vision that each team member has a role in the QI process.

Table 8-2: QI Coordinator Job Description*
1. Identify potential areas to monitor and evaluate
2. Coordinate and implement studies of specific issues and/or concerns
3. Direct data collection process and ensure accuracy of data
4. Analyze and interpret data
5. Formulate recommendations with QI committee including the following: ■ Changes to staff education, training, and development ■ Development and revisions of patient care standards, policies, procedures, and protocols
6. Oversee change process
7. Plan and organize QI committee meetings

*QI indicates quality improvement.

■■■■■■■■■■■■■■■■■■■■■■■■■■■■■■■■

Establishing a multidisciplinary QI committee provides the framework needed to set the goals, including meetings, attendance, and reporting mechanisms; oversee monitoring; establish ownership and commitment to the QI process; and recommend changes and determine the viability of the changes. The participants of this committee should include transport team members and personnel external to transport, such as additional medical advisors and quality improvement/administrative staff, and should report to the transport service management and to hospital administration.

There should be a clear understanding that a successful QI program is the ultimate responsibility of each member working as part of the team. Progress will occur when thoughtful communication is shared in a collegial, objective manner and responsive changes are made. Team members should continually analyze their practice in relation to the quality indicators and implement necessary changes. A staff-based approach is an effective method to improve compliance and accountability that can be incorporated into the peer review process. Creating a professional and safe atmosphere in which communication between team members is encouraged and supported and progress is emphasized will benefit the program overall.

Table 8-3 illustrates an application of the QI process from a representative transport program. It is not meant to be applicable in its entirety to each transport service. From the transport program's annual goals, key performance measures are identified as the first step in the QI monitoring process. Next, specific indicators and the data collection methods are noted in the action plan. The threshold for evaluation is agreed on. Results are noted and reported when a problem is identified and corrective action is taken with ongoing reevaluation. Overall, the QI process must show evidence of actions taken in identified problem areas and the evaluation of the effectiveness of that action. In addition, reporting the results through the established organizational structure to directly link the transport service with the base facility is vital. Monitoring may focus on a specific period, procedure, or population.

Table 8-3: Samples of Area-specific Indicators*

Category	Performance Measure	Rationale	Dimensions of Performance	Specific Indicators	Method for Data Collection	Multi-disciplinary Component	Assessment	Threshold
Patient care	Pain	■ High risk ■ High volume ■ Problem prone	■ Efficacy ■ Appropriateness ■ Availability ■ Timeliness ■ Effectiveness ■ Continuity ■ Efficiency ■ Respect and caring ■ Safety	■ Assessment noted on transport record—presence or absence of pain ■ If present, pain relief measure implemented and assessment of effectiveness documented ■ Use of pain scale	■ Review of transport record	■ No	■ Monthly	95%
Patient care	Safety	■ High risk ■ High volume ■ Problem prone	■ Efficacy ■ Appropriateness ■ Availability ■ Timeliness ■ Effectiveness ■ Continuity ■ Efficiency ■ Respect and caring ■ Safety	■ ID bands ■ Ambulance incident reports ■ Daily emergency equipment checks: storeroom check, defibrillator check, narcotic log check ■ Bimonthly: equipment bag check ■ Seatbelt and specific restraint use ■ Equipment secured to stretcher or isolette in vehicle	■ Review of occurrence reports ■ Review of occurrence reports ■ Weeklong survey ■ Review of occurrence reports ■ Review of checklists ■ Review of checklists ■ Weeklong survey ■ Weeklong survey	■ Risk Management ■ Medical director ■ Ambulance personnel ■ RN ■ RT	■ Monthly	100%
Patient care	Sedation	■ High risk ■ High volume ■ Problem prone	■ Efficacy ■ Appropriateness ■ Availability ■ Timeliness ■ Effectiveness ■ Continuity ■ Efficiency ■ Respect and caring ■ Safety	Documentation to include: ■ Presedation assessment of ABCs ■ Response to medication ■ VS monitoring in progress ■ Complications	■ Transport record review	■ Medical director ■ RN	■ Monthly	90%

Table 8-3: Samples of Area-specific Indicators,* continued

Category	Performance Measure	Rationale	Dimensions of Performance	Specific Indicators	Method for Data Collection	Multi-disciplinary Component	Assessment	Threshold
Patient care	Vascular access	■ High risk ■ High volume ■ Problem prone	■ Efficacy ■ Appropriateness ■ Availability ■ Timeliness ■ Effectiveness ■ Continuity ■ Efficiency ■ Respect and caring ■ Safety	Monitor: ■ Umbilical artery catheters ■ Placement documented per CXR ■ Assessment of pulses and perfusion distal to the line ■ Well secured to abdomen ■ Easily aspirates and flushes ■ Good arterial waveform per monitor ■ Umbilical venous catheters ■ Placement documented per CXR ■ Well secured to abdomen ■ IVF only (no meds) if tip below the diaphragm ■ IV or arterial line ■ Document assessment of site ■ Easily flushes (waveform, blood return)	■ Review of transport record	■ RN ■ Medical director	■ Monthly	90%
Documen-tation	Phone call record Transport record	■ High risk ■ High volume ■ Problem prone	■ Efficacy ■ Appropriateness ■ Availability ■ Timeliness ■ Effectiveness ■ Continuity ■ Efficiency ■ Respect and caring ■ Safety	■ Forms completed ■ Signature of RN present ■ If care suggestions given, individual receiving orders indicated ■ Time of interventions documented ■ VS on all patients docu-mented a minimum of every 15 min ■ Patient response to interventions documented	■ Review of transport record	■ No	■ Monthly	90%

Table 8-3: Samples of Area-specific Indicators,* continued

Category	Performance Measure	Rationale	Dimensions of Performance	Specific Indicators	Method for Data Collection	Multi-disciplinary Component	Assessment	Thresh-old
Documen-tation, continued				▪ ETT present Y / N ▪ ETT placement noted on x-ray and documented ▪ End-tidal CO_2 monitoring used for intubated patients (optional for neonates)				
Education	Mandatory yearly review	▪ High risk ▪ High volume ▪ Problem prone	▪ Efficacy ▪ Appropriateness ▪ Availability ▪ Timeliness ▪ Effectiveness ▪ Continuity ▪ Efficiency ▪ Respect and caring ▪ Safety	▪ Staff completion of yearly fire, safety, infection control, and critical clinical skills ▪ All transport team staff will attend yearly ambulance safety, helicopter safety, helipad fire safety, and altitude physiology classes. ▪ Staff will maintain current provider status in CPR, PALS, NRP, and ACLS. TNCC will be required by end 2002. Audit of ATLS encouraged. ▪ Staff will attend animal lab and demonstrate umbilical catheterization, needle aspiration of the chest and chest tube insertion (RNs), and intubation (RNs and RTs) a minimum of 3 times per year. ▪ RNs will obtain airway management experience in surgery at Westchester or on the main campus a mini-mum of 4 times a year (intubations on humans).	▪ Tracked in unit	▪ No	▪ Quarterly	100%

Table 8-3: Samples of Area-specific Indicators,* continued

Category	Performance Measure	Rationale	Dimensions of Performance	Specific Indicators	Method for Data Collection	Multi-disciplinary Component	Assessment	Thresh-old
Education, continued				▓ Completion of mandatory clinical education competencies, including child abuse, restraint policy, blood products administration, and age-specific competencies				
Satisfaction	Staff Patient and family Referring hospital personnel	▓ High risk ▓ High volume ▓ Problem prone		▓ Staff completion of yearly survey ▓ Review of parent satisfaction survey ▓ Referring hospitals to complete transport team service questionnaire	▓ Tally responses to referring hospital questionnaires. ▓ Press Ganey patient satisfaction survey; report given by CNE		▓ Yearly ▓ Monthly ▓ Quarterly	N/A
Patient care	Transport review indicators	▓ High risk ▓ High volume ▓ Problem prone	▓ Efficacy ▓ Appropriateness ▓ Availability ▓ Timeliness ▓ Effectiveness ▓ Continuity ▓ Efficiency ▓ Respect and caring ▓ Safety	▓ Multidisciplinary case review of transported patients. Patients whose cases will be reviewed include those with whom the following situations occurred during transport: death on transport; death within 24 hours of admission; unexpected need for the PICU within 24 hours of admission or backup bed not previously arranged; arrest; time at referring hospital: neonate, > 90 min, or pediatric, > 60 min; extubation;	▓ Use of transport review trigger form (preestablished criteria)	▓ Medical director ▓ RN ▓ RT	▓ Bimonthly	90%

144

Table 8-3: Samples of Area-specific Indicators,* continued

Category	Performance Measure	Rationale	Dimensions of Performance	Specific Indicators	Method for Data Collection	Multi-disciplinary Component	Assessment	Threshold
Patient care, continued				hypoxemia: saturation <95% for pediatric or <85% for neonate (excluding neonate for ECMO, suspected cyanotic CHD, use jet or oscillator vents); intubation (excluding neonate receiving PGE); needle thoracostomy; hypothermia; chest tube insertion; arrhythmias requiring drug therapy; hypotension; hypothermia; RN-transport only; initiation of vasopressor therapy; neonate receiving NO; helicopter transport				
Operations	Utilization appropriateness	▪ High risk ▪ High volume ▪ Problem prone	▪ Efficacy ▪ Appropriateness ▪ Availability ▪ Timeliness ▪ Effectiveness ▪ Continuity ▪ Efficiency ▪ Respect and caring ▪ Safety	▪ Coordination of transport from reception of request to liftoff/en route time: goal = 30" ▪ Number of transports completed ▪ Number of transports aborted owing to weather, maintenance, and patient condition	▪ Review of statistical reports	▪ No	▪ Monthly	90%
Operations	Utilization appropriateness	▪ High risk ▪ High volume ▪ Problem prone	▪ Efficacy ▪ Appropriateness ▪ Availability ▪ Timeliness ▪ Effectiveness ▪ Continuity	▪ Patients transferred to CMH ED by the transport service appropriately triaged before transfer to transport team vs ALS ▪ Medical need appropriate-	▪ Chart review of patients discharged from ED after transport; use of pre-established criteria will help determine	▪ No	▪ Monthly	90%

Table 8-3: Samples of Area-specific Indicators,* *continued*

Category	Performance Measure	Rationale	Dimensions of Performance	Specific Indicators	Method for Data Collection	Multi-disciplinary Component	Assessment	Threshold
Operations, continued			■ Efficiency ■ Respect and caring ■ Safety	ness of patients transferred to CMH by the transport service without IVs or oxygen, not transferred from a critical care service, scheduled transports, or interfacility to a lower level of care	appropriate use of transport service.			

*Example of Children's Memorial specific indicators. Reprinted with permission: Craig LaRusso, RN, Transport Team, Children's Memorial Hospital, Chicago, IL. ID indicates identification; ABCs, airway, breathing, circulation; VS, vital signs; CXR, chest x-ray; IVF, intravenous fluids; IV, intravenous; RN, registered nurse; RT, respiratory therapist; ETT, endotracheal tube; CPR, cardiopulmonary resuscitation; PALS, Pediatric Advanced Life Support; NRP, Neonatal Resuscitation Program; ACLS, Advanced Cardiac Life Support; TNCC, Trauma Nursing Core Course; ATLS, Advanced Trauma Life Support; CNE, chief nurse executive; N/A, not applicable; PICU, pediatric intensive care unit; ECMO, extracorporeal membrane oxygenation; CHD, congenital heart disease; PGE, prostaglandin E; NO, nitric oxide; CMH, Children's Memorial Hospital; ED, emergency department; and ALS, Advanced Life Support.

Role of the Medical Director(s) in the QI Process

Medical direction and the QI plan are intertwined. The medical director serves in various capacities as a resource, supervisor, moderator, evaluator, and educator. Activities that monitor quality may be prospective, concurrent, or retrospective.

Prospective activities include interviewing, hiring, educating personnel, developing treatment protocols, and directing overall transport operations. *Concurrent* activities oversee patient care during transport (online medical control) via direct communication such as radio, telephone, video, computer links, teleconferencing, or a combination of these. *Retrospective* activities review care after it has been provided, including chart review of documentation, review of transports when triggers were activated, recorded audio and/or video tapes, individual case review, and morbidity and mortality data. The medical director is also responsible for ensuring timely review of patient care, using the medical record and preestablished criteria.

The medical director must participate in the QI process if it is to be a viable component of the transport program. The medical director's influence on clinical decisions, efficiency, and safety supports the QI process. However, all transport-related disciplines should be included in the monitoring, review, and problem solving that can be used to provide a format for improving patient care.

Accreditation and the QI Process

In 2002, the JCAHO introduced its standardized core performance measures that allow rigorous comparisons between hospitals. Although JCAHO standards do not exist specifically for transport, the method of comparison and performance is notable. Performance measurement, comparison, and continual monitoring are key hallmarks of process improvement.

Within the transport arena, the Commission on Accreditation of Medical Transport Systems (CAMTS) is an accrediting body that aims to assist the transport community to provide a specific level of quality (see Chapter 19). Accreditation is a voluntary process in which an accrediting board of experts evaluates a program or institution against measurable standards or criteria. CAMTS has established the standards as a "blueprint for organizational planning" and marker of excellence.

▬▬▬▬▬▬▬▬▬▬▬▬▬▬▬▬▬▬▬▬▬▬▬▬▬▬▬▬▬▬▬▬▬▬

Summary

The QI program provides a positive mechanism to review all activities related to patient care, communication, and transport operations; identify problems; resolve identified problems; monitor the implementation of change; and provide ongoing reevaluation of strategies for process improvement.

A well-constructed QI program requires commitment at multiple levels: personal, clinical, financial, and administrative. A solid foundation (the transport program), a strong framework (the QI committee), and an insightful inspector (the QI coordinator) are the tools for a neonatal-pediatric transport program to maintain QI as one of its cornerstones. The transport program that continually strives to improve and promote safe, timely, appropriate, and quality patient care will be in a better position to market its services and will rise to the challenges of the future.

References

1. Plsek PE. Quality improvement methods in clinical medicine. *Pediatrics.* 1999;103 (1 suppl E):203-214
2. Bergman DA. Evidence-based guidelines and critical pathways for quality improvement. *Pediatrics.* 1999;103(1 suppl E):225–232
3. Emergency Medical Services for Children. *Quality Improvement in Emergency Medical Services for Children.* Available at: http://www.ems-c.org/downloads/doc/QI_EMSC.doc. Accessed April 2, 2004

Selected Readings

Agency for Healthcare Research and Quality. Quality and Patient Safety. Available at: http://www.ahrq.gov/qual/. Accessed January 13, 2006

Agency for Healthcare Research and Quality. *AHRQ Tools and Resources for Better Health Care.* Available at: http://www.ahrq.gov/qual/tools/toolsria.htm. Accessed April 28, 2004

Benson N. Quality assurance and continuous quality improvement. In McCloskey K, Orr R, eds. *Pediatric Transport Medicine.* St Louis, MO: Mosby; 1995:108–122

Commission on Accreditation of Medical Transport Systems. *Accreditation Standards of Commission on Accreditation of Medical Transport Systems.* 5th ed. Sandy Springs, SC: Commission on Accreditation of Medical Transport Systems; 2002

Deming WE, Shewart WA. PDCA cycle. Available at: http://www.asq.org/learn-about-quality/project-planning-tools/overview/pdca-cycle.html. Accessed January 13, 2006

Holleran RS. *Air and Surface Patient Transport: Principles and Practice.* 3rd ed. St Louis, MO: Mosby; 2003

Institute for Healthcare Improvement. "How to Improve..." Available at: http://www.ihi.org/IHI/Topics/Improvement/ImprovementMethods/HowToImprove/. Accessed January 18, 2006

Joint Commission on the Accreditation of Healthcare Organizations. *Agenda for Change Update.* Oakbrook Terrace, IL: Joint Commission on Accreditation of Healthcare Organizations; 1987

Langley GJ. *The Improvement Guide: A Practical Approach to Enhancing Organizational Performance.* San Francisco, CA: Jossey-Bass; 1996

McKeith JJ. Establishing a CQI program. E Medicine Available at: http://www.emedicine.com/emerg/topic668.htm. Accessed April 2, 2004

National Highway and Transportation Safety Administration. *A Leadership Guide to Quality Improvement for Emergency Medical Service Systems.* Washington, DC: National Highway and Transportation Safety Administration; July 1997. Available at www.nhtsa.dot.gov/people/injury/ems/leaderguide/index.html. Accessed January 13, 2006

Sayah AJ. EMS QA. E Medicine. Available at www.emedicine.com/emerg/topic719.htm. Accessed April 2, 2004

Questions

1. What objectives should be met in the QI plan?
2. Who are the responsible parties in the QI process?
3. Describe a systematic approach to quality improvement.

Answers

1. The objectives that should be met in the QI plan are determined for the program by team members and administrators involved with the transport program. As each area of concern is noted, comparisons with competitors are completed, and improvements and ideas are noted. Objectives should be formally written as noted in the tables provided in this chapter. Objectives with a focus on safety and clinical training are good places to start.
2. Each team member is responsible to participate in the QI process. The important aspect of QI is the continual, cyclical nature that requires each involved party to participate, oversee, and make changes and monitor improvements. When all participants are vested in the process, continuous QI becomes a natural process that reflects itself as a quality program.
3. PDSA, or PDCA: Plan, Do, Study (or Check), Act

Safety

Outline

- Environmental factors
- Safety policies
- Clothing
- Vehicle orientation
- Training for survival and emergency conditions
- Physical requirements
- Shift work and circadian disruption
- Teamwork training as a safety tool
- Safety responsibilities of the medical director and program director

Patient transport involves some risk to the patient and to transport personnel. Although the primary risks are medical, moving vehicles may pose unique hazards. The most extreme examples are rare, fatal vehicular crashes. However, less severe incidents can injure the patient, members of the transport team, or other occupants, resulting in permanent or temporary disability. In addition to the mental and physical discomfort experienced by the injured parties, there are monetary costs. The hospital or vehicle provider may be liable for workman's compensation claims and may become involved in civil litigation. Injured personnel may be unable to return to work for extended periods, forcing their organization to find and train temporary or permanent replacements. In many cases, the injuries and the costs can be avoided or mitigated by adequate attention to safety.

Environmental Factors

Transport medicine is greatly influenced by environmental conditions. In many cases, the acceptance or rejection of a transport is dependent on the weather. Weather conditions have their greatest effects on aircraft, but also are important for ground transport vehicles. Just as

■■■■■■■■■■■■■■■■■■■■■■■■■■■■■■■■■■■

foggy weather and high winds make aircraft operations dangerous, icy roads and heavy rain may make it imprudent to operate a ground ambulance. All teams should have clear guidelines delineating the minimal weather requirements for the vehicle(s) used, and these guidelines should be strictly followed. The rules may vary depending on the type of vehicle used and the local terrain. Aircraft may use visual flight rules (also called VFR) or, if more sophisticated, instrument flight rules (also called IFR) that allow safe flight in less-than-ideal (but not all) weather conditions. For ground operations, travel advisories issued by state and local authorities should be considered before a decision is made to proceed with the transport. In addition, the Commission on Accreditation of Medical Transport Systems (CAMTS) offers guidelines for minimal safe weather conditions. In all cases, the final decision rests with the driver or pilot and should be made based solely on the prevailing weather conditions along the entire route of travel. Neither patient severity or need nor pressures such as productivity or competition should influence the driver or pilot's decision. Furthermore, administrative personnel and the medical director should support these decisions. An expanded review and discussion regarding safety and mode of transport is included in Chapter 10.

Safety Policies

In addition to weather rules, the team should have policies dictating the safe conduct of transports based on the medical needs of the patient coupled with the safety of the patient and the team members. These policies should, for example, address if and when a ground ambulance can use lights and sirens to circumvent certain traffic regulations. In most cases, this practice is unnecessary because a potential few minutes saved does not justify the substantial risk of an emergency response. However, when the team lacks a clear policy regarding issues such as the use of lights and sirens and adherence to traffic regulations, the driver is free to use his or her judgment with potentially disastrous results. Other examples of necessary guidelines include the following: circumstances under which it is acceptable for a crew member to become unrestrained to care for the patient, standard precautions, use of hands-free communication technology by the driver or pilot, and transport of family members. There should be specific rules concerning team members who are impaired by drugs, alcohol, exhaustion, illness, or injury. All team members should be oriented to and understand the rules. Furthermore, personnel employed by contracted vehicle vendors must adhere to the transport team's safety policies unless those of the vendor company are more stringent.

Clothing

Clothing is an essential safety consideration. Some aeromedical teams wear helmets and fire-retardant clothing, whereas others, particularly those in very warm climates, do not. Aeromedical teams may require specialty neonatal and pediatric transport personnel to conform to their clothing rules. All teams, however, need to give attention to clothing. Attire that is appropriate and functional in the hospital may be hazardous during patient transport. Long or loose white coats, scarves, or other clothing can become tangled in equipment or in restraints. Clogs, popular among health care workers, are not appropriate for transport. They do not provide adequate traction on uneven surfaces or satisfactorily protect and support the foot and are less than ideal for walking long distances in remote environments. Certain types of jewelry, such as dangling bracelets, that may become caught in equipment or machinery may also be dangerous.

Clothing should, instead, be appropriate to the expected or potential environmental conditions, providing adequate warmth in the winter and preventing heat illness in the summer. Depending on the team's mission(s) and geographic location, options include flight suits, jumpsuits, and a standard uniform. Some teams providing on-scene care in hot environments wear short pants and short-sleeved shirts, although consideration must be given to universal safety protection as well as prevention of potential transport related issues (skin protection from heat, burns, sharp objects). Many teams choose uniforms that include pockets for extra equipment. Attention should also be given to appropriate eyewear. In addition to protection from prolonged sun exposure, protective eyewear is an essential component of standard precautions and can protect the eyes from debris when the team member is loading, unloading, or boarding a running

▪▪▪▪▪▪▪▪▪▪▪▪▪▪▪▪▪▪▪▪▪▪▪▪▪▪▪▪▪▪▪▪▪▪

helicopter. In addition, team members need to be cognizant of the possibility, however remote, of prolonged environmental exposure and ensure that they have appropriate protective clothing with them. A 1-hour flight may become a several-day ordeal if the aircraft is required to make an emergency landing in a wilderness location during the winter. Hospital scrubs and a light jacket would be inadequate under such circumstances. Environmental exposure also can occur under less extreme circumstances, for example, failure of the heating or air conditioning system in an ambulance. A team member with hypothermia will be unable to care for the patient or assist team members. Clothing choices should recognize these possibilities. During cold weather operations, layered clothing may be the best solution because it allows team members to remain comfortable across a range of temperatures. All protective clothing should also address the need to maintain standard precautions for protection of the crew from blood and body fluid exposure. Additional, more sophisticated protective equipment may be required for the transport of patients with toxic exposures or certain infectious diseases.

Vehicle Orientation

Every team member, especially those who infrequently participate in transports, should be oriented or reoriented to the transport vehicle(s) used by the team. For aircraft, the content of the orientation is mandated by the Federal Aviation Administration. Likewise, Department of Transportation rules govern the operations of ambulances. In addition, CAMTS offers transport programs the opportunity to be evaluated voluntarily against standards of quality and safety. The CAMTS standards include criteria for training in the safe use of transport equipment and vehicles. These issues are particularly important for neonatal-pediatric transport teams that occasionally fly with one or more unrelated aeromedical services. In such cases, the neonatal-pediatric team is expected to function as an integral part of the aeromedical team and is subject to the same rules and guidelines. The transport team should be fully oriented to all aircraft used and should understand how to safely approach the aircraft to board and to load and unload patients. Likewise, team members should be well versed in all emergency procedures. Although specific guidelines vary with the type of aircraft used, team members should be aware of the potential dangers associated with each type of aircraft, how to minimize these dangers, and how to respond if necessary. Helicopters pose the greatest hazards. Contact with the tail rotor blade or main rotor blades, which can dip several feet if turning slowly in high winds, is likely to be lethal. In addition, a landing helicopter can generate gale force winds that, like naturally occurring winds, will cause flying debris and can damage nearby objects and injure bystanders. Certainly, all team members should be familiar with and use restraint systems and ensure that the patient and all passengers are properly restrained. Equipment such as stretchers and isolettes must be properly restrained within the vehicle. Emergency evacuation procedures and appropriate responses to a vehicular crash, fire on board the vehicle, and other emergency situations should be well rehearsed. The more realistic the training, the more likely the crew is to survive an actual incident. With an estimated accident rate of approximately 1 in 1000 ground transports, it is likely that most transport teams will have experience with an adverse vehicular event.

Training for Survival and Emergency Conditions

Teams that travel over or through remote areas must have the training necessary to survive in these environments until rescued. Emergency and survival training should occur at regular intervals so that these skills are well understood by all team members. All such vehicles should carry survival equipment, including food and water. Personal flotation devices are mandatory for flights over water unless a safe glide to land can be assured. In many cases, the transport vehicle will serve as the crew's shelter; however, alternative arrangements should also be made in case the vehicle becomes unusable. In cold or cool environments, body heat can be lost quickly, and hypothermia is a risk for the crew and the patient. Crew members should have adequate clothing to withstand the weather, and a survival kit should include means of providing adequate warmth. Likewise, teams must have multiple methods of communication so that help can be contacted, if needed.

Physical Requirements

While survival training is important, it is even more important that team members and hospital administration understand that the transport environment requires physical capabilities beyond those expected of personnel who function only in a hospital or clinic. Team members may be required to lift patients or to carry heavy equipment, often with little or no help. Personnel need to be agile enough to maneuver within the confines of a transport vehicle and dexterous enough to perform procedures in a moving environment. In addition, they should not be unduly prone to motion sickness or should have mastered techniques to mitigate the effects of motion sickness. Most aircraft are subject to weight restrictions that vary with type of aircraft and the location and distance of the flight. These restrictions are likely to prevent very large team members from participating in at least some transports. Team members with certain chronic illnesses or disabilities may also be unable to perform all expected duties. Likewise, pregnancy may temporarily preclude participation and, at a minimum, medical clearance by the team member's obstetrician should be provided. In addition, certain medical conditions may permanently or temporarily preclude participation in transports. Unlike the situation in a hospital, the transport team has few options should a member become incapacitated while on duty. If the team member is suddenly unable to function, patient care and crew safety might be compromised. Therefore, rules precluding team participation under certain circumstances are reasonable. For example, team members with sinusitis or otitis media may be temporarily unable to fly, whereas those with uncontrolled seizures or brittle diabetes might be completely removed from transport duty owing to the risks to themselves and others. These issues are best addressed by a policy clearly and specifically stating the physical requirements for team membership (Figure 9-1). These policies should be drafted with the assistance of the human resources department and legal counsel. Team members should be encouraged to maintain physical fitness, and it is reasonable to make continued participation dependent on the results of regular (eg, annual) physical fitness testing.

Figure 9-1: Sample Team Participation Policy*
METHODIST HEALTHCARE SYSTEM
METHODIST CHILDREN'S HOSPITAL OF SOUTH TEXAS

TITLE:	Criteria for Transport Duty
EFFECTIVE DATE:	May 1997
REVISED DATE(S):	March 19, 2001
	May, 2002
REVIEWED DATE(S):	
AUDIENCE:	Children's Transport Services
APPROVED BY:	Coordinator

All standard policies and procedures represent our current knowledge and judgment regarding the issue covered by this policy. If you can think of a better way to handle the issue covered in this policy/procedure, or if this policy/procedure needs to be revised to reflect changes that have occurred, please "draft" a revision and give it to the transport coordinator or the team medical director so that we can consider improving this policy/procedure accordingly.

Policy:

1. On-duty team members will be physically and mentally able to manage a critical care transport. Criteria include, but are not limited to the following:
   - The team member is able to lift up to 50 lb.
   - The team member is able to withstand the potential stressors of the transport environment and transport activities. The team member is well rested—has had a minimum of 6 hours of sleep within the 24-hour period prior to on-duty status.
   - The team member is able to tolerate variances in diet.
   - The team member is not under the influence of medications that can cause excessive drowsiness or sedation.
   - The team member has not ingested alcohol within 8 hours of on-duty status.
   - The team member has not donated blood within the last 72 hours.

2. In the event of illness, injury, or personal difficulties that occur during a transport shift that would limit the team member's ability to adequately perform in the transport environment, the team member will notify:
   - Transport coordinator, clinical administrator or other supervisor
   If the team member cannot be replaced with in-house or on-call coverage such that a full team could still be mobilized, the "Closure of Transport Services" policy/procedure will be initiated.

Figure 9-1: Sample Team Participation Policy,* *continued*

3. Team members who have symptoms that would limit their ability to perform their duties on transport must notify the transport coordinator or respiratory therapy director/supervisor. The team member will be alert to the following conditions that are relative contraindications to aeromedical transport and may render them ineligible for duty:
   - Impacted sinusitis
   - Invasive dental work within 24 hours of on-duty status
   - Otitis media
   - Scuba diving within 24 hours of on-duty status
   - Any condition for which the employee health nurse has enacted work restrictions
   - Any condition for which the team member's physician has placed him/her on work restrictions
4. Any team member who has been placed on work restrictions is required to furnish a physician's statement clearing him/her for transport activities before returning to active duty status.
5. Team members who are aware they are pregnant are requested to notify the Transport Coordinator (as well as their manager/director) of their condition. Pregnant team members will be allowed to remain on active status until their first prenatal appointment with their MD. At the time of the first prenatal exam, they must obtain a letter/note from their MD clearing them for continuing active transport status. The pregnant transport provider assumes responsibility for informing her MD of the physical stressors of the transport environment and transport duties. She may provide her MD with a copy of this policy.

---

*MD indicates physician. Used with permission: Methodist Healthcare System, San Antonio, TX.

Shift Work and Circadian Disruption

In recent years, considerable attention has been given to the role of shift work and sleep deprivation in medical error, road collisions, and other types of incidents. Disruption of circadian rhythm is a key issue for many types of workers. Certainly, health care has always been a 24-hour business. However, transport teams have special problems related to sleep deprivation and shift work. First, unlike their colleagues in the hospital, transport team members may not be exposed to the stimulation of lights and personal interactions that contribute to remaining alert. In fact, they may be required to travel for many hours in a darkened vehicle performing relatively routine and monotonous tasks. Under such circumstances, vigilance and judgment may falter. Second, shifts can become lengthened with a prolonged transport, forcing the team member to work well beyond the scheduled end of the shift. For team members working several consecutive shifts, the result might be inadequate rest. In extreme cases such as international or cross-country transports, team members may be subject to jet lag, further disrupting sleep. There are few easy solutions to this problem. Certainly, all drivers and pilots should adhere strictly to regulations governing adequate rest before and after duty, even if this means that some transports must be delayed, divided into legs, or referred. Scheduling for team members should occur in a "circadian-friendly" manner, moving forward from day shifts to middle shifts to night shifts with adequate rest between the transition from nights to days. Dedicated transport teams (ie, the teams whose members have no other assigned or primary clinical duties when not transporting patients) may want to consider allowing team members to sleep during the night shift when not transporting patients. All teams should have rules dictating rest time before duty hours. Such rules should also address the minimum number of hours before duty that a team member can consume alcohol and certain medications.

Teamwork Training as a Safety Tool

It is becoming well understood that errors are minimized and safety is supported when the members of highly skilled teams function as a cohesive unit. The concepts were developed in the military and later were embraced by the aviation industry as "Cockpit Resource Management" and the evolution to "Crew Resource Management." More recently, they have been adapted for use in health care settings. At their core, these concepts place responsibility for safety on the entire team, and any member of the team, regardless of level of training or seniority, is empowered to voice safety concerns without fear of reprisal. In fact, team members are encouraged to address these issues candidly.

A complete discussion of these concepts is beyond the scope of this chapter (the reader is referred to the Selected Readings); however, the basic tenets will be summarized briefly. First, team structure is created and strengthened, and team members are assigned specific roles. Although one team member serves as the leader during each patient encounter, this role need not remain fixed across encounters; one member may serve as the leader for one transport with another member serving as the leader for a subsequent transport. Second, all team members are accountable to one another for performing their assigned duties and for asking for assistance when needed. Third (and a very important concept for teams that include a physician), team members must not be bound by traditional roles and are free to object to or question an order or a plan at least twice. This so-called 2-challenge rule is intended to force the leader to reconsider the action or order in question. Fourth, team members are encouraged to communicate in a specific manner. Orders are acknowledged and repeated by the recipient to ensure understanding. Unclear orders and plans are immediately questioned and clarified. Fifth, when errors or untoward events occur, as they surely will, they are discussed openly and in a spirit of system correction rather than individual blame.

Safety Responsibility of the Medical Director and Program Director

The ultimate responsibility for the adherence to safety policies lies with the medical director and the program director. These individuals should establish and enforce the physical requirements for the role. They are also responsible for delineating the safety policies of the team and should have the authority to require certain safety standards on the part of contracted vehicle vendors. Team members who knowingly violate safety policies are endangering themselves, their colleagues, and the patients. The medical director and program director should not tolerate such behavior. The medical director, the program director, or others in the organization are likely to receive occasional complaints from referring hospitals when transports are delayed or referred based on weather restrictions, crew fatigue, or other safety-related factors, and they should address these issues directly.

Selected Readings

Auerbach PS, Morris JA, Phillips JB Jr, Redlinger SR, Vaughn WK. An analysis of ambulance collisions in Tennessee. *JAMA*. 1987;258:1487–1490

Clawson JJ, Martin RL, Cady GA, Maio RF. The wake effect: emergency vehicle related collisions. *Prehosp Disaster Med*. 1997;12:274–277

Frazer R. Air medical accidents: a 20-year search for information. *AirMed*. 1999;5:34–39

Grogan EL, Stiles RA, France DJ, et al. The impact of aviation-based teamwork training on the attitudes of health-care professionals. *J Am Coll Surg*. 2004;199:843–848

Ho J, Casey B. Time saved with use of emergency warning lights and sirens during response requests for emergency medical aid in an urban environment. *Ann Emerg Med*. 1998;32:585–588

Hunt RC, Brown LH, Cabinum ES, et al. Is ambulance transport time with lights and siren faster than that without? *Ann Emerg Med*. 1995;25:507–511

King BR, Woodward GA. Pediatric critical care transport—the safety of the journey: a five-year review of vehicular collisions involving pediatric and neonatal transport teams. *Prehosp Emerg Care*. 2002;6:449–454

Kupas DF, Dula DJ, Pino BJ. Patient outcome using medical protocol to limit "lights and siren" transport. *Prehosp Disaster Med*. 1994;9:226–229

Levick N, Winston F, Aitkin S, Freemantle R, Marshall F, Smith G. Development and application of a dynamic testing procedure for ambulance paediatric patient restraint systems. *SAE Australia*. March/April 1998:14–15

Low RB, Dunne MJ, Blumen IJ, Tagney G. Factors associated with the safety of EMS helicopters. *Am J Emerg Med*. 1991;9:103–106

The National Transportation Safety Board Accident Database. Available at: http://www.ntsb.gov. Accessed January 13, 2006

Risser DT, Rice MM, Salisbury ML, Simon R, Jay GD, Berns, SD. The potential for improved teamwork to reduce medical errors in the emergency department. The MedTeams Research Consortium. *Ann Emerg Med*. 1999;34:370–372

Saunders CE, Heye CJ. Ambulance collisions in an urban environment. *Prehosp Disaster Med*. 1994;9:118–124

Seamster T, Boehm-Davis DA, Holt RW, Schultz K. *Developing Advanced Crew Resource Management (ACRM) Training: A Training Manual*. 1998. Available at: http://www.hf.faa.gov/docs/508/docs/DACRMT.pdf. Accessed January 13, 2006

Seidel JS, Greenlaw J. Use of restraints in ambulances: a state survey. *Pediatr Emerg Care*. 1998;14:221–223

Questions

1. Your transport team is called to a remote rural hospital to retrieve a critically ill neonate. The hospital has a level 2 nursery, and there are no level 3 nurseries closer to the rural hospital than your children's hospital. Without transport, the infant is unlikely to survive. A severe snowstorm is raging along your route of travel. The state department of transportation has issued a travel advisory recommending against road travel. Visibility is too poor for air transport. What is the best course of action?
2. Which types of clothing are best suited for transport in a cold climate?
3. What are the basic tenets of the teamwork model?

Answers

1. Although the needs of the patient seem compelling, several transport team members have been killed or injured attempting dangerous "rescues." The most appropriate course of action is to offer as much advice and support by telephone or telemedicine connection until a safe transport is possible.
2. Clothing should be appropriate to the environmental conditions that *could* be encountered *if* the heater fails, the ambulance skids into a snow bank and is disabled, or the helicopter makes an emergency landing in a remote area.
3. a. Creation of a team structure, designation of a leader (permanent or situational), and assignment of specific roles
   b. Mutual accountability
   c. Open communication and contribution; encouragement to voice concerns or objections
   d. Acknowledgment and repeating of orders to ensure that they are correct
   e. Frank discussion of errors and untoward outcomes with a goal of identifying and correcting problems rather than assigning blame

Transport Mode: Issues, Timing, Safety, Selection Criteria, Considerations, and Options

Outline

- Critical transport decisions
- Criteria for consideration of air vs ground transport
- General considerations
- Ground ambulances
- Helicopter air ambulances
- Fixed-wing air ambulances (airplanes)
- Vehicle operations
- Summary

The optimal transport of each neonatal and pediatric patient is facilitated when the personnel involved ensure the appropriate use of available resources, including staff, equipment, and vehicles. An increased awareness of transfer requirements has been highlighted by the federal Emergency Medical Treatment and Active Labor Act (EMTALA), which requires that all transfers be effected using qualified personnel and transportation equipment. Various medical and legal opinions have concluded that appropriate vehicle selection is no longer merely a patient care issue, but also an EMTALA compliance issue.

The selection of the most appropriate mode (vehicle) for neonatal-pediatric transport is influenced by numerous factors. The acuity and stability of the patient's condition and the need for unavailable local services (ie, a higher level of care) have major roles. Vehicle availability, weather, distance, geography, transport time, and transport "logistics" are also essential considerations. Transport logistics include the potential advantages and disadvantages of the various modes of transport.

Vehicles used in patient transport include surface (ground) and air ambulances. Air ambulances are rotor-wing (helicopter) or fixed-wing (airplane) aircraft. The transfer of a neonatal or pediatric patient between facilities may require one of these vehicles or a combination. Transport teams and program administrators commonly determine which of these vehicles best fits their particular mission profile. A fully integrated transport system would include all 3 mode types as options. At the time of a transport request, a triage decision should be made to determine the most appropriate vehicle (or combination of vehicles) for the particular mission. Unfortunately, but realistically, many transport teams have limited resources. Although it may be common for transport programs that serve large rural areas to provide helicopter and airplane transport, they may do few (if any) nonair transports. In these circumstances, the transports may be outsourced or coordinated with a program that provides ground transports. Programs that predominantly serve an urban area may provide only helicopter or ground ambulance transport.

Patient transfers may be 1-way, when a vehicle is dispatched directly from the referring facility to the receiving facility; however, for neonatal-pediatric transport, the transfer more commonly is 2-way, in which the vehicle and specialized transport team members are sent from the receiving facility to the referring facility to pick up the patient. In addition, transports also can be 3-way, in which a transport vehicle and team from neither the referring nor the receiving facility are requested to undertake the transport. Private ambulance companies (air and ground) and most community- or hospital-sponsored air-medical flight programs perform such 3-way transfers as needed or under the terms of an established transport agreement.

Vehicle purchasing and leasing decisions should be made with direct input from persons who are knowledgeable about the transport environment and the capability of the various vehicles. The planning group should include members of the transport team who are directly and routinely involved in transport decisions. The items presented in this chapter usually are considered when administrative and transport personnel decide which vehicle(s) will best fit the goals of their program.

Critical Transport Decisions

Before any transport, attention to the safety of the transport team and patient should always be the foremost consideration when determining the mode of transport. There are 4 subsequent critical decision steps necessary for each transport; consideration of these steps facilitates the selection of the optimal mode of transport.

The first step involves evaluation of the clinical status of the patient. It is important to know the patient's current medical condition and to anticipate the most serious complication reasonably possible during transport. This does not need to be based on a final diagnosis but on an accurate assessment of the patient's illnesses or injuries, present or potential. If a patient's medical condition is unstable, even a minimal shortening of the response time to the referring facility achieved by selecting one mode of transportation over another may be lifesaving. The emphasis on reducing the out-of-hospital transport time may be especially beneficial to patient outcome in situations such as surgical emergencies.

The second step is an evaluation of the medical care the patient requires before and during transport, including an evaluation of the available medical care at the referring facility or scene of an accident. Usually the primary consideration is the level of care required during transport. However, there also may be a need for urgent provision of a higher level of care or additional personnel at the referring facility, such as for certain types of airway or surgical emergencies.

The third step is to determine the urgency of the transport. For time-sensitive transports (eg, a need for urgent or locally unavailable interventions), the time required for a selected vehicle to reach the referring facility and to deliver the patient to the receiving facility should be considered. These considerations will take into account the distance between facilities, the mode of transportation, geographic characteristics of the area to be served, and the availability of vehicle options. If the transport is less urgent, the key consideration becomes the availability of an appropriate vehicle.

The fourth step involves some of the logistics of a patient transport (eg, local resources available for transport, weather considerations, and ground traffic accessibility). Depending on the type of vehicle selected, the number of staff may be affected. If a ground ambulance is used for a patient with a complex medical condition, staffing can potentially be increased as needed. Conversely, staffing additions may be limited in a small helicopter.

General criteria addressing the appropriate use of air-medical services can be divided into categories, which correspond to the aforementioned third and fourth steps. These criteria are summarized in the following section.

Criteria for Consideration of Air vs Ground Transport

Time and Distance Indicators

Distance. Distance to the closest appropriate facility is too great for safe and timely transport by ground ambulance.

Transport Time. The patient's clinical condition requires that the time spent out of the hospital environment, in transport, be as short as possible.

Timely Treatment. The patient requires a specific treatment or timely treatment that is not available at the referring facility (or scene) to minimize morbidity and mortality.

Transport Delays. The potential for transport delay that may be associated with the use of ground or air transport (eg, weather or weather-related obstacles, traffic congestion, construction, road obstacles, location of patient, and distance) is likely to worsen the patient's clinical condition.

Logistic Indicators

Critical Care. The patient requires critical care support (eg, monitoring, personnel, medication, special equipment) during transport that is not available from the local ambulance service.

Inaccessible Area. The patient is located in an area that is inaccessible to regular ground traffic, impeding ambulance egress or access to the scene owing to environmental obstacles or conditions, weather-related events (eg, floods, heavy snowfall), traffic congestion, wilderness rescue, or other geographic considerations.

Local Ground Resources. The use of a local ground transport service would leave the local area without adequate emergency medical service coverage, or local ground units are not trained or available for long-distance neonatal-pediatric transport.

Transport Times

When evaluating the time needed to undertake and complete a transport, many factors are involved beyond the speed of the vehicle and the distance between the referring and receiving facilities. The time-related considerations for transport include the following:

Mode of Transport

In an attempt to keep the out-of-hospital time to a minimum, consideration must be given to the distance between the referring and receiving hospitals. Comparing only the actual travel speeds, the airplane typically provides the fastest mode of transport and the ground ambulance the slowest. In a time-critical transport in remote geographic areas, the reduced travel time offered by a helicopter or airplane may be essential. However, in an urban setting, where much shorter distances may be traveled, the ground ambulance or helicopter may provide the best option. For transport over a moderate distance to or from locations without on-site helicopter access or landing facilities, direct ambulance transport may be as efficient as rotor wing.

Response Time

The length of time from receipt of a transport call until the transport team arrives at the referring facility or scene of an accident often is referred to as the *response time*. Transport services that respond directly to the scene clearly require a rapid response time. Similarly, in a true medical emergency, if a transferring facility cannot stabilize a patient's condition, the response time to the referring facility with a critical care transport team may be more crucial than the time in transit to the receiving facility after the patient's condition has been stabilized. Many variables enter into the response time equation. Following the initial contact, there is the time needed to accept the patient and to mobilize and dispatch the transport team. Dedicated ground and helicopter teams can often be on their way within 15 minutes, although specific guidelines and requirements may vary between programs and municipalities, as well as with specific patient populations (eg, scene response teams that depart in ≤5 minutes). The departure of a medical airplane usually takes longer, ranging from 30 minutes to an hour or more. The fixed-wing delay often is because the transport team and pilot may be on call rather than on-site at the airport. In addition, the pilot is required to file a flight plan before departure. The response time may be more prolonged if the airplane is not dedicated to patient transport and requires changes in the interior configuration.

The various response times and related logistics of the vehicle options may make the choice more difficult. A ground ambulance may be available immediately at a referring facility that could be en route to the receiving facility long before a distant helicopter could arrive at the referring facility. The ground ambulance, however, may have to contend with local terrain, traffic, construction, and other ground-related delays, and the local emergency medical services (EMS) team may not have the training, experience, or equipment required to manage the patient in transit.

If a helicopter is to be considered, the response time should include the availability of a safe and close helipad or landing zone. An on-site helipad or landing area near both facilities is advantageous. A distant landing zone that would require a 3-point transfer (an inter-mediary transfer between location and transport vehicle) may elimi-nate the advantage of the helicopter's speed by requiring additional ground time, increased patient risk, and transfers between vehicles to travel between the landing area and the referring facility. In most cases, the patient should not be delivered to a distant landing zone to meet the aircraft and transport team. During this period of transfer, the clinical care and monitoring of the patient may not be optimal, and a lack of interventional capability creates an unstable environ-ment. In addition to the potential for disruption of the care of the patient, any patient transfer between different types of vehicles may be challenging, especially if there are size limitations. Patient move-ments necessitated from multiple patient transfers may be detrimen-tal to the patient's medical condition. If the helicopter must land in a location away from the site of patient care, ideally, the critical care transport team will be transported to the patient rather than the patient to the air ambulance. Following their assessment, stabilization of the patient's condition, and preparation of the patient for transport, the ambulance will take the patient and team back to the helicopter. If a helicopter needs to land at a site distant to the receiving hospital, the air transport team members should accompany and continue to manage the patient until formal transfer of care occurs at the receiving facility. They should not, if at all possible, transfer care to an intermediary team or plan to do a sophisticated care transfer in the field. This practice of maintaining care and responsibility for the patient until the definitive care transfer helps maximize care consistency and minimizes potential information deficiencies.

If airplane vs helicopter transport is considered, in addition to the distance issues, the ability of the helicopter to arrive directly at the hospital or nearby landing zone must be evaluated and compared with the airplane landing at a more distant airport and the requirement for an ambulance to travel the distance between the referring facility and the airport.

The response times of any vehicle selected may be affected by the vehicle's availability and weather conditions. A local air-medical helicopter already may be committed to a transport or may be unable to fly because of adverse weather conditions or maintenance requirements. These considerations may require that an alternative vehicle be selected to avoid a significant delay in response time. Fixed-wing aircraft have the advantage of pressurized cabins; therefore, they are able to operate at higher altitudes to avoid weather and turbulence found at lower altitudes.

When promoting a neonatal-pediatric transport program, it is important to help the referring physicians understand the factors that can affect the response time and what the "routine" response time will be. Confusion may exist for referring physicians, who might anticipate response times from neonatal-pediatric transport programs to be identical to those of EMS agencies, local ground ambulance services, or other available transport teams.

Stabilization and Preparation Time

The amount of time spent by the transport team to stabilize the patient's condition and prepare the patient for transport is another important consideration related to vehicle selection. Compared with local ground ambulance services, critical care transport teams that arrive by air or ground often take more time to assess a patient and stabilize the patient's condition before transport. Critical care teams should have a minimum of 2 personnel accompany a critically ill patient. This may consist of a combination of a physician, nurse, respiratory therapist, and critical care technician (see chapters 3 and 4). A critical care transport team is an extension of an intensive care team. Sophisticated neonatal-pediatric assessment, evaluation, stabilization, and treatment of the patient are necessary. A helicopter transport service will need to consider these issues regarding potential prolonged downtime at the referring hospital, which may remove them from EMS or other responses and can add to the per capita cost for transport.

Out-of-Hospital Time

For a patient in unstable condition or for a time-critical transport, the out-of-hospital time may be the most important factor in the transport vehicle equation. In addition to the distance between the referring and receiving facilities, the total time spent between facilities in the transport environment will depend on the mode of transport and the related times and logistics necessary to get to and from the vehicle. Like the response time, the out-of-hospital time will be affected by off-site helicopter landing zones and travel to and from airports. The transfer of a patient from one vehicle to another is time-consuming and recognized as a particularly risky time in the transport of any critically ill or injured patient. Temperature instability may occur during the transfer. Equipment is most likely to become disconnected or fail during transfer between vehicles, and, as mentioned, monitoring of the patient's condition is more difficult. To enhance patient care and reduce transport times for critically ill patients, transfers between vehicles should be kept to a minimum. For patients in stable condition or patients whose conditions have been stabilized, the out-of-hospital time may not be a critical consideration.

The philosophy and practice of many neonatal-pediatric transport teams may lead to a different approach to the linking of the response time, stabilization time, and out-of-hospital time than is usual with other transport services. For example, to reduce the response time for transport of a critically ill patient, a team may be dispatched to a referring facility by helicopter but may return by ground ambulance after stabilizing the patient's condition, making the helicopter available for other transports during a sometimes prolonged stabilization period.

Vehicle Selection

Many makes and models of ground vehicles, helicopters, and airplanes used to transport patients are available. When evaluating a transport vehicle for neonatal-pediatric transport, specific aircraft or ground ambulance capabilities should be studied to ensure that the program uses the vehicles that best serve its mission. Vehicles should be assessed to determine the usable cabin space and available options for the medical configuration. The speed of transport and vehicle range also may be important considerations, and noise and vibration are inherent factors for all transport vehicles and the transport environment. If aircraft are under consideration, additional specifications to evaluate include single-engine versus multiengine, useful load (amount of weight that can be lifted), and cabin pressurization (airplanes). From an administrative and financial standpoint, the costs related to purchase or lease and operate transport vehicles should be evaluated carefully. Some organizations that provide transport contract with private service(s) for vehicle provision. Contract negotiations may include response time of the vehicle crew, vehicle configuration, and determination of billing services.

The ideal transport vehicle should be safe, fast, quiet, comfortable, and medically equipped to care for pediatric and neonatal patients. It should be large enough to transport 1 or 2 patients with 2 to 4 transport team members. The vehicle should be easy to load and should provide adequate access to the patient(s) from the various seats.

Safety

Safety must be the most important consideration in patient transport. A careful consideration of the risks and benefits of the different modes of transport should be completed before any patient transfer. This is also a requirement of the referring physician under EMTALA. Everyone involved with patient transport is responsible for overall safety in and around any transport vehicle. The selection of reliable and safe vehicles (ie, ground ambulances, helicopters, and airplanes) is as important as the training and experience of the pilots, drivers, and mechanics responsible for their operation. Only transport services (air or ground) with a demonstrated commitment to safety should be considered.

Accidents have occurred with all modes of patient transport. Collisions and crashes involving neonatal-pediatric transport teams are uncommon, but reported. Data obtained by King and Woodward[1] from neonatal and/or pediatric transport teams suggest that 1 collision or crash occurs for every 1000 patient transports. Collisions or crashes involving injury were less common and reportedly occur at a rate of 0.546 per 1000 transports. In their 5-year incident review, all 8 reported neonatal-pediatric transport personnel deaths occurred as the result of aircraft crashes. Ground ambulance collisions accounted for some moderate to severe injuries. The aircraft crashes usually resulted from pilot error or adverse weather conditions, whereas ambulance collisions were most often attributed to issues related to the driver, weather, mechanical breakdown, or a third party.

In January 2006, the National Transportation Safety Board (NTSB) issued the "Special Investigation Report on Emergency Medical Services (EMS) Operations" and included, in detail, the briefs of 7 EMS accidents.[2] It noted that 55 EMS aviation accidents occurred in the United States between January 2002 and January 2005, resulting in 54 fatalities and 18 serious injuries. Summary statistics for the 1990–2005 period showed 125 accidents, with 41 of those involving fatalities. During that period, there were 109 fatalities, 43 serious injuries, and 47 minor injuries reported. Although the number of flight hours increased from approximately 162 000 in 1991 to 300 000 in 2005, the accident rate also increased. The NTSB identified the following recurring safety issues: less stringent requirements for EMS operations conducted with patients on board; a lack of aviation flight risk evaluation programs for EMS operations; a lack of consistent, comprehensive flight dispatch procedures for EMS operations; and no requirements to use technologies such as terrain awareness and warning systems to enhance EMS flight safety. Their specific conclusions included the following: (1) The safety of EMS operations would be improved if the entire EMS flight plan operated under 14

Code of Federal Regulations Part 135 operations specifications; 35 of the 55 accidents in this special investigation occurred with crew members but no patients on board. (2) The minimal contribution of medical personnel to the safe operation of EMS flights is not sufficient to justify operating EMS positioning flights under the less stringent 14 *Code of Federal Regulations* Part 91 requirements. (3) The implementation of flight risk evaluation before each mission would enhance the safety of EMS operations. (4) Formalized dispatch and flight-following procedures, including a dedicated dispatcher with aviation-specific knowledge and experience, would enhance the safety of EMS flight operations by providing the pilot with consistent and critical weather information, assisting in go/no go decisions, and monitoring the flight's position. (5) The use of terrain awareness and warning systems would enhance safety of EMS flight operations by helping to prevent controlled flight into terrain accidents that occur at night or during adverse weather conditions. (6) If used properly, night vision imaging systems could help EMS pilots identify and avoid hazards during nighttime operations.

The specific recommendations to the Federal Aviation Administration included the following: (1) Require all EMS operators to comply with 14 *Code of Federal Regulations* Part 135 operations specifications during the conduct of all flights with medical personnel on board. (A-06-12). (2) Require all EMS operators to develop and implement flight risk evaluation programs that include training all employees involved in the operation, procedures that support the systematic evaluation of flight risks, and consultation with others trained in EMS flight operations if the risks reach a predefined level. (A-06-13). (3) Require EMS operators to use formalized dispatch and flight-following procedures that include up-to-date weather information and assistance in flight risk assessment decisions. (A-06-14). (4) Require all EMS operators to install terrain awareness and warning systems on their aircraft and to provide adequate training to ensure the flight crews are capable of using the systems to safely conduct EMS operations (A-06-15)

Further information is available at http://www.ntsb.gov/publictn/ 2006/SIR0601.pdf.

Transport Safety: Challenges, Innovation, and Future Direction

Safety is an extremely important yet complex issue in the patient transport environment, given the added dimension of providing emergency acute care, usually to a recumbent patient, while transport is underway in a nonuniform automotive vehicle. This occurs in a setting of fairly limited transport safety research data and rudimentary safety guidelines. It also has been the case that the world of state-of-the-art automotive safety research and development has been slow to embrace patient transport environments, and vice versa, although those bridges are now being built and defined.

The ground transport environment, while hazardous owing to its very nature, includes predictable and preventable occupant risks, particularly to the occupants of the rear compartment, which has been clearly demonstrated in safety crash test and epidemiology studies. Much of the sparse epidemiology and engineering literature has been published recently—however, it is now clear that application of even basic automotive safety principles is well overdue in ground patient transport vehicles. Crashworthiness in ground vehicle design, both interior structure and exterior structure; use of appropriate restraints (with monitoring) and safe placement for all occupants and equipment; and ergonomically and biomechanically appropriate interior designs with protective padding and the use of safety "intelligent transportation system" technologies are key to the safety of the occupants in patient transport vehicles. Intelligent transportation system technologies include hazard warning devices, vehicle stabilizing technologies, and crash prevention devices, to mention a few. An excellent overview of ergonomics and safety is described by Ferreira and Hignett,[3] highlighting the importance of this science to the field of patient transport and the limited available research data. There have been safety benefits demonstrated in the patient transport environment with the use of monitoring and feedback devices to augment driver safety performance (black boxes with audible real-time feedback) and in studies addressing personal protective equipment, including helmets, for ground vehicle personnel.

Oversight of safety, particularly in ground transport, has some substantive challenges. Although the FAA is required to investigate aviation EMS crashes, there is not a similar mandate for ground transport, with ground transport vehicles essentially exempt from federal motor vehicle safety standards. Even capturing data on ground transport safety and adverse events can be difficult. The 2006 American Society of Safety Engineers and American National Standards Institute Fleet Vehicle Safety Standard, ASSE/ANSI Z15.1, provides a valuable model for the development and design of ground vehicle safety oversight.[4] The purpose of this standard is to provide organizations with a document for the development of policies, procedures, and management processes to control risks associated with the operation of vehicles. This standard sets forth practices for the safe operation of vehicles owned or operated by organizations, and the scope of the standard specifically includes emergency vehicles. Each of the sections covered in the Z15 standard—management, leadership and administration, operational environment, driver and vehicle considerations, and incident reporting and analysis—provide clear structure relevant to the development of a comprehensive vehicle safety program. It should prove to be a useful tool to optimize the safety of the system.

Dissemination, acceptance, and implementation of best practices can be challenging in the rapidly changing, developing, and competitive area of transport medicine. The importance of including a focus on safety, when initial training is conducted and with continuing education, cannot be overstated. It is important to ensure that the material provided is accurate and reliable, ideally from appropriate peer-reviewed medical and/or engineering publications or from experts in the field who have relevant experience and data-based information. Automotive safety is a science, and the laws of physics prevail. Web-based portals for patient transport safety information are avaiable (eg, www.objectivesafety.net) and are useful resources for the rapid dissemination of peer-reviewed and state-of-the-art safety information. User caution is advised with public access portals, to ensure that the information is reliable, accurate, and objective.

It is important to continue to advance the field of patient transport safety and to reevaluate the design of transport vehicles and practice policies with multidisciplinary teams, including EMS providers, automotive engineers, ergonomists, and public health researchers. Restraint techniques that have been demonstrated in engineering safety testing to enhance patient transport safety should be used. Injury-mitigating interventions that have been demonstrated to be safe need to be included in the specifications for ambulance vehicles. Personal protective equipment options during transport should be presented to EMS providers in training courses. Standards specific for ambulance vehicle occupant safety need to be developed and supported by ambulance safety testing designed to simulate the real-life setting and practice. Technologies that have been demonstrated to be effective, such as high-visibility clothing, head protection, and black box monitoring and feedback devices, should be encouraged for all patient transport services.

General Considerations

Cabin Space

Space is limited in transport vehicles. Although vehicles come in different sizes, shapes, and configurations, the available patient care area in the transport environment is more limited than in the hospital setting. In choosing a vehicle to support a transport program or to perform a particular transport, several space considerations should be assessed. It is important to determine the number of patients and transport team members that can be transported at one time, the medical configuration, and the amount and type of medical equipment that can be carried. Many vehicles, especially helicopters, are capable of transporting only 1 patient, whereas other vehicles may accommodate 2. The cabin space may be so cramped that the optimal number and type of personnel may be unable to accompany the patient, and assessment and procedures are limited owing to restricted access to the patient.

An important issue related to cabin space is the consideration for family members accompanying a neonate or child during transport. Parental presence often is beneficial when transporting an anxious child (see Chapter 12: Family-Centered Care). In the tight confines of some vehicles, this may not be possible or recommended. Increased size, however, will raise the cost of purchase and operation.

Medical Configuration

Most states have regulations that establish the minimum medical equipment required for ground transport vehicles. Some state regulations also address medical configuration, whereas the Federal Aviation Administration (FAA) regulates how built-in equipment must be installed and secured in aircraft. Adherence to local and federal regulations is required for ground and air ambulances. The design of the medical interior is usually left to the owners and/or operators of the vehicles and the transport personnel who use them.

The medical configuration goes beyond the location of equipment and the number and location of patient litters and seats for transport team members. Easy access to the vehicle's patient care area is critical and must be addressed. Doors must be wide enough to accommodate a transport isolette or patient litter (gurney) with all attached medical equipment. Two personnel should be able to maneuver the equipment easily into and out of the vehicle without excessive rotation or tilt from the horizontal plane. A hydraulic lift device on a ground ambulance is helpful for reducing lifting injuries. Adequate access to the patient while in the transport vehicle is essential, and easy access to the patient's airway and visualization of the patient's upper torso must be possible at all times.

The medical configuration must be designed with the safety of the patient and transport team in mind. Equipment should never be installed in proximity to a person's head. During a crash or severe turbulence, the head strike area must remain clear to avoid a head injury. This is true for air and ground ambulances. In addition, the transport team members, patient, and all equipment must be secured during any vehicle movement. Unsecured or improperly secured equipment may become projectile during a crash or a sudden extreme movement of the vehicle, possibly resulting in significant injury to the transport team members, patient, or the pilot or driver, with potentially devastating consequences. All equipment must be secured, and all responsible personnel must be properly instructed in procedures to secure all on board.

At a minimum, vehicle equipment requirements that should be evaluated include medical gas storage and supply, suction, built-in or portable medical equipment, supply cabinets, electrical outlets, cabin lighting, climate control, and communications equipment.

Oxygen and Air

All patient transport vehicles should have built-in and portable gas sources with the ability to provide oxygen in concentrations from 21% to 100%. Sufficient medical gas must be carried to meet the estimated duration of the longest anticipated trip, with a recommended reserve of approximately 2 times the trip length. Vehicles that may transport 2 patients should have separate medical gas supply systems for each patient. Portable medical gas tanks should be available to back up the built-in system and to safely accomplish the transfer between the vehicle and facility or between vehicles.

Suction

Suction capability is essential in the transport environment. Built-in suction is generally recommended, with a portable system for backup. The suction should be regulated with a maximum of -300 mm Hg achievable as needed. As with the medical gas, vehicles that will transport 2 patients should have duplicate suction capabilities.

Medical Equipment

Most medical equipment used during transport should be portable to allow the equipment to go with the patient, bedside to bedside. This also eliminates the need for the primary monitors, ventilators, infusion pumps, and other devices to be built into the vehicle. However, it may be prudent to have equipment built into the vehicle or as portable devices as backups in case of battery power loss or equipment failure. If possible, rotation of the devices between the patient bedside and the ambulance allows efficient charging and use. Regardless of the number of devices used, it is necessary to configure the vehicle to properly secure all equipment.

Supply Cabinets

Whenever possible, adequate cabinet space should be built into a vehicle for the storage of routine and necessary supplies during transport. Cabinets for these on-board supplies should be easily accessible to the transport team members from a seat-belted position. The cabinets should be closed and secured during transport. Interior vehicle configurations and certain equipment may vary; however, they are subject to safety policies mandated by local or state regulations.

Electrical Outlets, Power Inverters, and Demand Inverters

Although portable medical equipment usually is supported by battery reserve, it is often preferable to conserve battery life during transport. The transport vehicle should provide an alternating current inverter and electrical outlets in sufficient numbers for the equipment used. Many vehicles also are equipped with a "shore line," allowing portable equipment to be plugged into outlets in the vehicle so that the batteries can charge while the air or ground ambulance is stationary between transports.

Cabin Lighting

Adequate cabin lighting, allowing continuous assessment of the patient and necessary treatment en route, is essential. The lighting should be adjustable to meet the needs of each transport situation. Patient care compartments should have illumination to 400 lux, with high-intensity directional lighting of 1000 to 1500 lux available for procedures. In addition, barriers should be available to protect the driver or pilot from the bright patient cabin light that could interfere with night vision.

Climate Control

Patient transport has the potential to expose the vehicle, patient, and transport team members to significant temperature variation, which may result in clinical and operational complications. This is true for ground and air transport with regard to seasonal and geographic considerations. Flying at higher altitudes also results in significant temperature changes.

Neonatal and pediatric patients have large surface/mass ratios and, therefore, can become hypothermic or hyperthermic rapidly. For the transport team members, marked deviation from the normal comfort zone may result in impaired performance. Therefore, the environment of the patient cabin should be controlled and monitored easily.

■■■■■■■■■■■■■■■■■■■■■■■■■■■■■■■■■■

Communications Equipment

Every transport vehicle should be equipped with adequate communication equipment. At a minimum, the transport team members in the
vehicle should be able to contact the communications center or base
of operations and medical control. In addition, aircraft crew members must be able to talk to the FAA control tower personnel and
personnel in other aircraft. Cellular phones are, however, prohibited
by the FAA and the Federal Communications Commission in airborne
aircraft because of potential interference of aircraft navigational aids,
especially those on the ground that send radio signals to planes to
help pilots stay on course. An option available for aircraft is satellite
technology. Satellite phones (which are FAA approved) do not interfere
with avionic equipment and have an extensive coverage area that is
larger than most commercial cellular systems.

It is advantageous to have multiple communication modalities
in ambulances. In ground ambulances, cellular phone technology is
permitted. Ground ambulances are often equipped with 2-way radios
having very high frequency (VHF) and/or ultrahigh frequency (UHF)
capabilities. Therefore, the transport team can contact its base hospital, medical control, or the receiving hospital via the dispatcher of the
ambulance vendor. Similar methods can be used with aircraft pilots
communicating with their dispatcher or air traffic control. Helmets
outfitted with avionics can be used by helicopter transport personnel
who can communicate with the pilot who, in turn, can transfer information to an appropriate recipient. Ideally, specific medical information is relayed directly to the intended recipients and not through
a nonmedical intermediary. Communication can also be achieved
by other modes such as alpha-numeric paging, fax machines, and
computer-based programs (ie, Internet).

Speed

In a time-critical situation or when out-of-hospital time must be
kept to a minimum, the speed of the transport vehicle may be important. Ground ambulances may be limited to the legal speed limit, and
there is little difference between the different types of ambulances
with regard to capabilities for speed. The speeds for helicopters and
airplanes, however, vary by make and model. Helicopters can fly

▪▪▪▪▪▪▪▪▪▪▪▪▪▪▪▪▪▪▪▪▪▪▪▪▪▪▪▪▪▪▪▪▪▪▪

between 100 and 180 mph, and airplane speeds range between 120 and 450 mph, depending on the manufacturer and model of the aircraft.

Range

The *range* of a vehicle is defined commonly as the total distance it can travel without refueling. Ground ambulances and helicopters often have a functional range between 0 and 150 miles (although it can be farther), whereas airplanes and jets commonly used for medical transport may have a range up to 2000 miles.

Service Area

There is a direct correlation between the anticipated service area of a transport program and the range and speed for the chosen vehicle. Beyond distances of 100 miles, a ground ambulance may become inefficient, costly to operate, and time-consuming. Programs with helicopters generally operate within a radius up to 150 miles from the base of operations, although this may be expanded in some programs with refueling or long-range capabilities, whereas programs with airplanes may be regional, cross-country, or international.

Costs

Financial considerations are addressed in Chapter 15; however, a few points deserve emphasis in this chapter. The cost varies greatly based on the type of vehicle chosen and whether the vehicle is dedicated to patient transport and/or to only 1 transport team. The helicopter is the most expensive (cost per mile) vehicle for transportation from the operational standpoint and with regard to patient charges. Airplane transport also may be costly but becomes more economical for greater distances.

It also is likely that a dedicated vehicle will be more expensive than a vehicle that can be used on an as-needed basis. A dedicated vehicle may or may not be feasible for a particular transport service. If it is impractical for a neonatal-pediatric transport team to have its own dedicated vehicle, involvement of other transport teams to share the vehicle and the high costs involved in its operation and upkeep may be necessary. If a dedicated vehicle cannot be justified, it is recommended that the team select one or more vehicle operators who can provide the appropriate vehicle(s) for use within an established timeframe.

Ground Ambulances

Ground ambulances are the primary means of prehospital patient transport and the most common vehicle used for interfacility transport. As with selection of any vehicle for neonatal-pediatric transport, consideration of the potential advantages and disadvantages of the mode of transport is important.

Ground vehicles offer many advantages over air ambulances. More ground ambulances are routinely available to serve a given geographic area. Although the scope of services (critical care, advanced life support, and basic life support) and availability of ground ambulances may be limited in many rural areas, urban and suburban areas usually have large numbers of ground vehicles in their service areas. If an ambulance breaks down, other ambulances are likely to be available for backup. Parts and maintenance also are more readily available, so that a disabled ambulance can be back in service without extensive delays. Diesel fuel or gasoline also is more readily available than aviation fuel.

The ground ambulance can operate in weather conditions that often restrict safe air operations. Thus, the transport team members determining the mode of transport will have a reliable vehicle that should be readily available in a wide range of weather situations.

The transport environment of the ground ambulance may be more user-friendly and functional for the transport team than other vehicles. The cabin usually is larger than cabins in aircraft, and many vehicles are able to accommodate 2 to 4 transport team members and 1 or 2 patients, depending on the configuration of the vehicle. There also are fewer restrictions to the size, weight, and amount of equipment that can be taken on a ground transport. Unlike aircraft, especially helicopters, there usually are not significant weight issues in ground transport for the amount of equipment that can be carried or the location of the equipment during transport. Another advantage is that the transport team can easily "pull over" and interrupt a transport in an emergency situation to facilitate patient assessment and intervention. If necessary, the ground ambulance also can be easily diverted to the closest hospital if the patient's condition deteriorates or supplies have been exhausted.

Ground ambulances provide door-to-door service, with no need for a helipad, landing zone, or runway. The patient or isolette is secured on the stretcher, which is then secured in the ambulance for transport directly to the receiving facility. The patient does not need to be moved from vehicle to vehicle. Keeping transfers between vehicles to a minimum is always desirable.

Many health care professionals believe that it is easier to educate personnel for ground transport than to educate them for air-medical transport. Medical personnel can be oriented more quickly to ground safety procedures and to the location and proper use of supplies and equipment. However, medical personnel unfamiliar with the world of "mobile medicine" may still find this environment most challenging.

In times when cost, use, and reimbursement are important issues, the ground ambulance remains the most affordable vehicle to operate. The approximate cost of a medically configured ground ambulance is $150 000 to $350 000, depending on the manufacturer and model selected. The annual maintenance and fuel costs might range from $10 000 to $25 000 per vehicle. Costs vary depending on annual use of the vehicle. Compared with the costs for helicopters and airplanes, the ground ambulance costs considerably less to operate, purchase or lease, maintain, and insure.

There are 3 basic types of ground ambulances. A type I ambulance is a modular or box-type unit mounted on a conventional cab and chassis. Unless specifically modified, the crew and patient compartments are not connected by a passageway. Type II is a standard van in which the body and cab are continuous. A type III ground ambulance is a larger modular-type vehicle with a walk-through between the cab and the patient compartment.

A decision about the type of ground ambulance for a transport system should be based on numerous factors. Most important are safety, expected patient population, and the maximum number of transport team members and patients to be transported at one time. In addition, it is important to consider the amount, type, and size of medical equipment that will be taken on transport.

Although there are many advantages to the ground ambulance, there also are limitations. Ground vehicles have a high potential for a rough ride owing to the type of vehicle suspension, narrow wheel base, high center of gravity, and bad roads. The bouncing may be painful or potentially detrimental to certain patients, including those with vertebral fractures and other orthopedic injuries.

Another common problem is the possibility of motion sickness for the patient, family member, and transport team members. This usually is a result of various factors, including a confined space, poor ventilation, sideways seating, poor road conditions, a lack of visual references (the horizon), and a loss of orientation to the direction of travel. The smell of gasoline or diesel fuel may be an aggravating factor for people experiencing motion sickness. Medication to prevent or alleviate motion sickness may be beneficial. Transport team members should, however, be concerned about the potential adverse effects of any medication taken, especially drowsiness. Optimal vehicle ventilation, visual fixation on a distant object, and other nonpharmaceutical approaches have proved helpful.

Ground ambulances have significant time, distance, and access constraints. They may be unable to proceed into remote or restricted areas. Their speed is limited, and traffic congestion, construction zones, detours, inclement weather (eg, rain, floods, fog, ice, and snow), and inaccessible terrain can delay or halt ground transport. With lengthy trips or long distances and prolonged out-of-hospital times, there may be a greater risk of patient complications and fatigue of the transport team members. When the number of ground ambulances is limited, the dispatch of one unit on a distant transport may cause other areas to be underserved temporarily.

Overall, although ground ambulances have their limitations, they remain the dominant vehicle in patient transport and often the preference for critical care transport.

Helicopter Air Ambulances

Helicopters have a definite role in patient transport, but they are not the single solution to all patient transfers. Like any other vehicle, their strengths and weaknesses must be considered carefully when making a selection.

Generally speaking, when one thinks of a medical helicopter, it usually is synonymous with experienced transport team members who provide advanced medical skills using specialized medical equipment. The vehicle itself, however, provides significant advantages over other modes of patient travel.

Helicopters provide rapid transport at speeds of 120 to 180 mph, depending on the type of helicopter, weather, altitude, and weight load. Traveling via medical helicopter often equates to a transport time of one third to one fourth that required for an equivalent distance by ground transport, making the helicopter very beneficial when time is critical. The service area of helicopter programs usually is up to 150 miles from the base of operations; most helicopters are able to cover this distance in 1 to $1^{1}/_{2}$ hours.

The speed of travel is only one unique capability of the helicopter. The helicopter does not need a runway to land; it requires only a relatively small, flat area (~100×100 ft) that is clear of obstructions. The helicopter has the ability to avoid common traffic delays and ground obstacles and can fly into locations that are inaccessible to other modes of travel. This may be beneficial when roads become impassable owing to traffic, flood, snowstorm, tornado, or other disaster. Like the ground ambulance, the helicopter has the ability to go door-to-door when there are on-site helipads or landing areas at the referring and receiving facilities.

Although helicopters have distinct advantages as patient transfer vehicles, they also have inherent disadvantages. The limitations of helicopter transport may vary with the type of helicopter considered for use. In many helicopters, the patient cabin may be considerably smaller than the cabin in ground ambulances. In small and medium-sized helicopters, cramped patient compartments and weight limitations may be disadvantages for optimal patient care. In larger helicopters, access to patients may be limited after they have been loaded into the aircraft.

Weight and balance are extremely important considerations for every helicopter flight, regardless of the size of the aircraft. Every helicopter has a maximum lift capability, from which a useful payload can be calculated. The combined weight of the pilots, transport team members, patient(s), and equipment must be considered. High ambient temperatures and high humidity reduce the useful load that a helicopter can carry. Commonly in these conditions, pilots may choose to carry less fuel (and thereby decrease their range) to maintain an adequate payload for each medical mission. Larger helicopters may have fewer restrictions, but the same principles apply.

Landing zone requirements for helicopters are a disadvantage compared with ground ambulances, but they offer an advantage over the airport requirements of fixed-wing aircraft. If a helipad is not readily available, the time needed to prepare or access the landing zone may diminish the helicopter's advantage of speed.

Weather considerations can significantly limit the availability of helicopter transport. These conditions include low-lying clouds (decreased ceiling), limited visibility (eg, fog, sleet, heavy snowfall, and heavy rain), high winds, and lightning. Most helicopter programs operate under visual flight rules (VFR), but travel under instrument flight rules (IFR) is becoming more common. Additional, recurrent pilot training and specialized aviation equipment are necessary for IFR missions, which may make this option costly. However, in some areas where poor visibility and low ceilings cause a significant number of missed flights, IFR may be an important consideration. The majority of IFR flights are airport to airport, but global positioning system technology is making possible IFR medical missions direct to a medical facility helipad. IFR flights are subject to Federal Aviation Regulations (FAR). A pilot cannot initiate an instrument approach procedure to a designated landing zone unless the airport has a weather reporting facility operated by the US National Weather Service or a source approved by the US National Weather Service and the latest weather report issued by the weather reporting facility indicates that weather conditions are at or above the authorized IFR landing minimums for that airport. Interference and distraction from noise, vibration, and turbulence usually are more severe in helicopters than in other forms of transportation. Helmets or headsets should be worn by the transport team members, and a headset can be given to awake patients to facilitate communications in flight and/or protect hearing (earplugs can be used for small infants). Altitude and flight physiology can be factors affecting helicopter transport, as noted in Chapter 11.

Transport by helicopter is significantly more expensive than travel by ground. The costs related to purchasing or operating a helicopter indicate why dedicated helicopters may be cost-prohibitive to many transport programs. In addition, the recurrent controversy surrounding the use of twin- or single-engine aircraft goes beyond cost. Although twin-engine helicopters are more expensive, they have an inherently larger safety margin than their single-engine counterparts. Further discussion on this complicated issue is beyond the scope of this chapter.

The purchase price of a medically equipped single-engine helicopter (eg, Eurocopter A-Star [European Aeronautic, Defense and Space Company Germany, Spain, France, USA] or Bell 407, Textron, USA) averages approximately $2 million. A light twin-engine helicopter (eg, Eurocopter EC 135 or Twin Star 355) may cost twice as much. The new Eurocopter EC145 and Bell 430, both medium-sized, twin-engine helicopters, cost between $4 and $6 million, and a large twin-engine helicopter, such as the Eurocopter Dauphin 365N-2, the Bell 412, or the Sikorsky SR76, costs about $1 to $2 million more. Of course, these prices are only for the helicopter and do not include other aviation-related expenses. Pilot salaries range from $60 000 to $85 000 annually; a staff of 4 is required to cover 1 helicopter 24 hours, 7 days a week. If the helicopter is IFR-capable, the pilot salary budget can double because of the need for 2 pilots for IFR missions. Financial concerns include fixed and variable (hourly) costs. Fixed costs include insurance, taxes, pilot and transport team member costs, overhead, interest, hangar fees, and capital equipment. These costs are irrespective of the number of hours the helicopter has flown and vary with the type of helicopter. Variable (hourly) costs or direct operating costs vary directly with the number of hours flown. These costs include fuel and oil, scheduled maintenance labor, unscheduled maintenance labor, engine overhaul, airframe overhaul, and airframe items with a limited life span.

Looking only at the aviation-related expenses for a leased medical helicopter (eg, aircraft lease, pilots, mechanics, flight time, and fuel), the annual operating expense typically starts at more than $1 million for a single-engine helicopter and increases to almost $2 million for a large twin-engine helicopter.

Fixed-wing Air Ambulances (Airplanes)

Fixed-wing aircraft travel at greater speed, cover a greater service area, and offer several other advantages over the ground ambulance and the helicopter. The patient cabin often is larger than the cabin in helicopters. Many airplanes can transport 2 patients and allow room for 2 or more transport team members or additional family members, although the transport of 2 critically ill patients may result in space limitations. Each patient may require individual transport teams, monitors, and other medical equipment. Weight restriction, weather, noise, vibration, and turbulence are less of a factor with fixed-wing travel than with helicopter travel. Airplanes have the ability to fly above or around inclement weather conditions on long-distance transports. The cost per mile for long-distance, fixed-wing transport is often less than for helicopter transport. As a general rule, for transports more than approximately 150 miles, programs should consider the use of an airplane or jet rather than a helicopter.

Certain makes and models of airplanes have the capability to provide a pressurized cabin, which helps combat the effects of altitude on the physiologic functions and provides for a safer and more comfortable transport environment. Smaller fixed-wing aircraft typically are not pressurized and are limited to flying at lower altitudes. Pressurized aircraft, flying at actual altitudes of 30 000 to 40 000 feet usually can simulate a cabin altitude of 7000 to 8000 feet (or even lower, although this feature is not often used because of effects on efficiency and cost). When transporting patients with significant respiratory compromise and for whom altitude-related hypoxia is a concern, it may be beneficial to fly at lower altitudes, allowing cabin pressure to approach that of sea level.

The greatest limitation to the use of fixed-wing aircraft is the necessity to land at an airport, which may be distant from the referral and/or receiving facilities. The length of the runway needed depends on the type of aircraft used. Generally speaking, jets require longer runways than propeller airplanes. Also, with fixed-wing transports, patients require multiple transfers—from facility to ambulance and ambulance to airplane. Stresses of flight, discussed in Chapter 11, are of significant relevance when flying at altitudes above 8000 feet and are especially important with pressurized aircraft that may fly at an altitude of 30 000 to 40 000 feet. Although a pressurized cabin is extremely beneficial, a loss of cabin pressure at altitude can be very hazardous.

Although most ground ambulances and medical helicopters are dedicated and properly designed for patient transport, the same is not always true with airplanes. There is a potential that fixed-wing "ambulance" providers (or any type of ambulance provider) promote their patient transport capabilities in what could be considered a less than ideal medical transport environment. The patient litter, oxygen tanks, and medical equipment may not be secured properly. The medical gas and electrical systems may be inadequate for long transports. Before using any fixed-wing provider, carefully inspect the airplane and the medical configuration to be certain that the emphasis is on safety and appropriate medical capabilities and that appropriate FAA certifications have been received. Professional air-medical organizations such as the Association of Air Medical Services and the Commission on Accreditation of Medical Transport Systems also can provide service information.

The cost of operating fixed-wing aircraft can be substantially higher than that of operating a ground ambulance but often less than a helicopter program. Fixed-wing vendors may use their aircraft for nonmedical transports. This business venture defrays some operational costs (see "Vehicle Operations") of the plane. On the other hand, aircraft availability may be limited when the plane is on a business flight and an urgent fixed-wing transport is pending. The transition of the interior of a plane to a medically configured format may also delay transport; thus, delivery of urgent medical care is compromised.

The purchase price of new fixed-wing aircraft may be prohibitive for a particular transport team or hospital system budget. Used fixed-wing aircraft prices are more reasonable. These prices can range from $3 million for a Beechcraft King Air turboprop (Raytheon, Kansas) to $10 million for a Learjet (Bombardier Aerospace USA, Canada, Ireland). General estimates of annual aviation expenses include pilot and copilot salaries (approximately $60 000 each), hangar fees ($24 000), insurance ($28 000), training ($20 000), and computerized maintenance ($10 000). Total direct operation costs can vary depending on the number of hours of flight annually. For example, a Lear 36 jet with 200 annual hours of flight time will have direct operating costs at approximately $200 000; at 400 annual hours, approximately $400 000; and at 600 annual hours, approximately $600 000. However, owing to these operational constraints, the airplane is not practical for transports of less than 150 miles, unless traveling to an island or similarly isolated area.

Vehicle Operations

Various options are available for neonatal-pediatric transport teams to obtain the vehicle of choice. A hospital can decide to operate the entire medical ambulance program independently. The vehicle(s) can be purchased or leased, and the personnel (pilots, drivers, and mechanics) can work directly for the base facility (usually a hospital). The base facility is then financially and legally responsible for compliance with all state and federal regulations. This option places all the financial and legal risk on the base facility, and expenses and liabilities are less predictable than with other options. If the transport program is well managed, the base facility can save a significant amount of money, but if poorly managed, the endeavor can be very costly.

Another option is for the base facility to enter into a contractual agreement for the entire air or ground operation. The contract operator usually will assist the base facility with vehicle selection and medical configuration. The entire operation (vehicle maintenance, backup vehicle, nonmedical personnel, and regulatory compliance) becomes the responsibility of the operator, and all of the base facility's costs are determined by the contract. This option is often the most expensive, but the financial and legal risk belongs to the operator. Under this option, annual expenses are much more predictable.

The base facility may select another option—buy or lease the vehicle(s) and have an operator manage the entire operation. The base facility gains the benefit of owning or leasing and retains a purchased vehicle if operators are changed.

A fourth option is for a transport team to enter into agreements with other air and/or ground ambulance services that then transport the neonatal-pediatric transport team when a transport request is received. Depending on the volume of transports, this option may be the most cost-effective and is the practice of many helicopter and airplane programs that make their aircraft available to several transport teams.

Any contract between a base facility and an operator or an agreement between a transport team and an outside transport service should address several important issues. A commitment to safety must be evident, and the safety record should be reviewed carefully. The qualifications, experience, training, and licensure of the pilots, drivers, and mechanics must be known. Vehicle specifications and capabilities should be discussed, and there should be a plan for backup when maintenance is required on the vehicle or when personnel are on vacation. Vehicles should be dedicated and configured specifically for the needs of the transport team. Availability (ie, 24 hours per day, 7 days a week, except when the vehicle is already on a transport) and response times (ie, within 30 minutes of the contact call) should be defined. Provision of liability limits and insurance verification data for all transport vehicles and vehicle operators should be mandated.

Summary

Transport of neonatal and pediatric patients requires appropriate planning, personnel, medical equipment, and vehicle selection. Many types of helicopters, airplanes, and ground vehicles are available for transporting patients, and no single vehicle will be ideal for all patient transports or all transport teams. Rather, it is essential to determine the appropriate mode of transport (air or ground vehicle) based on the mission profile of the neonatal-pediatric transport team and the unique needs of each patient.

References

1. King BR, Woodward GA. Pediatric critical care transport—the safety of the journey: a five-year review of vehicular collisions involving pediatric and neonatal transport teams. *Prehosp Emerg Care.* 2002;6:449–454
2. National Transport Saftey Board. Special Investigation Report on Emergency Medical Services Operations. Washington, DC. Available at: http://www.ntsb.gov/publictn/2006/sir0601.htm. Accessed March 15, 2006
3. Ferreira J, Hignett S. Reviewing ambulance design for clinical efficiency and paramedic safety: *Appl Ergon.* 2005;36:97–105
4. ANSI/ASSE Z15.1-2006 American National Standards Institute. Safe Practices for Motor Vehicle Operations, February 2006. Available at: http://www.asse.org/press523.htm, Accessed March 15, 2006

Selected Readings

Becker LR, Zaloshnja E, Levick N, Li G, Miller TR. Relative risk of injury and death in ambulances and other emergency vehicles, *Accid Anal Prev.* 2003;35:941–948

Bell Helicopter Web site. Available at: http://www.bellhelicopter.ch. Accessed January 13, 2006

Best GH, Zivkovic G, Ryan GA. Development of an effective ambulance patient restraint, *Soc Automot Eng Australas.* 1993;53:17–20

Bottner J, Schiera T. Aircraft capabilities for air medical transport. In: Rodenberg H, Blumen IJ, eds. *Air Medical Physicians' Handbook.* Salt Lake City, UT: Air Medical Physician Association; 1999:IV-2:1–10

Brink LW, Newman B, Wynn J. Air transport. *Pediatr Clin North Am.* 1993;40:439–456

Brown J, Tomkins K, Chaney E, Donovan R. Family member ride-alongs during interfacility transport. *Air Med J.* 1998;17:169–173

De Graeve K, Deroo KF, Calle PA, Vanhaute OA, Buylaert WA. How to modify the risk-taking behaviour of emergency medical services drivers. *Eur J Emerg Med.* 2003;10:111–116

European Committee for Standardization. Medical vehicles and their equipment. Road Ambulances. BS EN 1789:2002

Federal Aviation Regulations. Part 91, 135, 121. Available at: http://www.gpo.gov/nara/cfr/waisidx_01/14cfr91_01.html; http://www.gpo.gov/nara/cfr/waisidx_01/14cfr135_01.html; http://www.access.gpo.gov/nara/cfr/waisidx_02/14cfr121_02.html. Accessed August 18, 2006

General Services Administration Federal Supply Service. Federal Specification for Ambulances KKK-A-1822E, 2002. Available at: http://fss.gsa.gov/vehicles/buying. Accessed August 18, 2006

Heick R, Peek-Asa C, Zwerling C. Occupational injury in EMS: does risk outweigh reward. Paper presented at: 133rd Annual Meeting of the American Public Health Association; December 10–14, 2005; Philadelphia, PA.

Joint Standards Australia/Standards New Zealand Committee ME/48 Restraint Systems in Vehicles, Standards for Ambulance Restraint Systems, AS/NZS 4535:1999

SELECTED READINGS

Kahn CA, Pirrallo RG, Kuhn EM. Characteristics of fatal ambulance crashes in the United States: an 11-year retrospective analysis, *Prehosp Emerg Care*. 2001;5:261–269

Levick NR, Better AI, Grabowski JG, Li G, Smith G. Injury hazards in pediatric ambulance transport [abstract]. *Pediatr Res* 2000;47(suppl):113A. Abstract 662

Levick NR, Donnelly BR, Blatt A, Gillespie G, Schultze M. Ambulance crashworthiness and occupant dynamics in vehicle-to-vehicle crash tests: preliminary report, Enhanced Safety of Vehicles, Technical paper series; paper 452, May 2001. Available at: http://www-nrd.nhtsa.dot.gov/pdf/nrd-01/esv/esv17/proceed/00012.pdf. Accessed April 28, 2006

Levick NR, Garigan M. Head protection: are there solutions for emergency medical service providers. Paper presented at: 133rd Annual Meeting of the American Public Health Association; December 10–14, 2005; Philadelphia, PA

Levick NR, Yannaccone JR, Gupta P, Gillespie GP. Biomechanics of the patient compartment of ambulance vehicles under crash conditions: testing countermeasures to mitigate injury. Technical paper 2001-01-1173, March 2001. Presented at: Society of Automotive Engineering 2001 World Congress; March 2001; Detroit, MI

Levick NR, Li G, Yannaccone J. Development of a dynamic testing procedure to assess crashworthiness of the rear patient compartment of ambulance vehicles, Enhanced Safety of Vehicles, Technical paper series; Paper 454. Presented at: 17th International Technical Conference on the Enhanced Safety of Vehicles; June 4–7, 2001; Amsterdam, The Netherlands: Available at: http://www-nrd.nhtsa. dot.gov/pdf/nrd-01/esv/esv17/proceed/00053.pdf. Accessed April 28, 2006

Levick NR, Swanson J. An optimal solution for enhancing ambulance safety: implementing a driver performance feedback and monitoring device in ground emergency medical service vehicles. *Annu Assoc Adv Automo Med*. 2005;48:Proc 35–50

Levick NR, Winston F, Aitken S, Freemantle R, Marshall F, Smith G. Development and application of a dynamic testing procedure for ambulance paediatric restraint systems. *Soc Automot Eng Australas*. 1998;58:14–15

MacDonald MG, Miller MK, eds. *Emergency Transport of the Perinatal Patient*. Boston, MA: Little Brown & Co; 1989:appendices 8 and 9

Maguire BJ, Hunting KL, Smith GS, Levick NR. Occupational fatalities in emergency medical services: a hidden crisis. *Ann Emerg Med*. 2002;40:625–632

McCloskey KA, Orr RA. *Pediatric Transport Medicine*. St Louis, MO: Mosby; 1995

McGinnis K, Judge T: Air Medicine: Accessing the Future of Health Care. Alexandria, VA: Foundation for Air-Medical Research and Education, 2006

The Official Helicopter Blue Book, The Official Helicopter Specification Book and Helicopter Equipment Lists and Prices (HELP). Vol 25. 2nd Issue, Lincolnshire, IL: Helivalue$, Inc; 2003

Schneider C, Gomez M, Lee R. Evaluation of ground ambulance, rotor-wing, and fixed-wing aircraft services. *Crit Care Clin*. 1992;8:533–564

Questions

1. Which of the following is *false* about transport vehicle selection?
   a. After selecting the mode of transport, patient and transport team safety should be considered.
   b. Equipment should never be installed in proximity to a person's head.
   c. Cabinets containing on-board supplies should always be easily accessible to transport team members from a seat-belted position.
   d. When selecting a transport vehicle vendor, only air or ground transport services with a demonstrated commitment to safety should be considered.

2. When selecting a mode of transport, which of the following is *false* regarding a helicopter ambulance?
   a. Helicopters can provide rapid transports at speeds of 120 to 180 mph.
   b. The service area of helicopter programs is typically more than 250 miles from the base of operations.
   c. Weather can significantly limit the availability of helicopter transport.
   d. Similar to ground ambulances, the helicopter ambulance has the ability for door-to-door transport.

3. Which of the following is *false* regarding fixed-wing transports?
   a. The cabin of a fixed-wing ambulance cannot be simulated to a lower pressure altitude when flying at 30 000 to 40 000 feet.
   b. Fixed-wing transport program operational costs are usually less than those of a helicopter program.
   c. The airplane is not usually practical for transports of less than 150 miles.
   d. Weight restrictions, weather, noise, and vibration are less a factor with fixed-wing travel than with helicopter travel.

Answers

1. a. Attention to patient and transport team safety should be done *before* the mode of transport is selected. Weather and traffic conditions have a vital role in determining the mode of transport. A transport team member's head strike area must remain clear to avoid head injury in cases of an accident or severe turbulence; therefore, equipment should never be secured near a person's head. For obvious safety reasons, transport team members should always be restrained properly during transport. Therefore, cabinets should be easily accessible from a seat-belted position.

2. b. Depending on the type, helicopters can fly at speeds up to 180 mph. Many other factors such as weather, altitude, and weight load can affect the top speed of a helicopter. The service area of a helicopter ambulance is typically ≤150 miles (although it can be more in some cases) from the base of operations, and most helicopters can cover this distance in 1 to 1½ hours.

Answers, continued

Weather considerations such as low-lying clouds, lightning, high winds, and limited visibility due to fog, sleet, heavy rain, and snow limit helicopter transport. If on-site helipads or landing areas are present at the referring and receiving facilities, door-to-door transports are possible with helicopter transports.

3. a. Many models of airplanes have the capability to provide a pressurized cabin. At 30 000 to 40 000 feet altitude, pressurized aircraft can simulate a cabin altitude of 7000 to 8000 feet. Pressurizing down to sea level, however, requires a great amount of energy from the aircraft. Therefore, physiologic gas laws need to be considered when treating patients before , during, and after transport. Flying at lower altitudes is required for smaller, unpressurized, fixed-wing aircraft.

Transport Physiology and Stresses of Transport

Outline

- The atmosphere
- Physical gas laws
  a. Boyle's law
  b. Dalton's law
  c. Henry's law
- Cabin altitude
- Stresses of flight
  a. Barometric pressure
  b. Hypoxia
  c. Noise
  d. Vibration
  e. Thermal considerations
  f. Humidity and dehydration
  g. Gravitational forces
  h. Fluid dynamics
  i. Fatigue
- Self-imposed stress

Perhaps nothing is more challenging than trying to provide optimal critical care in the poorly controlled confines of a mobile environment during air and ground medical transport. This situation poses many unique challenges and demands on neonatal-pediatric transport teams, especially with regard to altitude and flight physiology. However, this chapter addresses more than just *altitude* and *flight* physiology. It also addresses the stresses of transport so that team members can consider their effects during patient assessment and treatment and on themselves.

Altitude physiology and the stresses of flight may have their greatest impact during fixed-wing transport; however, helicopter transport is not immune to these stresses. An understanding and knowledge of many of the same factors is also beneficial for transport teams who use ground ambulances.

Despite these generalities, an in-depth understanding of the unique features of altitude physiology is essential to allow the transport team to provide optimal patient care in the aviation environment, especially when transporting a child or infant whose condition is already compromised. The patient, the flight crew, the transport team members, and some medical equipment may be affected by the changes in the partial pressures of gases at altitudes above sea level.

It is necessary to have the background knowledge pertaining to the atmosphere, physical gas laws, and cabin altitude. A general understanding of these topics is needed to know how the human body responds to atmospheric changes and the various stresses of flight.

The Atmosphere

The atmosphere is composed of a variety of gases. To an altitude of approximately 70 000 ft, these gases exist in a uniform percentage. Nitrogen constitutes the largest percentage (78.08%), followed by oxygen (20.95%). Argon, carbon dioxide, hydrogen, neon, and helium, all in very small percentages, represent the remaining gases in the atmosphere.

The atmosphere can be characterized by the *physiologic zones* that predict the effects of altitude on the human body. Many of these predictable effects are based on atmospheric properties that can be observed at any given altitude. Atmospheric pressure, or barometric pressure, is the force or weight exerted by the atmosphere at any given point. Temperature and volume changes will also be observed at the varying altitudes. Table 11-1 summarizes altitude-related properties.

There are 4 physiologic zones that compose the earth's atmosphere. These zones are characterized by the pressure changes that take place within the altitude boundaries and their physiologic effects on the human body.

The *physiologic zone,* or the *efficient zone,* extends from sea level to approximately 12 000 ft. Within this zone, the barometric pressure decreases from 760 to 483 mm Hg. This is the most acceptable zone for normal physiologic functioning unless a person acclimatizes to a higher altitude or supplemental oxygen is used. With prolonged exposure, only minor problems may occur, especially if the person continues to ascend, exerts himself or herself, or stays too long at the higher altitude.

A dramatic drop in barometric pressure and temperature is seen in the *physiologic deficient zone.* From 12 000 to 50 000 ft, the barometric pressure drops from 483 to 87 mm Hg. Normal physiologic function is seriously impaired at the upper limits of this zone if there is no appropriate intervention. Most commercial aviation occurs in this zone, whereas the majority of private aviation occurs in the physiologic zone.

The *partial space equivalent zone* and the *total space equivalent zone* represent the final 2 physiologic zones of the atmosphere. The partial space equivalent zone extends from 50 000 ft to 120 miles, where a pressurized environment is mandatory to compensate for the barometric changes that can affect the body. Beyond 120 miles above sea level is the total space equivalent zone, where weightlessness occurs in "true space."

Physical Gas Laws

Boyle's Law

Boyle's law relates to the expansion of gases in the earth's atmosphere. It states that the volume of a given gas varies inversely as its pressure. The formula for Boyle's law is as follows:

$$P_1V_1 = P_2V_2$$

P_1 equals the initial barometric pressure; V_1, the initial volume of gas; P_2, the final barometric pressure; and V_2, the final volume of the enclosed gas.

As an aircraft ascends, the ambient (surrounding) barometric pressure decreases and, according to Boyle's law, the volume of gas within an enclosed space expands (Table 11-1). As the aircraft descends, the reverse is true.

■ ■

Table 11-1
Altitude-related Effects in the Earth's Atmosphere

Altitude (ft)	Barometric Pressure, torr (mm Hg)	Temperature °C	°F	Gas Expansion Ratio
Sea Level (0)	760	15.0	59.0	1.0
2000	706	11.0	51.8	1.1
5000	632	5.1	41.2	1.2
8000	565	-0.9	30.4	1.3
10 000	523	-4.8	3.4	1.5
15 000	429	-14.7	5.5	1.8
18 000	380	-20.7	-5.2	2.0
20 000	349	-24.6	-12.3	2.4
25 000	282	-34.5	-30.1	2.7
30 000	228	-44.4	-47.9	3.3
40 000	141	-56.5	-69.7	5.4
50 000	87	-56.5	-69.7	8.7

By using Boyle's law, gas expansion ratios can be calculated for different altitudes. At the altitudes that helicopters usually fly (up to a few thousand feet above ground level, except in mountainous regions), the amount of gas expansion will be relatively small (10% to 15%). At 8000 ft above sea level, the gas expansion will be 30%. This altitude is an important consideration for unpressurized aircraft and also represents the effective cabin altitude for many pressurized aircraft flying at 35 000 to 40 000 ft.

Boyle's law can affect any medical equipment or body cavity that has an enclosed air space. Intravenous flow rates, the pressure in medical antishock trousers (or MAST), and endotracheal tube cuff expansion can be altered. Body cavities that can be affected include the stomach, intestines, middle ear, sinuses, and a closed pneumothorax. Other potential areas of involvement include the intracranial space and brain (pneumocephalus), bowel wall (pneumatosis), the abdominal cavity (pneumoperitoneum), and skin (subcutaneous emphysema). The respiratory rate and volume of gas exchange may be affected.

Dalton's Law

Dalton's law of partial pressure describes the pressure exerted by gases at various altitudes, stating that the total pressure of a gas mixture is the sum of the individual or partial pressures of all the gases in the mixture. Mathematically, Dalton's law can be represented by the following equation:

$$P_t = P_1 + P_2 + P_3 \ldots P_n$$

P_t is equal to the total pressure, and P_1, P_2, and so forth represent the partial pressure of each gas in the mixture containing "n" gases (Table 11-2).

Table 11-2
Partial Pressure of Gases in the Earth's Atmosphere

Gas	Percentage Within the Atmosphere	Partial Pressure (torr)			
		at Sea Level	at 2000 ft	at 5000 ft	at 10 000 ft
Nitrogen	78	593	551	493	408
Oxygen	21	160 (159)	148	133	110
Other gases	1	7	7	6	5
Total	100	760	706	632	523

Within a mixture of gases, each gas exerts a pressure equal to its own percentage of the total gaseous concentration. At sea level, where the total barometric pressure is 760 mm Hg, the percentage of oxygen is equal to 20.95%. The partial pressure of oxygen (Po_2) at sea level can be calculated as follows:

$$Po_2 = 20.95\% \times 760 \text{ mm Hg} = 159.22 \text{ mm Hg}$$

From sea level to 70 000 ft, the percentage of each gas within the atmosphere remains constant. As the altitude increases and the total barometric pressure decreases, the partial pressure of the gaseous components decreases, exerting less pressure. At an altitude of 10 000 ft, the atmospheric pressure is 523 mm Hg. The percentage of oxygen remains 20.95%, but the Po_2 will decrease as follows (Table 11-3):

$$Po_2 = 20.95\% \times 523 \text{ mm Hg} = 109.57 \text{ mm Hg}$$

████████████████████████████████████

Table 11-3
Effects of Altitude on Oxygenation

Altitude (ft)	Barometric Pressure (mm Hg)	Po_2 (mm Hg)	Pao_2 (mm Hg)	Pao_2 (mm Hg)	$Paco_2$ (mm Hg)	Oxygen Saturation (%)
Sea Level (0)	760	159.2	103.0	95	40.0	98
2000	706	148.0	93.8	86	39.0	97
5000	632	132.5	81.0	73	37.4	95
8000	565	118.4	68.9	61	36.0	93
10000	523	109.6	61.2	53	35.0	87
15000	429	89.9	45.0	37	32.0	84
18000	380	79.6	37.8	30	30.4	72
20000	349	73.1	34.3	26	29.4	66
22000	321	67.2	32.8	25	28.4	60

*Po_2 indicates partial pressure of ambient oxygen; Pao_2, partial pressure of alveolar oxygen; Pao_2, partial pressure of arterial oxygen; and $Paco_2$, partial pressure of arterial carbon dioxide.

Pao_2 varies with underlying pathophysiology and, therefore, may require periodic or continuous monitoring. Almost all neonates have pulmonary systemic shunts of varying magnitudes. Therefore, the data in the column labeled Pao_2 should be considered an approximation only. The data are presented for illustrative purposes. The actual equation is as follows:

$$A-a\,(O_2) = (FIO_2\%/100) \times (P_{atm} - 47 \text{ mm Hg}) - (Paco_2/0.8) - (Pao_2)$$

$A-a\,(O_2)$ is the difference between the alveolar (A) and arterial (a) oxygen; FIO_2, the fraction of inspired oxygen; P_{atm}, the barometric pressure in mm Hg; and 47 mm Hg at 37°C represents the partial pressure of water at body temperature. Because carbon dioxide displaces oxygen in the alveoli, the estimated alveolar carbon dioxide must be subtracted. The alveolar carbon dioxide is estimated by dividing the arterial $Paco_2$ by a "respiratory quotient fudge factor" of 0.8. Some authorities prefer to multiply the $Paco_2$ by a respiratory quotient fudge factor of 1.25. The net result is the same.

Henry's Law

Henry's law is another important gas law affecting air-medical transport and explains the solubility of gases within a liquid. According to this law, the amount of gas dissolved in a liquid is determined by the partial pressure and the solubility of the gas. With a significant change in barometric pressure, nitrogen gas bubbles can form in the blood. The *bends,* a decompression sickness, is a clinical condition exemplifying this law.

There is no specific altitude threshold to predict a clinical response to Henry's law and the probability of developing a decompression sickness. However, there is evidence of altitude decompression sickness occurring in healthy people at altitudes below 18 000 ft who have recently been scuba (self-contained underwater breathing apparatus) diving. Exposure to altitudes between 18 000 and 25 000 ft has shown a low occurrence of a decompression sickness, and most cases occur among people exposed to altitudes of 25 000 ft or higher. The higher the altitude of exposure, the greater the risk of developing a decompression sickness.

Cabin Altitude

The first protection against the influences of a changing altitude is the creation of an artificial atmosphere or *cabin altitude.* In a pressurized fixed-wing aircraft, compressed air is pumped into the cabin to maintain a cabin altitude significantly less than the flight altitude. The cabin altitude that can be maintained in various ambient altitudes varies with aircraft. Helicopters are unpressurized and, therefore, cannot create an artificial atmosphere. Therefore, these vehicles offer nothing to prevent the effects of a changing altitude because the cabin altitude will be the same as the actual flight altitude.

Although airplane travel is clearly affected by flight physiology and the stresses of flight, helicopter transport is also susceptible. It is often thought that flying at altitudes only above 8000 ft affects the patient, transport team, or flight crew, but this is not always the case. According to Boyle's law, team or flight crew members or patients flying with sinus problems, ear problems, or upper respiratory infections may feel the effects of barometric pressure changes with as little as a 1000- to 2000-ft change in altitude.

Smaller unpressurized airplanes offer no benefit over helicopters in combating the effects of the gas laws and, therefore, are generally limited to altitudes less than 10 000 ft. Pressurized fixed-wing aircraft, however, can fly higher while counteracting the negative effects of

■■■■■■■■■■■■■■■■■■■■■■■■■■■■■■■■■■■■■

altitude. At flight altitudes of 30 000 to 40 000 ft, pressurized aircraft can often create an internal cabin altitude of 7000 to 8000 feet. This corresponds to an interior cabin pressure equal to approximately 3/4 atm (565 mm Hg), which also prevents pressurized airplanes from expanding and contracting too much as they change altitude. By flying at lower altitudes, high-differential cabin-pressure aircraft have the ability to create a cabin pressure that simulates ground altitude pressures. This may be beneficial when transporting a patient with a decompression illness.

Up to 25% of people who rapidly ascend to an altitude of 8000 ft (cabin altitude of 8000 ft or actual attitude of 8000 ft in an unpressurized aircraft) will become symptomatic. Nearly everyone abruptly exposed to an altitude of 12 000 ft will have symptoms commonly referred to as *altitude sickness.*

A malfunction of the pressurization equipment or aircraft structural damage from a cracked window or foreign object may result in a loss of cabin pressure or *decompression.* When this happens, the pilot will attempt to rapidly descend to a lower altitude. The transport team must be prepared to deal with the effects of decompression, which will depend on several factors: total cabin volume, size of the structural defect in the hull, flight altitude, and the pressure differential between the flight altitude and the cabin altitude.

During a *rapid decompression,* objects move toward the structural defect and will be affected by the gravitational forces of a rapid descent. At the same time, there is a sudden drop in the cabin temperature. This causes the aircraft to fill with fog, owing to moisture condensation in the expanding cabin atmosphere. This fog may be mistaken for smoke in the cabin. Hearing becomes impaired secondary to noise and to effects of the rapid decompression on the middle ear. The most important clinical consequence of rapid decompression at high altitude is a rapid drop in the cabin PO_2, which can quickly lead to hypoxia in the flight crew, transport team, and patient. Supplemental oxygen for the pilot, transport team members, and patient is essential, and the window of time for effectiveness of this intervention can be very short before unconsciousness ensues. A loss of cabin pressurization may result in a variety of decompression sicknesses as gas dissolved in the blood is released. Another clinically significant event is the rapid expansion of air within an enclosed space. If decompression occurs, all catheters, chest tubes, and nasogastric tubes should be unclamped (Table 11-4).

Table 11-4
Prevention of Complications During Air Transport of Neonatal and Pediatric Patients *

Gas Expansion

1. Insert orogastric or nasogastric tubes open to air in every infant and child who may experience gastrointestinal symptoms or may be at risk for vomiting.
2. If a cuffed endotracheal or tracheostomy tube is in place, carefully monitor cuff pressure or consider replacement of air with water to prevent expansion of the cuff with altitude changes.
3. Ensure that chest tubes, endotracheal tubes, and other artificial vents are patent.
4. Suction airway well before and during transport, as needed.
5. Reevaluate frequently for presence of extrapulmonary air.
   a. Carry a portable transillumination device (for neonates).
   b. Have a needle thoracentesis set available.
6. Request that, if possible, the pilot fly at a lower altitude or increase the cabin pressurization (to simulate a lower altitude) when transporting a patient with trapped gas (eg, pneumothorax, pneumoperitoneum, or bowel obstruction).

Decreased PO_2

1. Before leaving the referring hospital:
   a. Ensure that the child is optimally oxygenated.
   b. Correlate arterial PO_2 and CO_2 measurements with cutaneous pulse oximetry and $ETCO_2$ (in-line or nasal) and/or blood gas values by using point-of-care testing.
   c. Check placement and stabilization of the endotracheal tube.
2. En route:
   a. Use a cutaneous oxygen saturation monitor for all patients requiring oxygen or assisted ventilation (along with frequent careful assessment of the color of skin and mucous membranes).
   a. Increase FIO_2 as needed to maintain adequate oxygenation saturation.
   a. The oxygen adjustment equation can be used to calculate the FIO_2 required at any cabin altitude or destination altitude as follows:

$$\frac{(FIO_2 \cdot BP_1)}{BP_2} = FIO_2 \text{ Required}$$

   where FIO_2 is the fraction of inspired oxygen the patient is receiving; BP_1, the current barometric pressure; and BP_2, the destination or altitude barometric pressure.

---

*$ETCO_2$ indicates end-tidal carbon dioxide.

██████████████████████████████████████

Stresses of Flight

Two types of stresses are associated with the transport environment and air-medical transport: the stresses of flight and self-imposed stresses. These stresses are *cumulative* and may lead to significant emotional and physiologic compromise. Many of these stresses also affect ground transport. Therefore, even neonatal-pediatric transport teams that never participate in helicopter or fixed-wing transport will benefit from a basic knowledge of the stresses.

Several authors and organizations have identified various stresses of flight: barometric pressure, hypoxia, noise, vibration, thermal changes, decreased humidity, dehydration, gravitational forces, fluid leakage out of intravascular spaces (third spacing), fatigue, spatial disorientation, flicker vertigo, and exposure to fuel vapors and exhaust. Patients, transport team members, and pilots may all be affected by the stresses of flight. Vibration, noise, and turbulence are generally more severe in helicopters than in other forms of transportation. The stresses that may have the greatest effect on ground transport are noise, vibration, temperature, gravitational forces, and fatigue.

Any significant altitude change exposes the patient, pilots, and transport team members to additional physiologic stresses. There are 3 major factors that influence the incidence, onset, and severity of complications that can be experienced during air transport: rate of ascent (or descent), the altitude achieved, and the length of stay at that altitude. Varying severity of complications occurs when any of these factors or a combination of them exceeds a person's ability to adapt to the new environment. Young children, because of their physiologic differences from adults, are at greater risk for the development of many altitude-related illnesses. Although the severity of symptoms decreases with increasing age, it is essential to watch for the onset of symptoms during all neonatal-pediatric transports.

Barometric Pressure

The effects of changing altitude during air-medical transport may be related directly to the physical gas laws. The effect of barometric pressure changes can affect the transport team, patient, and equipment in many ways.

There are 3 mechanisms by which barometric pressure affects the body. The first follows Boyle's law, dealing with gas within an enclosed space and changes in ambient pressure. If air is unable to escape, positive pressure develops that may result in a rupture or the compression of adjacent structures. The second mechanism follows Henry's law, when gas dissolved in blood is released. The third mechanism applies to barometric changes in an underwater environment (ie, scuba diving) and addresses abnormal tissue concentrations of various gases.

Disturbances of the middle ear (barotitis media) may result from barometric pressure changes. As altitude increases, gas expands in the middle ear behind the tympanic membrane. As altitude decreases, the gas within the middle ear contracts, pulling the tympanic membrane inward. Gas usually will pass through the eustachian tube (actively or passively), allowing for equalization of pressures. However, if a person has allergies, an upper respiratory infection, or sinus problems or is a small infant, the eustachian tube may be obstructed and equalization may be restricted. Encouraging a small infant to suck a pacifier or older children to swallow during *descent* helps to maintain patency of the small eustachian tubes and to prevent pain. If the patient is paralyzed, equalization of pressure requires active assistance during descent.

Normally, air can pass easily in and out through the air-filled sinus cavities. If a person has an upper respiratory or sinus infection, swelling of the mucous membrane lining may result. This trapped air expands as altitude increases, causing barosinusitis. Symptoms include severe sinus pain and epistaxis.

Special attention should be given to patients with suspected or documented pneumothorax. It is optimal that the pneumothorax be diagnosed and treated before transport because a pneumothorax is prone to further expansion at higher altitudes.

The stomach and the intestines normally contain a variable amount of gas (up to 1000 mL in an adult) at a pressure approximately equivalent to the surrounding atmospheric pressure. The stomach and large intestine contain considerably more gas than does the small intestine. On ascent, symptoms of bloating may develop. At 18 000 ft, the volume of gas in an enclosed expandable space will double, but symptoms usually do not become severe until an altitude of 25 000 ft, when the volume of gas triples. Crying children and infants who are feeding tend to swallow a substantial amount of air. In addition, eating large meals, ingesting a large amount of a carbonated beverage, chewing gum (and swallowing air), and preexisting gastrointestinal problems may also increase the volume of gas in the intestines. As gas expansion occurs, a person may experience discomfort, nausea, vomiting, shortness of breath, and hyperventilation.

Changes in atmospheric pressure may affect any medical equipment with air enclosed in a given space. Endotracheal tube balloons should be evaluated to prevent rupture or excessive pressure on the tracheal wall during ascent and for an inadequate air seal on descent. Replacing the air in the endotracheal tube cuff with water eliminates this potential complication during air-medical transport. The air in intravenous containers expands on ascent, resulting in an increased flow of the intravenous fluid. On descent, the flow of the intravenous fluid slows when the air volume is decreased. Pneumatic splints and MAST also may be affected by pressure changes, resulting in hypotension on descent or distal circulation compromise during ascent. Ventilators not tested for use in the flight environment can also malfunction because of pressure changes.

Henry's law predicts that gases will move from an area of higher concentration to that of lower concentration. Clinically, a drop in barometric pressure may result in the release of gas dissolved in blood. When a scuba diver ascends too quickly, nitrogen gas bubbles can form in the blood. Special precautions should be taken for decompression victims who must be transported by helicopter. In some cases, even a minimal altitude increase can cause significant gas bubble formation. It is advised that patients with a decompression illness be transported at an altitude of not greater than 1000 ft above the diver's ascent site in nonpressurized aircraft.

Hypoxia

During air-medical transport, the most threatening aspect of hypoxia is its insidious onset. The transport team may be involved in patient care activities and may not notice the early onset of signs or symptoms in the patient or in themselves. No one is exempt from the effects of hypoxia, although the onset and severity of symptoms may vary among individuals. Some people may tolerate a few thousand feet more altitude than others. However, all patients, pilots, and transport team members will begin to experience symptoms of hypoxia if exposed to a high enough altitude.

The results of available research suggest that no significant risk is associated with air-medical transport of a pregnant woman and her fetus. The arterial partial pressure of oxygen in the fetus is significantly lower than that of the mother. A healthy fetus at sea level has arterial oxygenation (PaO_2) of 32 mm Hg in the umbilical arterial circulation, whereas the PaO_2 of the mother will be approximately 100 mm Hg. At an altitude of 8000 ft, the PaO_2 of the mother will drop to 64 mm Hg, corresponding to an oxygen saturation of approximately 90%; the fetal PaO_2 will drop only from 32 to 25.6 mm Hg. In addition to the lower PaO_2 in the fetus, the oxygen dissociation curve for fetal hemoglobin differs from that for mature hemoglobin. Consequently, fetal hemoglobin is more fully saturated at a lower PaO_2 than is the hemoglobin of the mother.

Neonates, especially preterm neonates, are more likely than adults to develop hypoxia as the partial pressure of alveolar oxygen falls during ascent. Although the usual alveolar-arterial oxygen difference in adults is approximately 10 mm Hg, the difference in neonates is much larger (approximately 25 mm Hg). Therefore, a modest drop in partial pressure of alveolar oxygen will result in hypoxia in neonates.

Many factors may influence a person's susceptibility to hypoxia. Children and people with low tidal volumes and increased oxygen consumption are less able to respond to the hypoxic insult and, therefore, are more prone to the development of related complications. Many pediatric medical illnesses are exacerbated at altitude, including pneumonia, acute asthma, pneumothorax, shock, and blood loss. Numerous social factors also have an important role in susceptibility. Physical activity, physical fitness, metabolic rate, diet, nutrition, emotions, and fatigue influence the response to hypoxia. A physically fit person normally will have a higher tolerance to altitude-related problems, although an acute increase in physical activity will raise the body's demand for oxygen and cause more rapid onset of symptoms. A person's metabolic rate will increase with exposure to temperature extremes, increasing oxygen requirements and, therefore, reducing the hypoxic threshold.

Although altitude-related hypoxia in patients is a concern, the routine use of pulse oximetry and supplemental oxygen minimizes this hazard. In the setting of hypoxemia, increasing FIO_2 levels and, in some circumstances, the addition of positive end-expiratory pressure easily compensates for the hypoxic effects of altitude. However, in rare patients already receiving maximal oxygen support, flight at lower altitudes may allow the artificial cabin pressure to approach that of sea level, maintaining an acceptable PO_2.

Hypoxia is also a concern for pilots and transport team members who generally are not monitored. During air-medical transport at high altitudes, it may be advantageous to check oxygen saturation values of the pilots and transport team members. In addition, the Federal Aviation Administration (FAA) has specific regulations addressing the use of oxygen. The FAA regulations require pilots to use supplemental oxygen if they are flying at cabin altitudes above 10 000 ft for more than 30 minutes and at all times when above 12 000 ft. At cabin pressure altitudes above 15 000 ft, each occupant of the aircraft must use supplemental oxygen.

Noise

Noise and vibration may represent the most difficult and troublesome stresses encountered in the air and ground transport environments. Excessive noise may interfere directly with patient care.

During transport, it may be impossible to accurately auscultate the lungs or blood pressure. As a result, the transport team must rely on other means to monitor and assess patient condition. Close observation for alteration in the patient's respiratory rate, chest expansion, level of consciousness, discomfort, and abdominal distention may detect a possible change in the patient's condition. Blood pressure can be monitored by using invasive or noninvasive devices. Pulse oximetry provides valuable information about the patient's oxygenation and respiratory status, and carbon dioxide detectors or monitors are helpful when assessing tracheal tube position and patency.

As with many of the stresses of flight, there is individual variation in tolerance and effect of noise. The longer the exposure and the more intense the noise, the greater the potential damage.

Prolonged and intense exposure to noise may generate discomfort, headaches, fatigue, nausea, visual disturbances, vertigo, temporary or permanent ear damage, and deterioration in performance of tasks. During aircraft operation, hearing protection (ie, ear plugs, headsets, or helmets) should be worn by the flight crew, transport team, and patient.

Vibration

Vibration is inherent to all transport vehicles and may interfere with patient assessment and some routine physiologic functions. The most common sources of vibration during air-medical transport are the aircraft engines and air turbulence. During helicopter transport, vibration is most severe during transition to a hover or during turbulent weather conditions. In fixed-wing transport, vibration increases during high-speed, low-level flight and during cloud penetration in turbulent weather. In ground ambulances, poor road conditions, tight vehicle suspensions, narrow wheelbases, and high centers of gravity predispose to rough and unstable rides that may be detrimental or excessively painful to patients with spinal cord injury, intracerebral hemorrhage, and orthopedic injuries.

Exposure to moderate vibration results in a slight increase in metabolic rate and can cause fatigue, shortness of breath, motion sickness, chest pain, and abdominal pain. Vibration from the aircraft also may interfere with normal body thermoregulation and with the operation of some invasive and noninvasive electronic patient monitoring equipment.

Little can be done by pilots or in-flight crew members to eliminate or decrease the amount of vibration in the aircraft. This also is true of the ambulance drivers and ground transport personnel in ground vehicles. To minimize the effects of vibration, efforts should be made to avoid or reduce direct contact with the vehicle's frame. Padding should be placed on any part of the frame that may come in contact with people on board. Adequate padding in the form of cushioned seats and stretcher pads should be used. Direct contact with the

▪▪▪▪▪▪▪▪▪▪▪▪▪▪▪▪▪▪▪▪▪▪▪▪▪▪▪▪▪▪

bulkhead of the vehicle should be avoided by placing blankets or other cushions appropriately. Patients and transport team members should be properly restrained at all times to minimize the effects of vibration. In ground transport vehicles, careful attention also should be given to correct loads, tire pressures, appropriate shock absorbers, and overall vehicle maintenance.

Thermal Considerations

During helicopter, fixed-wing, and ground transport, the patient, pilots, and transport team may be exposed to a significant temperature variation that may result in clinical and operational complications. These temperature changes may be due to inherent seasonal changes, geographic factors, and altitude variation.

Exposure to extremes in temperature can result in increased metabolic rate and oxygen demand and consumption, which may further compromise an already hypoxic patient. Prolonged exposure also can result in motion sickness, headache, disorientation, fatigue, discomfort, irritability, impaired performance, and reduced ability to cope with other stresses, such as hypoxia.

Many factors can exacerbate or mitigate exposure to temperature variation, such as air circulation, duration of exposure, condition and type of clothing, and physical status. Whenever possible, the transport team should take steps to prevent potential complications related to thermal stress. The cabin should be kept at a comfortable temperature, minimizing exposure to ambient environmental extremes. To prevent hypothermia, appropriate layers of clothing or blankets should be used to limit heat loss. In addition, wet clothing or moist dressings should be removed. Prolonged exposure to high temperatures may require increased oral or intravenous fluids to prevent dehydration. The use of increased ventilation, cool water mist, or moist dressings may be of benefit.

No matter which medical transport vehicle is used, it is recommended that the transport team members be "dressed for the weather." In the summer, it may be appropriate for transport team members to undertake a transport wearing scrubs and a short, nonflowing hospital lab coat, as long as these articles can be safely worn in that environment. As the temperatures get colder, however, this would not be adequate because they should be prepared for prolonged, unexpected exposure to the elements owing to an accident, vehicle breakdown, remote locations, and changes in environmental controls. In the winter, appropriate attire includes a winter coat, gloves, hat, appropriate footwear, and layered clothing.

Humidity and Dehydration

As altitude increases and the air cools, the amount of moisture in the air drops significantly. Therefore, a pressurized aircraft that draws its fresh air from the outside dry atmosphere results in a pressurized cabin with an extremely low humidity level, and dehydration becomes another concern. In addition, dry medical oxygen will further predispose the patient to dehydration.

The decrease in humidity is particularly important as it relates to patient airway secretions. Dried airway secretions can lead to airway obstruction, atelectasis, and hypoxemia. Providing humidified medical oxygen helps to prevent airway obstruction due to dried secretions.

To prevent dehydration, fluid intake (oral or intravenous) should be monitored carefully, and all patients should receive humidified medical oxygen. These recommendations are especially important during long transports.

Gravitational Forces

During routine flight operations, gravitational forces will not significantly affect the patient, pilots, or transport team. However, an understanding of the relevance of gravitational forces to positioning of the transport team and patient within the aircraft and to their safety and survival is needed. One "g" represents the force that a person exerts when seated and is a result of gravitational force imposed on the body. Gravitational forces are applied to the body during ascent and descent and during a change in speed or direction.

During any sudden or excessive change in direction or speed, a person or object is subjected to the effects of gravitational forces. During deceleration of an air or ground vehicle, an unrestrained or improperly restrained person in a forward-facing seat may be injured or ejected from the seat. In contrast, a rear-facing seat may provide better restraint during crash deceleration.

In theory, patient positioning within the aircraft may enhance or minimize the effect of gravitational forces during takeoff (acceleration) and landing (deceleration). For patients with cardiac disease, myocardial perfusion is improved during acceleration by positioning the patient with the head toward the back (aft) of the aircraft. As negative gravitational forces increase, pooling of blood occurs in the upper part of the body. In head-injured patients or patients with fluid overload, augmentation of positive gravitational forces, which would pool blood in the lower extremities, may be desirable. This is accomplished by positioning the patient with the head toward the front (fore) of the aircraft. In a head-injured patient, positioning the head toward the front of the aircraft may reduce the risk of a transient increase in intracranial pressure during takeoff.

Fluid Dynamics

Long-distance or high-altitude air-medical transport may precipitate third spacing of fluid. A decrease in barometric pressure may cause this leakage that also may be aggravated by temperature extremes, vibration, and gravitational forces. Signs and symptoms include edema, dehydration, increased heart rate, and decreased blood pressure. Other stresses of flight or preexisting medical problems, such as preexisting capillary leak, cardiac conditions, and nephrotic disease, may aggravate the onset and complications of third spacing.

Fatigue

Although fatigue is considered one of the stresses, it also may be considered an end product of the contributing factors already discussed. Hypoxia, gravitational forces, barometric changes, and dehydration contribute to fatigue. It also is regarded as one of the self-imposed stresses.

Self-imposed Stress

A transport team member's self-imposed stresses can greatly influence physiologic performance during medical transport. Most of these stresses may be applicable to the flight crew and transport team members; their application to pediatric patients may be limited.

However, a clear understanding of these stresses is important to be able to provide optimal patient care.

Self-imposed stresses may greatly influence physiologic response during air or ground medical transport. Therefore, having a clear understanding of these factors is important for optimal transport safety and patient care. The acronym "DEATH" may be helpful to remember the components: Drugs, Exhaustion (fatigue), Alcohol, Tobacco, and Hypoglycemia (diet/dehydration; see Chapter 22)

Prescription and nonprescription medications and the medical conditions for which they are taken may interfere with performance, perception, decision making, and motor skills. Transport team members must be aware of the adverse effects, overdose reactions, allergic responses, and synergistic effects of medications they are taking.

All transport team members, as well as ambulance drivers and aircraft pilots, should avoid exhaustion and fatigue to prevent errors in judgment, poor attention span, and decreased work capacity and performance. Concerns and controversy regarding fatigue in health care providers received a great deal of attention in recent years and also was a concern for aircraft pilots and teams that use resident physicians. As a result, pilots are regulated by the FAA with regard to maximum duty hours. The Federal Aviation Regulation (FAR) requirement, Part 135, requires a pilot to have a minimum of 10 hours of uninterrupted rest within every 24-hour period. "On-call" time, when the pilot is required to carry and respond to a pager, is counted as "duty time" and cannot be included in the minimum 10 hours of required rest. Similarly, as of July 2003, the Accreditation Council for Graduate Medical Education limits resident physicians (fellows also are governed by these rules) to a maximum of 80 hours per week and 30 hours on duty at a time. Residents are required to have a minimum of 10 hours off between shifts and 1 day off in 7. Unfortunately, there are no other uniformly accepted work rules to govern transport teams and prevent fatigue. Many dedicated teams routinely work 24-hour shifts, and some team members may work several jobs or shifts back to back. Systems should be in place to audit duty time and to ensure the availability of backup personnel in case of fatigue.

The effects of alcohol ingestion tend to be exacerbated by altitude, as discussed in Chapter 22. Ingesting 1 alcoholic beverage at 10 000 ft is equivalent to ingesting 2 or 3 times as much at sea level. Similarly, the effects of tobacco are magnified during flight. The carbon monoxide by-product of smoking at sea level may result in mild hypoxia similar to that seen at an altitude of 8000 ft. This may occur with smoking as few as 3 cigarettes in rapid succession.

Diet is the final self-imposed stress. An inadequate or improper diet can result in nausea, headache, lightheadedness, dizziness, errors in judgment, and loss of consciousness. Precautions should be taken to avoid the development of hypoglycemia and dehydration.

Conclusion

Transport-related stresses create a significant challenge to personnel providing medical care to critically ill or injured children or neonates. An in-depth knowledge of flight physiology, stresses of flight, and self-imposed stresses enables the transport team to provide optimal patient care in the unique environment. The team must anticipate and prevent potentially serious complications by vigilant monitoring of the patient's condition and the initiation of appropriate treatment.

Selected Readings

Ackerman N. Aeromedical physiology. In: McCloskey KA, Orr RA, eds. *Pediatric Transport Medicine.* St Louis, MO: Mosby; 1995:143–157

Blumen IJ. Altitude and flight physiology: a reference for air medical physicians. In: Rodenberg H, Blumen IJ, eds. *Air Medical Physicians' Handbook.* Salt Lake City, UT: Air Medical Physician Association; 1999:V-1, 1–24

Blumen IJ, Dunne MJ. Altitude physiology and the stresses of flight. In: York D, ed. *Flight and Ground Transport Nursing Core Curriculum.* Denver, CO: Air & Surface Transport Nurses Association; 2006

Blumen IJ, Rinnert KJ. Altitude physiology and the stresses of flight. *Air Med J.* 1995;14:87–100

Bose CL. The transport environment. In: MacDonald MG, Miller MK, eds. *Emergency Transport of the Perinatal Patient.* Boston, MA: Little Brown & Co; 1989:194–211

DeHart RL, Davis JR, eds. *Fundamentals of Aerospace Medicine.* 3rd ed. Philadelphia, PA: Lippincott Williams & Wilkins; 2002

Elliott JP, Trujillo R. Fetal monitoring during emergency obstetric transport. *Am J Obstet Gynecol.* 1987;157:245–247

Federal Aviation Regulations, Airman's Information Manual: Part 91.17. Renton. Available at: http://www.access.gpo.gov/nara/cfr/waisidx_06/14cfr91_06.html. Accessed August 11, 2006

■■■■■■■■■■■■■■■■■■■■■■■■■■■■■■■■■■

Guidelines for Air Medical Crew Education. Alexandria, Va: Association of Air Medical
   Services; Dubuque, IA: Kendall/Hunt; 2004
Scholten P. Pregnant stewardess: should she fly? *Aviat Space Environ Med.* 1976;47:77–81
Holleran RS, ed. Transport physiology. In: *Air and Surface Patient Transport: Principles
   and Practice.* 3rd ed. Mosby, St Louis, MO; 2003:41–66

Questions

1. Describe Boyle's law and how it can affect patient transport.
2. What are the stresses of flight, and which of them may have the greatest
   effects on ground ambulance transport?
3. Why is hypoxia a major concern in air-medical transport?

Answers

1. Boyle's law relates to the expansion of gases. As an aircraft ascends, the volume of gas within an enclosed space expands. This expansion can affect any
   medical equipment or body cavity that has an enclosed air space, including
   the stomach, intestines, middle ear, sinuses, closed pneumothorax, intravenous flow rates, MAST, and endotracheal tube cuff.
2. Stresses of flight: barometric pressure, hypoxia, temperature, dehydration,
   noise, vibration, gravitational forces, fluid leakage out of intravascular spaces
   (third spacing), and fatigue. The stresses that may have the greatest effect on
   ground transport include noise, vibration, temperature, gravitational forces,
   and fatigue.
3. During air-medical transport, the most threatening aspect of hypoxia is its
   insidious onset. In addition, no one is exempt from the effects of hypoxia,
   although the onset and severity of symptoms vary among people.

CHAPTER 12

Family-Centered Care

Outline

- Key elements in FCC
- Benefits of FCC
- Other FCC issues during transport
- Transition to inpatient FCC

Family-centered care (FCC) is a philosophy of care that recognizes and respects the pivotal role of the family in the lives of children. It helps providers support families in their natural caregiving roles by building on their unique strengths as individuals and as families. Family members and professionals are viewed as equals in a partnership committed to excellence at all levels of health care. The practice of FCC redefines the relationship among patients, families, and health care providers. Family-centered care has been shown to improve patient and family satisfaction. Patients with complex and chronic conditions and their families benefit from an interdisciplinary approach to care. The interdisciplinary team effects the best outcomes by consistently using FCC in practice. In transport medicine, FCC manifests as accommodating the common and understandable request for the family to be with the patient.

Key Elements in FCC

The essential elements for providing FCC are as follows:

1. Recognition that the child is a member of a family with parents, siblings, and/or others who are the constants in the child's life
2. Consideration that the parents and the child are experts on the child's illness experience, response to treatment, and likelihood of success of care plans
3. Recognition that health professional personnel and expectations vary between systems and sometimes within institutions

4. Parent and professional respect and collaboration at all locations and levels of health care
5. Recognition of the profound influence of family strengths and individual values and needs on the success of the care plan and the ultimate outcomes for children and families
6. Provision to parents of unbiased and complete information about their child's care on an ongoing basis in an appropriate and supportive manner
7. Facilitation of parent-to-parent and sibling-to-sibling networking and support
8. Incorporation of the developmental needs of infants, children, adolescents, and their families into health care systems
9. Adoption of policies and programs that provide emotional and spiritual support for the families of chronically ill and critically ill or injured children
10. Flexible and accessible provision of health care that is responsive to family needs

Benefits of FCC

The American Academy of Pediatrics has identified the following benefits of FCC:
1. Improved health care outcomes for the child
2. Greater child and family satisfaction with their health care
3. A stronger alliance with the family in promoting each child's health and development
4. Improved clinical decision making on the basis of better information and collaborative practice
5. Improved follow-through when the plan of care is developed collaboratively with the family
6. Greater understanding of the family's strengths and care-giving capacities
7. More efficient and effective use of professional time and health care resources
8. Improved communication among members of the health care team
9. A more competitive position in the health care marketplace

10. An enhanced learning environment for future pediatricians and other professionals in training
11. A practice environment that enhances professional satisfaction

The transport team fulfills a crucial role in the initiation of FCC for critically ill and injured children. Principles used in the inpatient environment are no different from those used in the transport environment. However, the acuity of the patient's condition and the need for rapid mobilization and transport may lead to the parent's separation from the child at a time that the child is at risk of dying, which is understandably difficult for parents to cope with or even comprehend. Handing the care of an ill child to strangers who are taking the child to an often unknown destination is likely to create and intensify feelings of helplessness, fear, and loss. For these reasons, parents should be given the opportunity to discuss their child's management with transport team members at the earliest time possible. Parents need to know that their intimate knowledge of the child's history and reactions to illness and health care interventions is valued and will be incorporated into the plan of care, that they will continue to have access to their child, and that their child is in the care of competent staff.

It must be noted that, despite evidence of the benefits, there is not yet universal acceptance and implementation of FCC in clinical settings, including transport. Transport team members have cited the following reasons for excluding parents: (1) anticipated difficulty caring for the patient should the parent need attention, (2) potential trouble dealing with emotional or distraught parents, (3) difficulty controlling a child with the parent present, and (4) general team member anxiety about providing care and performing interventions with a parent watching.

By addressing the needs and concerns of the parent, the likelihood of parents becoming out of control is lessened dramatically. Moreover, the expertise of the parent can ease the clinical care; parents of chronically ill children may know where the easiest intravenous access is, parents of injured children may be able to calm the child by singing a favorite song, and parents of suddenly and overwhelmingly ill children may fight to be with their child over all objections owing to a sense that the child may die during the

████████████████████████████████████

transport and their desperate desire to provide support to their child that no one else can. It may, in fact, be much easier to care for the child with the parent present. By incorporating the parent, the energy and concern of the parent can be directed to the therapeutic goals and ease the burdens of the child and transport team. It is the responsibility of the neonatal-pediatric transport system to define a standard of FCC for the transport of ill and injured children.

Offering families the option to be present during the provision of emergency and critical care is a cornerstone of FCC. Family presence during resuscitation continues to gain widespread support. Many studies have shown that this practice allows families to remain as therapeutic allies in the care of their children, even in the most dire circumstances. In Woodward and Fleegler's[1,2] investigations of family presence in a large transport system at a children's hospital, parents were cooperative and did not create difficulties for transport team members or the patients. Furthermore, family presence at attempted resuscitations enabled them to see, first hand, that the team members did their best for their child and also treated the child with respect, dignity, and empathy throughout the process, which is proven to enable the family to more smoothly begin the inevitable grieving process.

Some responders are concerned that personalization of care occasionally leads to the creation of emotional bonds with families, which potentially can be difficult for all involved. This is most common with families of critically or terminally ill children. It is important to note that parents testifying to the Institute of Medicine Committee on the Care of Children Who Die often related that first responders were the most loving and empathic of all health care providers they encountered; memories of these personnel and their efforts sustained these parents in the darkest days of their bereavement. However, not everyone is capable of giving so much of himself or herself. It is important that each transport team member know his or her own limitations and ensure that at least one member of each team is able to provide emotional support to parents. Transport team members need support to address the inevitable reactions and concerns generated by being exposed to devastating scenarios, and they should have the opportunity to work with such concerns individually or in a group forum, based on their sense of what helps most. When necessary, assistance should be solicited from critical incident stress management teams or mental health professionals.

Other FCC Issues During Transport

Team safety should always be considered. All vehicle occupants should wear appropriate restraints. Children should never be transported in a parent's lap or arms. Spatial concerns also must be addressed. Family members should be provided with an explanation if it is unsafe or problematic for them to ride in the transport vehicle or in a specific location within the vehicle.

Prehospital providers will come in contact with families with diverse health beliefs, customs, and practices, including the use of alternative and uncommon treatment methods. Eliciting this history is important, and thorough documentation is beneficial to the overall care of the child. Strategies to overcome language and cultural barriers must be developed and made available to all transport team members.

Transition to Inpatient FCC

The principles of family-centered prehospital care ideally should be practiced throughout the transport process, from on-scene treatment, through the transport, to the transition of care to in-hospital health care providers. Because of this continuum, all members of the health care team, including emergency medical services prehospital personnel, should be involved in the development of strategies to implement and practice FCC from initial patient contact.

One of the essential elements of these protocols is a "point person" who will be the main communication contact among the family and transport and hospital staff. This person needs to be reliably and consistently available and provide frequent communication. The point person prepares and provides information to the family about the anticipated clinical management of their child during the transport and about any anticipated or potential complications. The mode of transport and relevant equipment and procedures should be explained. In addition, the point person assists in arranging ongoing family access to the patient.

The point person should offer the family the opportunity to accompany the child whenever possible. The legal and insurance coverage ramifications of accompaniment (in case of accident), if any, should have been identified before transport and discussed with parents as indicated. Because not all families will want to (or be able to) participate this intimately, they should receive detailed information about their child's destination. This should include the name of the receiving physician and clinical service, the telephone numbers of the hospital and the specific inpatient care unit, and driving directions and parking information for the receiving hospital. On arrival at the receiving facility, the child and family should be introduced to the new health care team. The transport team, if available, can assist with this clinical transfer. A new point person should be identified who will be responsible for providing ongoing information within the hospital setting.

The therapeutic alliance gained by implementing an FCC philosophy is important throughout the child's health care experience and is nowhere more important than in potentially life-threatening chronic and critical illnesses. These challenging situations often begin with a medical transport and the opportunity to create an alliance with the child and family.

References

1. Woodward GA, Fleegler EW. Should parents accompany pediatric interfacility ground ambulance transports? The parents' perspective. *Pediatr Emerg Care.* 2000;16:383–390
2. Woodward GA, Fleegler EW. Should parents accompany pediatric interfacility ground ambulance transports? Results of a national survey of pediatric transport team managers. *Pediatr Emerg Care.* 2001;17:22–27

Selected Readings

American Academy of Pediatrics Committee on Hospital Care: Family-centered care and the pediatrician's role. *Pediatrics.* 2003;112:691–696
Boudreaux EO, Francis JL, Loyacano T. Family presence during invasive procedures and resuscitations in the emergency department: a critical review and suggestions for future research. *Ann Emerg Med.* 2002;40:193–205
Edgington BH. Transporting the family and other concerned parties aboard air medical aircraft. *J Air Med Transp.* 1992, 11:11–13
The Institute for Family-Centered Care. Available at: http://www.familycenteredcare.org. Accessed January 13, 2006

Jaimovich DG, Vidyasagar D. *Handbook of Pediatric and Neonatal Transport Medicine.* 2nd ed. Philadelphia, PA: Hanley and Belfus; 2002

Lewis MM, Holditch-Davis D, Brunssen S. Parents as passengers during pediatric transport. *Air Med J.* 1997;16:38–43

National Association of Emergency Medical Technicians. Family-centered prehospital care: partnering with families to improve care. Fact Sheet. 2002 Available at: http://www.ems-c.org/downloads/doc/876FactSheet.doc. Accessed January 13, 2006

Shelton TL, Jeppson ES, Johnson BH. *Family Centered Care for Children With Special Health Care Needs.* Washington, DC: Association for the Care of Children's Health; 1987

Tucker TL. Family presence during resuscitation. *Crit Care Nurs Clin North Am.* 2002; 14:177–185

Questions

1. Describe the benefits of family-centered care (FCC) during transport.
2. Do all families want to be present with their child throughout the continuum of care?
3. Describe the role of the point person during transport.

Answers

1. FCC decreases parental anxiety and loss of control. Optimal outcomes for the child and family can be achieved through collaboration between transport team members and family.
2. No; however, they should be provided with the opportunity and, if present during the transport, receive ongoing information throughout the experience.
3. Provide ongoing communication and assist in arranging family access to the child

Marketing the Neonatal-Pediatric Transport Team

Outline

- Current trends influencing a transport program
- Program assessment
- Marketing research
- Development of the marketing plan
- Implementation of the marketing plan
- Maintenance of the marketing plan

Current Trends Influencing a Transport Program

The last decade has seen numerous changes in the provision of health care. There has been an increase in outsourcing and contracting with outside vendors for services such as laundry, security, laboratory, and blood banking. Health care alliances have changed affiliations, and satellite facilities have been established in an effort to reach a broader share of the market. An emphasis on reimbursement from third-party payers and tighter cost-containment strategies has dominated the efforts of health care administrators as they continue to position their institutions for the changes of the future. As a result, the concept of marketing hospital services has evolved dramatically. Competition in the health care arena has given greater focus to marketing strategies used by these facilities as health care providers continue to use many mediums to reach their markets. Although not all transport systems function in directly competitive environments, attention to the principles and practices described herein should improve positioning and potentially improve current services.

■■■■■■■■■■■■■■■■■■■■■■■■■■■■■■■■■■■■

Marketing is an established concept in the retail world of goods and services. *Marketing* is defined as a process whereby individuals and groups obtain what they need and what they want by creating and exchanging products and value with others. Businesses have learned that marketing is a necessary tool to maintain and gain customers. In health care, the marketing cornerstones of the 4 Ps (product, place, price, and promotion) as well as the 4 Cs (competence, convenience, cost, and communication) have penetrated every aspect of the provision of patient care. Goals noted by the Institute of Medicine state that high-quality care should be provided in a safe, effective, timely, efficient, equitable, and patient-centered manner.

Marketing a neonatal-pediatric transport program poses a unique challenge to achieve these goals and integrate the cornerstones of marketing. Neonatal-pediatric transport teams should be aware of factors that are important to the users of their services. Successful transport programs have learned and implemented strategies for success in providing and maintaining business. Despite emphasis on the need for safe, specialized transport services for neonatal and pediatric patients, various trends and factors determine referral practices.

Competition, market share sought through affiliation agreements, government regulations, and cost-containment measures are some of the variables that affect how a transport program positions itself now and in the future. The key determinants remain understanding the need and demand (Table 13-1) for transport services and maintaining and marketing a safe, quality program. Understanding the type of demand will help new and established transport programs evaluate whether the need for service exists or continues and determine possible changes needed in the program to meet the specific type of demand.

Table 13-1: Examples and Types of Demand*

Negative demand
Product or service is disliked
Example: Poor service and reputation

No demand
Target consumers uninterested or indifferent to product or service
Example: Other transport opportunities (programs) are effective and preferred

Latent demand
No existing product or service exists that can satisfy the consumer
Example: No current neonatal-pediatric transport services for a certain area

Falling demand
Decline in interest in product or service; goal is to restimulate the demand or develop
   new target markets
Example: Decrease in referrals owing to new (effective) competition in area

Irregular demand
Variations in overwork or idle capacity, seasonal work
Example: Team workload with no transport demand or during high-volume periods

Full demand
Pleasing volume of business; task is to maintain level of demand despite competition and
   changing consumer preference, keep quality, and measure consumer satisfaction
Example: Transport requests are completed by teams in a timely manner, and there are
   enough teams to accommodate the requests.

Overfull demand
Requires finding ways to reduce demand
Example: Too many transport calls, and pediatric and neonatal intensive care unit and
   specialty care beds are full; integration and teamwork with other transport venues
   and services

Unwholesome demand
Involves discouraging a product or service
Example: Demand for critical care and/or certain modes of transport for routine
   patient transfer

*KOTLER, PHILIP; KELLER, KEVIN LANE, MARKETING MANAGEMENT: ANALYSIS, PLANNING, IMPLEMENTATION AND
CONTROL, 12th Edition, © 2006, p. 10. Adapted by permission of Pearson Education, Inc., Upper Saddle River, NJ

Program Assessment

The initial program assessment should critically review the program's
strengths and weaknesses and specifically identify the current and
planned marketing efforts implemented by transport management
and operational personnel. A common method to evaluate the
internal and external environments is SWOT analysis (Strengths,
Weaknesses, Opportunities, and Threats; Table 13-2).

As applied to a neonatal-pediatric transport program, SWOT might identify the following:

Table 13-2: Sample SWOT Analysis

S (Strengths)
- Good reputation among users; demonstrates expertise
- Solid relationship with air and ground vendors

W (Weaknesses)
- High cost structure
- Location of receiving facility

O (Opportunities)
- New technology
- Ground ambulance vendor willing to put logo on ambulance
- Possible merger with other facility

T (Threats)
- Tighter regulations
- New transport program in referral area (competitor)
- Other programs have superior access to referral facilities

Specific services provided by the referral and receiving facilities, such as tertiary neonatal or pediatric care, burn care, transplant services, and level 1 trauma services, imply a demand for specialized transport services. A needs assessment of the medical facility, demographics, and emergency medical services providers will offer a basis for long-range planning and marketing.

The questions listed in Table 13-3 identify pertinent areas to evaluate as part of the program assessment. Evaluating market share is often neglected if the transport program is the only one in the region. However, other transport programs may want to expand into the same catchment area. Program evaluators should identify the present and potential service or referral areas. There may be areas that are underserved or inefficiently served, which can be determined by a thorough program assessment. Team management can review its own and regional statistical information, such as the number and type of transports and the originating individual referral and receiving facilities and their frequency of transport contact as a basis for improving transport operations.

The marketing evaluators need to consider third-party payer issues, affiliate relationships, transfer agreements and contracts, and

██ ██

Table 13-3: Sample Program Assessment Questions

1. Who are the current users?

2. What internal marketing strategies are used within the institution to inform attending physicians about the services provided within the institution?

3. What external marketing strategies are used outside the institution to promote the services provided?

4. What are the receiving institution's strengths that can be used to identify the target market (eg, pediatric trauma center, liver transplant program), and do these target markets reflect the current users of the program?

5. What growth is expected in the receiving institution and the transport program?

6. How do users contact the program and why?

7. What facets or attributes do the users like about the program?

8. For institutions not contacting the program, why do they not use the services provided?

9. Who is the competition?

10. What is the relationship of the program with the competition?

11. What does the program do that is different from other programs?

12. What features exist in the program that are worthy of acknowledgment?

13. Does the program offer a quality and reputable service?

14. How is quality measured by the service?

15. Are safety, equipment, and training standards up-to-date, and how are these conveyed to users?

16. How are other highlights or distinguishing features of the program currently conveyed to the users?

17. What is the marketing budget?

18. Are current strategies effective?

19. What obstacles exist that may hinder growth?

20. How can these obstacles be overcome?

21. What opportunities exist to attract future users?

state-mandated regionalization. All participants in the marketing process should be provided with an appreciation of the public relations and cost-benefit analyses of the various transport options.

Geographic considerations, weather patterns, response time, and traffic patterns in urban, suburban, and rural service areas and available modes of transport should be considered in any marketing strategy. Recognized limitations of the program should be publicized to prevent unrealistic expectations by potential users (ie, potential litigation).

Marketing efforts may be subtle and amount to common and courteous activities such as follow-up letters to staff involved in each transport. Transport programs must be mindful of Health Information Portability and Accountability Act restrictions, and consents should reflect the release of certain aspects of patient information before sending follow-up letters. Additional marketing efforts to highlight special activities can produce even more recognition. Notable transport team and personnel activities should be disseminated to local media, including radio, television, and newspapers. Providing surveys by Web page links and electronic mail to program users or potential users is another avenue to assess the program. There are currently several Web sites with extensive links dealing with emergency medical services and air and ground transport activities (Appendix E). Proactive action plans involving the community (eg, mock disaster drills, open houses, health fairs, and safety fairs), emergency services providers, and local health care personnel (eg, hosting no-cost advanced life support training programs and in-service courses) are a means of achieving continuous visibility.

A program assessment provides an opportunity to determine the effectiveness and efficiency of current marketing strategies. A review of new and existing transport programs permits the marketing evaluators to determine whether there is a need for expansion of services. Consideration should also be given to eliminating certain types of infrequent or high-risk transfer operations. In addition, the program's evaluation should include marketing strategies implemented by competing programs in the service area. If possible, it is recommended that a national comparison with other programs of similar background, mission, and volume be included. Comparisons with other local, regional, and national services and databases can facilitate program introspection. Program organizations, such as the Commission on Accreditation of Medical Transport Systems (see Chapter 19), may be of assistance during a comprehensive review.

Marketing Research

Knowledge of, attitudes toward, and satisfaction with the transport service and areas for expansion or modification of the transport program should be evaluated and identified through the marketing research process. Market research specifies the information necessary to address program issues, data collection methods, implementation, analysis, and communication of the findings and their implications.

A systematic approach to the marketing research process includes the following steps:

- Define the problem.
- Determine how data will be obtained.
- Select a sampling method.
- Decide how data will be analyzed.
- Determine the budget and timeframe.
- Obtain the data.
- Analyze and check the data.
- Communicate the findings.

Evaluators (team leaders, administrative personnel, or others) should identify the target market or respondents to solicit for the survey. Internal markets may be composed of attending physicians, administrators, and departments within the institution who interface with the program. External target markets may include referring physicians and administrative managers from emergency departments, nurseries, and pediatric units at the referral institutions. Depending on the program's mission, other respondents might include third-party payers, fire and police departments, emergency medical services, and clinics.

The most critical element in obtaining data is the development of data collection instruments. Each question on a form must have a known purpose. Questions should be unambiguous, and forced choices should be used to assist in data analysis and qualitative and quantitative data presentation.

There are many traditional data collection techniques that can be used to reach users or potential users of the transport program. Telephone interviews with preidentified persons should be performed by appointment. It is recommended that convenient times be pre-arranged for the telephone call and that the respondents receive the questions before the telephone call so they can be properly prepared and expedite the survey process.

Other techniques involved in marketing surveys include a written survey or questionnaire. A properly designed instrument with review by personnel outside of transport, as well as a pilot testing process, is very important. This process can ensure that the survey presentation, content, and length are appropriate; that questions are properly presented and not leading; and that the responses will provide the desired information. If internal resources are not available, there are professional organizations that can assist with this process. The survey can be mailed, providing the respondent an opportunity to review questions and develop answers. Evaluators can design the survey to query specific areas and convey the reason for the questionnaire. Questions should be carefully designed to elicit the data that one desires to examine. Written surveys may solicit referral patterns, satisfaction, and referral needs. Written surveys should be accompanied by a cover letter introducing the survey, and anonymity should be assured to survey respondents. Return of this letter by the postal service to the sender indicates an incorrect address that can be corrected so that the survey form (and other potential communications) reaches the intended target. Preaddressed, postage-paid return envelopes increase response rates by permitting easy return of the survey form. Offering a fax number or e-mail contact address may also provide a convenient method for return of the survey. Regardless of the response rates, written and telephone follow-up is useful to determine reasons for lack of response (eg, a survey form that was too complex or lengthy or included potential respondents who had no interest in the service). Telephone and written surveys should be followed with a letter of appreciation for the respondent's insight and participation.

The Internet has created many new opportunities for market research. Surveys can be conducted by electronic mail or attachments. Web pages or links can be set up for users to respond to a survey via a specific Web site. Although many opportunities exist for obtaining data, personal contact is also appreciated and offers an opportunity for developing relationships and networking with users or potential users of the program.

Development of the Marketing Plan

The marketing plan is the written blueprint detailing how the message will be communicated to the consumer or user of the product or services. It identifies target markets and areas for growth and details the strategies that will be necessary to successfully penetrate, capture, and maintain the market share of the program's referral area.

Key elements of the marketing plan include the following: (1) mission statement of program; (2) market research and analysis; (3) the establishment of program goals, marketing strategies, and integration with other program plans; (4) the establishment of action plans; and (5) the evaluation process.

After the pertinent data are obtained, a decision should be made about how to use the information. Priorities should be identified and categorized in order of importance or necessity. Whether program services must change or advertising strategies are needed, program decision makers must prioritize the potential effect of each strategy and whether it is organizationally and financially feasible. Using resources from within the institution or contracting consultant services may be a consideration in the prioritization process. It is crucial for the program to carefully coordinate efforts in order to maximize the impact of the data collected. Emphasis may include the rapid availability of a dedicated ground ambulance or helicopter, the program's safety record, and the expertise of specialty teams that have extensive training in neonatal and pediatric transport. Media communication and written materials should be reviewed by administration and the public relations department to ensure compliance with the institution's overall plan for consistent and effective communication.

Focus should also be applied to the anticipated costs of available marketing strategies so that options can be weighed and resources can be identified. Consideration of return on investment to sponsors is important. Cost issues could move the plan forward or bring it to a halt. In addition, decision makers should request feedback to identify areas of concern and excellence as identified by the transport team. Important concepts include measurement strategies to obtain and communicate information, metrics of assessment and internal comparison, and the ability to benchmark against other local, national, and other similar services or institutions. Once the plan has met with the approval of the transport program director, reviewing with senior hospital administration is advisable to secure a firm level of institutional support and a financial commitment.

There are many types of marketing strategies (Table 13-4). Each strategy should be evaluated carefully in relation to probable benefit, potential obstacles and risks, and timeframes for implementation.

Table 13-4: Sample Marketing Strategies

Personal Contact

- Visit referral hospitals, and offer tours of the helicopter, ground ambulance, or both.
- Invite referring facility personnel to open houses or anniversary celebrations.
- Conduct a telephone survey of referring facilities and units.
- Sponsor local transport meetings and conferences.
- Offer presentations to fund-raising groups that support the hospital and team.
- Call back the referring facility staff about patient follow-up and to thank them for their assistance.
- Develop name recognition with staff at facilities that are regular users.

Written Contact

Coordinate all distributed materials with hospital or team logo, including:

- Business cards
- Rotary cards
- Form letters
- Brochures about the team and how to initiate a transport
- Newsletters
- Comment and response cards
- Mail survey to solicit information
- Follow-up letters and notes
- Internal advertising of team to hospital staff via hospital publications with accomplishments, statistics, and other newsworthy information
- Team phone number noted on promotional items such as pens, notepads, and magnets
- Static display

Media Contact

- Arrange media spots on TV or radio.
- Share special interest stories via newspaper with testimonials or transport profile.
- Sponsor public safety announcements via TV or radio.
- Develop a video marketing presentation.
- Create a team Web site with available services, team description, and phone numbers, photos, service area, and e-mail addresses.

Customer-oriented Services

- Hotline or toll-free phone number
- Outreach: offer educational conferences or courses such as a neonatal resuscitation program or pediatric advanced life support
- Offer safety in-service class to all personnel involved with helicopter and ground ambulance programs
- Ride-along program
- Preceptorship
- Transfer agreements
- Volume discounts
- Telephone accessibility for consultation
- Telemedicine links for regular or affiliate users

Program leadership should identify the strategies that:

- offer the most to the team in terms of a clear and consistent message,
- use resources identified,
- conform to the budget plan,
- are most cost-effective, and
- highlight the program's specialty services as noted during the data collection and market research processes.

A sample marketing plan as applicable to a transport program is depicted in Table 13-5.

Table 13-5: Sample Marketing Plan

Action Program	Cost	Responsible Department	Start Date	Completion Date	Maintenance Requirements	Evaluation
Access to transport team: toll-free number						
Logo on ambulance						
Brochures						
Safety fair						

Implementation of the Marketing Plan

The marketing message must be presented to each level of the administrative and clinical team involved with the transport program (and base facility) to ensure that it is incorporated into the patient referral process.

Visibility is a key marketing tool. Consistency in logo, colors, and uniforms is helpful to identify an institution or service. Using a slogan or a visual image that is consistent with the referral hospital's corporate identity also can reinforce the marketing plan.

The transport team's expertise, professional affiliations, safety awards, speeches, or recognition can be highlighted in newsletters or marketing brochures. Team members who actively attend or lead educational offerings or obtain special certifications may lend credence to the transport program's unique expertise.

Maintenance of the Marketing Plan

Ultimately, the goal is to keep consumers satisfied based on program responsiveness, service excellence, and cost-effectiveness. A program can respond optimally to its consumers only if there is awareness of their needs and their perception of the services provided. The importance of follow-up must be stressed. Providing immediate follow-up to the referring facility's staff about the transported child is a successful marketing technique. Follow-up letters can serve as a source of continuing education to the referral institution by communicating the patient's outcome to those who provided care. This must be done with consent and confidentiality as dictated by the Health Insurance Portability and Accountability Act and can occur via telephone, note card, letter, or fax provided that consent and confidentiality are maintained. Communication with expression of appreciation for the referral is an immeasurable professional courtesy. The influence of "word of mouth" advertising should not be underestimated.

Another method used to evaluate the effectiveness of the marketing plan is data comparison with statistical analysis. This requires ongoing data entry of all calls received and missions and transport accomplished. Analysis may include the following:

- Frequency of referral from certain institutions during a specified period
- Review intervals (eg, 3 and 6 months and 1 year)
- Diagnostic categories, transports, response times, and consultations
- Volume assessment for time of day and day of week

Comparisons can identify areas of change such as increased referrals (or decreased demand) from a particular hospital or unit. Monitoring and reassessment should be consistent and ongoing. After careful study, the marketing plan can be revised, taking into consideration the changing needs and environment.

The critical elements of the marketing process include emphasis on the quality of service and the importance of customer relations. Providing an excellent service, maintaining current data on the demand for service, sustaining a sound relationship with program users, and using consistent and quality promotion strategies are the key components of an effective marketing plan. Evaluation and measurement of the marketing plan's success can be used to provide valuable feedback to the transport program about its effectiveness.

Suggested Readings

Alward RR, Camunas C. *The Nurse's Guide to Marketing.* Albany, NY: Delmar Publishers; 1991

Collett HM. Marketing an aeromedical transport system in emergency transport of the perinatal patient. MacDonald MG, Miller MK, eds. Boston, MA: Little Brown & Co; 1989:112–123.

Holleran RS, ed. *Air and Surface Patient Transport: Principles and Practice.* 3rd ed. St Louis, MO: Mosby; 2003

Kotler P, Keller KL. *Marketing Management: Analysis, Planning, Implementation and Control.* 12th Edition. Upper Saddle River, NJ: Pearson Education, Inc.; 2006:10

Kotler P, Armstrong G. *Principles of Marketing.* 10th ed. Englewood Cliffs, NJ: Prentice Hall; 2003

Questions

1. What types of trends have influenced transport teams?
2. What are the types of demand?
3. What is a method to analyze the internal and external environments of a program?

Answers

1. Trends that have influenced transport programs include an increasing use of outside vendors, more institutions creating health care alliances and agreements, and the constraints of health care financial resources. An emphasis on cost containment and competition directly influences the forces affecting marketing of the transport program.

2. The types of demand applicable to transport programs include falling demand, irregular demand, full demand, and overfull demand. Falling demand would indicate a decline in the need for the service or factors such as competition that are creating a lesser volume. Irregular demand is when there are variations in overwork or idle capacity. Overfull demand is when there is too much demand for service, and the transport program has difficulty accommodating requests. Full demand is when there is a pleasing volume of transports.

3. Internal markets are the markets (customers) within the institution such as attending physicians who refer patients to the program or administrators who support the service. External markets relate to the groups or individuals outside the program or institution who exchange products or services with the program. These markets could be referral hospitals, equipment vendors, and helicopter and ambulance services.

■ Outreach Education ■

Outline

■ Outreach education
■ Benefits of outreach education
■ Learning styles
■ Educational content
■ Objectives and implementation

Outreach Education

An outreach educational program should be a key component of all transport programs. The medical, social, and legal complexities of interfacility transfer of critically ill or injured neonates and pediatric patients make fertile ground for continuing education activities, which are also of benefit to marketing efforts (see Chapter 13). The outreach education program objectives also integrate and overlap with the marketing strategies of the transport program (Table 14-1). The ultimate goal of effective outreach education is to improve patient outcome. Frequently asked questions regarding transport outreach education are included in Figure 14-1.

When considering developing a transport program, it is imperative that the transport leadership team spend time marketing the program to the hospitals in the local community and meeting the medical directors and medical and nursing staffs of the emergency departments and inpatient pediatric and neonatal units. This initial contact not only introduces the team, but also is an ideal opportunity to further assess the need for and offer outreach education.

An educational and training assessment, often part of a marketing survey, permits targeting of necessary and sought-after (the two are not always the same) education and training activities. Developing relationships with department educators and clinicians will assist in

Table 14-1: Objectives of Transport Outreach Education

- Ensure knowledge of basic stabilization principles for neonatal and pediatric patients
- Teach recognition of neonatal and pediatric illness that requires transfer to a higher level of care
- Delineate how to access the transport system and obtain consultation and recommendations for stabilization
- Upgrade understanding of the physiologic basis for initiating care and stabilization for the unique transport environment before team arrival at the referring facility
- Develop a system to provide follow-up information on patient progress and outcome (Constructive advice about patient care at the referring facility is helpful.)
- Arrange for seminars and other educational activities on topics relevant to transport (see Table 14-2 and Appendix E)

determining institution-specific educational needs. An assessment of institutional resources should be included when developing teaching goals and needs. There are many different types of educational offerings that may be of interest to referring hospital staff. Written surveys may be developed, with a checklist of specific courses or individual lectures or skills content that are areas of expertise for the transport team members. Transport teams also can determine educational opportunities in a more informal setting, through conversations with physicians, educators, or individual staff members and when the transport team medical director and/or coordinator continue the marketing and public relations sessions with small groups at the referring centers. Quality improvement reviews and identification of perceived deficiencies may direct the focus of education.

Informal discussions during initiation of transport, at the referring facility, and during the completion of the transport at the receiving facility also can assist in determining the required and requested education and training from people who will be attending the training sessions and applying the information to the transport environment. As the referring facility personnel become more comfortable and develop relationships with the transport team, they are more willing to approach transport team members, ask questions, and verbalize specific educational needs. Transport team members can gauge and influence the competency of referring personnel by participating as instructors in formal certified training programs (activities), such as the Pediatric Advanced Life Support (PALS), Pediatric Education

Figure 14-1
Frequently Asked Questions About Outreach Education

1. **Why should my transport program become involved in outreach education?**
   It gives transport team members an opportunity to meet and interact with staff from referring institutions without the added stress of a critically ill or injured neonate or child. Staff at referring institutions want to know how to best care for their patients until a transport team arrives. Meeting that need and providing a low-stress environment in a learning environment and sharing the expertise of your team members is something the referring institutions will remember when faced with a critically ill or injured neonate or child. Outreach education is also an excellent marketing tool for any transport team.

2. **What are the important steps in developing an outreach program within your institution?**
   - First, the leadership of the transport program needs to understand the concept of outreach education and the ultimate benefit to the team.
   - Next, consider your resources. Who on your team is trained, experienced, and excited about teaching? What specific "expertise" exists or is needed in specific topics, diseases, and management? Who has experience speaking to small and large groups?
   - Once you have identified resources within your institution or program, you are ready to consider marketing outreach education.

3. **Who should be involved in an outreach program?**
   Any and all members of the transport team, as well as staff within the hospital (emergency department [ED], pediatric and neonatal intensive care units [PICU and NICU]). Some institutions may have an outreach coordinator who will help with the logistics, contact institutions, set up activities, and perhaps be an active member of the educational team.

4. **What should we do before our first outreach program?**
   - Start local and small. Consider your geographic location. Are there multiple transport programs in your area?
   - What is unique about your program, and how can you best market your specialty?
   - With the assistance of your public relations department, you may develop a marketing strategy. Are there institutions in your geographic area that are not referring ill or injured children or neonates to your hospital at this time? Are there institutions that have been identified by members of your transport team as possibly benefiting from educational opportunities your team members could provide?
   - Now it is time to make the initial contact to these "targeted" institutions, clinics, and offices. Consider contacting the medical and/or nursing director of the department (eg, ED, NICU). Introduce yourself, and offer the services of your team for outreach education. Has this physician or nurse identified an educational need among staff? Was there a specific case that referring staff might like your team to present with patient follow-up and possibly "lessons learned" or how to better manage the patient until the transport team arrives?

5. **What about the national certification/resuscitation courses? How are they a benefit to an outreach program?**
   Nationally recognized programs can be a definite asset to any outreach program. All of these programs offer continuing education units for participants, and many also offer a verification card that is valid for 2 to 4 years, depending on the curriculum.

Figure 14-1
Frequently Asked Questions About Outreach Education, *continued*

Many hospitals offer some type of financial bonus for their staff who successfully complete the curriculum. In many areas of the country, there are not enough courses offered to meet the requests from staff. Many community hospitals pride themselves and market to their own community that 100% of their nurses on a specific unit (eg, ED, NICU) are certified in a particular area. These courses are another way for your transport staff to meet the need for staff education in community hospitals and clinics, which also can become a marketing tool for that community hospital. Most national courses require instructors to have taken the provider course and then an instructor course before being able to teach.

6. **How do you measure success in an outreach educational program?**
   - Measuring success depends on many factors. Ideally, we would all like to see improved care delivery and new and increased referrals from the hospitals that were targeted for outreach educational efforts. This, however, may be unrealistic because not all neonates and children need the services of a transport team.
   - Evaluation forms provide immediate feedback of the learners' perception of success of the teaching program.
   - Knowledge change can be measured with a pretest and posttest design.
   - Patient outcome may be measured by morbidity and mortality reviews before and after the educational offering.
   - Before starting an outreach program, your team and institution may want to obtain baseline data about current referral patterns, potentially targeting other institutions that are not referring or do not often refer patients to your facility.
   - Reevaluate after a specified timeframe (6–9 months) to determine whether there has been an increase in referrals from individual institutions or requests from new institutions.
   - Your outreach program may be considered successful when your team is able to report that the staff at the targeted hospitals was able to better stabilize the condition of and prepare a neonate or pediatric patient for transfer.
   - Success in outreach education also can be measured in the trust and professional relationships that are developed over time between the transport team and community agency staff. Hopefully, when a critically ill or injured neonate or pediatric patient is admitted to their institution, the staff members will be able to manage the patient while they call your team for transport.

7. **Why is it important to consider outreach educational activities to prehospital providers (EMS providers)?**
   There is a great need for neonatal and pediatric education in the prehospital setting. There is limited time devoted to neonatal and pediatric topics in any initial prehospital curriculum (basic life support [BLS], cardiac rescue technician [CRT], advanced life support [ALS]). Depending on the population, some EMS providers may transport few patients in any year, and the patients may or may not be critically ill or injured. These providers may benefit from the same type of educational opportunities as the staff at community hospitals and clinics. Many states have prehospital continuing education conferences annually.

Figure 14-1
Frequently Asked Questions About Outreach Education, *continued*

We know that neonatal and pediatric patients may have subtle manifestations of serious, even life-threatening conditions. Sharing your expertise with EMS providers will sharpen their assessment skills and teach them to take neonatal and pediatric patients to the right hospital at the right time.

8. **What are the financial issues to consider with an outreach program?**
   - The financial commitment will vary depending on your program goals and plans. Some transport teams include participation in outreach education as one of the requirements to be on the transport team. In this environment, the transport budget may include time for individual team members to prepare and present outreach topics.
   - The financial commitment also will depend on whether you have a dedicated educational coordinator as part of the leadership of your team.
   - If you do not have outreach education as a requirement for your team members, your institution's mission statement might include an educational component or an expectation that staff will participate in some volunteer efforts.
   - Your commitment might need to include paying staff salaries for preparation, time presenting the educational curriculum, and travel expenses.
   - Individual transport programs and institutions also can be creative in supporting outreach educational efforts by offering incentives to members who assist in outreach education.

9. **What is the benefit to the referring agency to participate in an outreach educational program?**
   Referring institutions and agencies benefit because they have the opportunity to learn from and ask questions of transport team members who have expertise in specific areas, diseases, and management. Also, from case reviews, they have the opportunity to learn and be better prepared for the next neonates and children who need transport.

---

for Prehospital Professionals (PEPP), Advanced Pediatric Life Support (APLS), and Neonatal Resuscitation Program (NRP) courses (see Appendix E).

Many times, referring facility personnel are interested in specific lectures or a combination of lectures and psychomotor skill practice. Topics might include basic ABCs (airway, breathing, and circulation), preparation and stabilization for transport, respiratory diseases, intravenous access with practice, conscious sedation, resuscitation, medication calculation and administration, management of diabetic ketoacidosis, management of seizures, pediatric assessment, and trauma. Faculty for this type of educational session can include a combination of physicians, nurses, and paramedics.

The need for well-prepared and experienced instructors is paramount. The initial impression of transport team members as outreach educators can be a lasting one. Meeting the educational needs of many individuals also can be a challenge. As the transport team begins educational opportunities with individual health care facilities, the relationship with the team and the team's institution is strengthened. Transport teams should collaborate with their own marketing department in selecting specific promotional items bearing the team logo and contact information that can be distributed at educational sessions. These may include pens, pencils, key chains, note pads, posters, and drug dosage cards. One popular item is a small magnet, in the shape of an ambulance, with the team logo and contact information. Many referring facilities have magnetic patient tracking boards, and these magnets are used by the referring facility to "mark" transport patients when a transfer is in progress.

Benefits of Outreach Education

Education and training activities provide an opportunity to discuss issues associated with transport and expand the knowledge base of referring hospital personnel when stabilizing the condition of a neonatal or pediatric patient for transport. Many times, referring hospital personnel are anxious to learn more about the disease process and current management, as well as how they can better care for the patient until the transport team arrives. This is also a good opportunity for a team to learn about its customers, their needs, and the transport team's performance and perception in the community. Delivering a well-developed case study with highlighted topics and care interventions of representative infants or children transported (or not) from a referring hospital provides an open forum for multidisciplinary discussion and possible improvements of care while strengthening community ties. Instructors must be trained, however, to avoid alienating the audience with perceived or real criticisms of care and personnel and to be able to solicit and graciously accept constructive criticism of their transport service. The outreach educator should always emphasize what was done well by the referring hospital and its staff.

Outreach education also benefits transport team members by refreshing their own knowledge base when preparing educational offerings. They may develop a better understanding of what referring facilities may be faced with when presented with a critically ill patient (few referring facilities will have the pediatric subspecialists and equipment immediately available that may be considered routine and necessary at the transport team's base facility). Increasing regional awareness of the transport team, its capabilities, and how to access the service will further enable overall program success. Most important, pretransport patient care may be improved, as may the overall patient outcomes.

Learning Styles

When implementing outreach education, adult learning styles need to be considered. Adult learners have accumulated knowledge and experience that serve as a foundation for future learning experiences. They are internally motivated to learn and seek application for the knowledge they gain. The education program needs to be consistent with the learners' current knowledge base and skills.

When contemplating outreach education, take into consideration the experience level of the learners and the topic to be presented. The educator should have a strong knowledge base for the topic to be presented. Being aware of the knowledge base of the learners on the topic to be presented can help the educator tailor the presentation of material to the level of training and experience of the attendees. An interactive approach may facilitate retention of material presented and elicit enthusiasm toward learning from the participants. Case studies can be an effective method of building on the knowledge base of adult learners. Information is presented in a manner in which learners can listen and visualize; then the information is applied in the case study by the learners and facilitated by the educator. Case-based discussions, with specific identifiers removed and presented in an educational, nonjudgmental manner can be useful, especially with cases from the referring institution. Although presentations with paper-based handouts have been the traditional teaching method, other methods of facilitating learning may be more effective for adult learners.

■■■■■■■■■■■■■■■■■■■■■■■■■■■■■■■■■

Simulation-based training is an excellent method of facilitating interactive learning. The learner is placed in a realistic environment and actively participates in a medical scenario and a postsimulation debriefing. Technology-intensive, simulation-based training may be limited by availability and financial constraints. However, similar medical scenarios can be created with less expensive mannequins and the educator facilitating the scenario. This interactive, hands-on method allows learners to attain experience and gain confidence in a lower-stress environment. When distance, financial, and time constraints limit the number of educational offerings, videoconferencing may provide the opportunity to effectively reach a larger audience.

Referring hospital-staff rarely have the opportunity to view transport operations from the transporters' viewpoint. If your program permits, ride-along programs are a creative means of sharing the transport experience with clinical and managerial staff at the receiving and referring hospitals.

Education Content

Appendix E lists multiple certification courses that could be used for transport-related outreach education efforts. Table 14-2 lists more detailed topics for consideration. Members of the transport team should be encouraged to become qualified instructors of national certification/resuscitation courses and to teach these whenever possible. Transport team members should participate in the courses taught as community outreach. This may aid the transport team members in bedside teaching skills and confidence, an integral part of the educational process, and it should help maintain consistency in education.

Not all education topics listed in Appendix E and Table 14-2 can be offered to every referring facility. However, even if a transport team does not provide the course, it can encourage participation in national courses. For specific topics, the team can make suggestions or defer to the topics the referring facility considers the most important. When presenting selected topics, team members can leave references, scripts, videos, or summaries that supplement the information presented. When the team provides a brief (1- to 4-hour), nursing-focused outreach education program, it is helpful to offer it more than once in 1 day to reach staff from different shifts.

Table 14-2: Sample Topic List for a Transport-related Outreach Education Program

- General topics (eg, stabilization of the patient's condition for transport)
- Respiratory (eg, upper and lower airway disease, structural anomalies such as diaphragmatic hernia, tracheoesophageal fistula)
- Cardiovascular (eg, shock, congenital heart disease, arrhythmias)
- Neurologic (eg, coma, seizures)
- Poisonings
- Trauma (accidental, nonaccidental, birth-related)
- Metabolic (eg, diabetic ketoacidosis, congenital metabolic disorder)
- Hematologic-oncologic emergencies (eg, sickle cell crisis, primary and secondary hemorrhagic diathesis)
- Infection-related emergencies (eg, sepsis, meningitis)
- Renal (eg, renal failure)
- Surgical emergencies in addition to those involving the respiratory system
- Transport case reviews
- Management of accompanying and nonaccompanying family members

---

Objectives and Implementation

It is important to approach outreach education as an opportunity for positively influencing care for children. Transport team members may be concerned about criticizing the management by referring hospital staff and the potential effects on future referrals. It is recommended that "ground rules" be presented and agreed on by all participants, including the confidentiality of any discussions held during case reviews. Education should be provided in a nonjudgmental manner, and the participants should be encouraged to offer their own experiences and cases and to point out to others any unique or unusual capabilities or configurations of their own facility.

Communication among transport team members and referring facility personnel at the time of a stressful neonatal or pediatric stabilization can be difficult. Professionals, often previously unknown to each other, must work together and trust each other in the interest of optimal patient care. The value of advanced preparation through outreach education cannot be overemphasized. There is a different quality of cooperation (hopefully improved) and mutual trust when a team member and staff member recognize each other from a previous nonstressful encounter.

Outreach education should not be limited to referring health care facilities. The transport team members are experts in pediatric and neonatal care. Developing relationships with local, regional, and/or state emergency medical services agencies also should be an important outreach activity. Well-prepared prehospital providers will become more comfortable with smaller patients and able to provide better care to pediatric and neonatal patients. Many EMS agencies offer regular continuing education conferences throughout the year, and the transport team members (physicians, nurses, respiratory therapists, and paramedics) can be the experts to bring some of the same formal courses or individual lectures and skills to prehospital providers at these conferences. Members of the transport team (physicians, nurses, and paramedics) also may be invited to participate on regional or state-wide prehospital committees, as advisors, and to share their expertise in developing and/or refining protocols.

Outreach education programs are an essential component of a successful transport program. This is especially true in pediatrics because referring facility staff may be less well trained, inexperienced, and/or uncomfortable when faced with a critically ill neonate or child. Outreach education benefits the patients, transport team personnel, referring hospital personnel, and receiving hospital. Better stabilization of the patient's condition may occur, communication will improve, and referrals may increase.

Selected Readings

Aehlert B. *ACLS Quick Review Study Guide.* 2nd ed. St Louis, MO: Mosby, Inc; 2002

Cummins RO, ed. *ACLS Provider Manual.* Dallas, TX: American Heart Association; 2002

Dieckmann RA, ed. *American Academy Pediatrics Pediatric Education for Prehospital Professionals (PEPP).* Sudbury, MA: Jones & Bartlett Publishers; 2000

Emergency Nurses Association. *Course in Advanced Trauma Nursing (CATN)-II: A Conceptual Approach to Injury and Illness.* 2nd ed. Dubuque, IA: Kendall/ Hunt Publishing Co; 2002

ENPC: Emergency Nursing Pediatric Course Instructor's Supplement. 3rd ed. Des Plaines, IL: Emergency Nurses Association; 2004

ENPC: Emergency Nursing Pediatric Course Provider Manual. 3rd ed. Des Plaines, IL: Emergency Nurses Association; 2004

SELECTED READINGS

Forrest S. Learning and teaching: the reciprocal link. *J Contin Educ Nurs.* 2004;35:74–79

Gauche M, ed. *APLS: The Pediatric Emergency Medicine Course Instructor Manual.* 4th ed. Elk Grove, IL: American Academy of Pediatrics; 2004

Hazinski MF, Cummins RO, Field JM, eds. *Handbook of Emergency Cardiovascular Care for HealthCare Providers.* Dallas, TX: American Heart Association; 2002

Hazinski MF, Zaritsky AL, Chameides L, Pedersen, AJ, Adirim, T. *American Academy of Pediatrics and American Heart Association PALS Provider Manual.* Dallas, TX: American Heart Association; 2002

Hotz H, Henn R, Lush S, Hollingsworth-Fridlund P, eds. *Advanced Trauma Care for Nurses Provider Manual 2003 Edition.* Santa Fe, NM: Society of Trauma Nurses; 2003

Karlsen K. *The S.T.A.B.L.E. Program Learner/Provider Manual.* 2006. Available at: http://www.stableprogram.org. Accessed January 13, 2006

Kattwinkel J, Zaichkin J, eds. *Instructor's Manual for Neonatal Resuscitation.* 3rd ed. Elk Grove Village, IL: American Academy of Pediatrics and American Heart Association; 2000

Kattwinkel J, Cook LJ, Nowacek G, et al. Regionalized perinatal education. *Semin Neonatol.* 2004;9:155–165

Linares AZ. Learning styles of students and faculty in selected health care professions. *J Nurs Educ.* 1999;38:407–414

Loewen L, Seshia MM, Askin DF, Cronin C, Roberts S. Effective delivery of neonatal stabilization education using videoconferencing to Manitoba. *J Telemed Telecare.* 2003;9:334–338

TNCC: Trauma Nursing Core Course Instructor Supplement. 5th ed. Des Plaines, IL: Emergency Nurses Association; 2000

TNCC: Trauma Nursing Core Course Provider Manual. 5th ed. Des Plaines, IL: Emergency Nurses Association; 2000

Yaeger KA, Halamek LD, Coyle M, et al. High-fidelity simulation-based training in neonatal nursing. *Adv Neonatal Care.* 2004;4:326–331

Subcommittee on Pediatric Resuscitation. *American Academy of Pediatrics and American Heart Association Pediatric Advanced Life Support: Instructor's Manual.* Dallas, TX: American Heart Association; 2001

Questions

1. The products of outreach education are:
   a. Better community image
   b. Improved initial care
   c. Improved communications
   d. Potential increase in market share
   e. All of the above
2. The following are all true *except:*
   a. Only the most senior transport team personnel should participate in outreach education.
   b. Outreach efforts should be determined by request and perceived need.
   c. Outreach educators should be trained in effective adult learning techniques.
   d. Case reviews should be focused and nonjudgmental.
   e. Learning can occur by the transport team educators and by the participants in the educational sessions.
3. Outreach education should be considered an optional component of a pediatric transport system.
   a. True
   b. False

Answers

1. e
2. a
3. b

CHAPTER 15

Financial Considerations

Outline

- Review of the financial equations included in transport
- Billing, coding, and reimbursement
- Contractual options and vendor relationships
- Nonfinancial components of the transport service (goodwill, exposure, and branding)
- Carve-out options
- Economies of scale and scope

Transport capabilities are a necessity for regional pediatric centers. Stand-alone or unit-based transport teams may not be financially desirable if evaluated as independent entities. The contribution of the transport service to the additional charges and revenue (including diagnostic, procedural, personnel, global, and ancillary charges) generated for the health care system by transported patients needs to be considered when evaluating the financial impact of a transport program. The value of a reliable and efficient transport system cannot be overstated with respect to community perception and public relations. *Goodwill,* defined as an intangible asset that provides a competitive advantage, such as a strong brand or reputation or high employee morale, and an altruistic attitude, however, are not enough to keep a transport team solvent. Because most neonatal-pediatric transport teams exist as subsidiaries of larger organizations, it is important that transport team management personnel become and remain familiar with fiscal issues germane to transport and program management. In this chapter, a number of budgetary and fiscal issues are discussed. This is not an exhaustive review, and readers are encouraged to explore the noted references, readings, and other resources.

■■■■■■■■■■■■■■■■■■■■■■■■■■■■■■■■■■■■

Table 15-1: Transport Costs

■ Fixed Costs
1. Facility costs
   ✧ Utilities
   ✧ Maintenance
2. Personnel costs (salaried employees)
   ✧ Fringe benefits
   ✧ Wages
3. Planned and scheduled equipment maintenance
4. Durable equipment depreciation and replacement
   ✧ Transport vehicles (owned or leased by the institution)
   ✧ Monitoring equipment
5. Contract requirements

■ Variable Costs
1. Disposable supplies
2. New equipment and preventive maintenance
3. Nonsalaried, variable personnel costs
   ✧ Wages (hourly employees)
   ✧ Fringe benefits (hourly employees)
   ✧ Overtime wages
4. Vehicle usage costs
   ✧ Unscheduled vehicular repair
   ✧ Mileage costs
   ✧ Fuel costs

Review of the Financial Equations Included in Transport

Budgeting is an important part of planning for a transport program's organizational structure and resources. The budget is probably the most fundamental financial document any division of a health care organization develops and may be the first encounter that a health care manager has with accounting information. The budget is a basic tool for tying together the planning and implementation functions of management.

The budgeting process and the results of the approved budget plan serve to allocate limited organizational resources among competing users. Comparing actual results with budgeted results helps to evaluate the performance of individuals, contractual agreements, and system operations and illustrates the relative revenues and expenses and their respective variances.

When establishing a budget, managers should consider the fixed and variable costs of a transport program (Table 15-1). Fixed costs include buildings, utilities, compensation of salaried employees (including administrative personnel), physical plant maintenance, owned or leased transport vehicles, and existing equipment. Variable costs include supplies, new equipment, wages of part-time or registry employees, vehicle maintenance, mileage and fuel costs, and overtime wages.

To best understand the transport service's financial position, a comprehensive financial analysis is necessary to evaluate the strengths and weaknesses of the current transport team contracts. Each payer's contracted reimbursement rate needs to be evaluated and compared with the transport team's cost/charge ratio.

Transport team revenue and margins by payer class, segmented by Medicare, Medicaid, commercial, managed care, and self-paid categories, should be delineated. Transport cost/charge ratio trends and statistical comparisons with industry benchmarks should be developed. Collaboration with established experts within the institution will be important to understand and strategize regarding the impact of financial data.

Furthermore, transport costs per adjusted (a financial calculation and comparator that includes all of the hospital's inpatient and outpatient services) discharge and adjusted patient transport should be ascertained in addition to a statement of operations analyses and balance sheet analyses. Depending on the employee status of the transport team and the physicians at the institution, the highest reimbursement per transport may be if all charges (physician, nurse, nurse practitioner, respiratory care practitioner, supplies, and equipment) are billed to the patient and collected directly by the institution. The institution should evaluate whether the revenues will be sufficient to support the number of full-time-equivalent positions necessary to provide the coverage required for the transport team.

Billing, Coding, and Reimbursement

Transport teams can establish various types of relationships with institutions in the region they serve. One approach is interfacility agreements, which the institutions enter into with the understanding that the patient's transfer to the tertiary institution will be streamlined, as long as there are no insurance or other operational restraints.

A second type of arrangement can be made whereby a tertiary transport team may contract with other institutions that have smaller units and may not have the volume necessary to maintain the skills or to make a transport program cost-effective. These contractual agreements may be made on a fixed dollar amount per transport or prorated on an hourly rate plus replacement of supplies.

When establishing a fixed rate per transport or an hourly rate, actual costs, depreciation of equipment, goodwill, and missed opportunities need to be accounted for and factored into the respective charges. The tertiary institution must be thorough and well versed on the appropriate billing codes, charges, and reimbursement opportunities for critical care transport. Depending on the transport team staff, there may be different potential charges that can be applied to each transport. There are essentially 5 levels of charges that can be billed for each patient. If there is an attending physician present on the transport, there are specific *Current Procedural Terminology (CPT®)* transport codes that can be applied; they are noted here and summarized in Table 15-2:

- 99371–99373: Telephone consultation or coordination of management with providers before arrival of the transport team
- 99288: Physician direction of emergency medical services, emergency care, or advanced life support used for directing the transport staff from a hospital or facility using 2-way communication
- 99289: Physician constant attention of the critically ill or injured patient, younger than 24 months of age, during an interfacility transport (the first 30–74 minutes of direct contact [face-to-face] with the transport patient). Care of less than 30 minutes should not be reported with this code (instead use appropriate evaluation and management code).
- 99290: Physician constant attention of the critically ill or injured patient, younger than 24 months of age, during an interfacility transport (for each additional 30 minutes of direct care with the transport patient; use in conjunction with 99289)
- 99291: The first 30 to 74 minutes of critical care services provided by a physician to a patient older than 24 months. Care of less than 30 minutes should not be reported with this code (instead use appropriate evaluation and management code).

Table 15-2: *Current Procedural Terminology* Codes for Transport Physician Involvement

Code	Service Provided	Time	Requirements to Bill for Service*
99373	Telephone consultation before team arrival		Documentation of interaction
99288	Physician direction of team		2-way communication during transport
99289	Physician presence during transport (patient <24 mo of age)	30–74 min	Constant physician attention during transport
99290	Physician presence during transport (patient <24 mo of age)	Additional 30 min after 74 min	Constant physician attention during transport
99291	Physician-provided critical care (patient >24 mo of age)	30–74 minutes	Constant physician attention; patient condition described as critical
99292	Physician-provided critical care (patient >24 mo of age)	Additional 30 min after 74 min	Constant physician attention; patient condition described as critical

Adapted from *CPT 2006: Current Procedural Terminology.* American Medical Association. Chicago, IL: AMA Press; 2005.

*The supervising physician cannot code the actual procedures and interventions provided by the team in the field unless the physician is physically present with the team during the transport. Billable care begins when the physician assumes primary responsibility for the patient's care at the referring hospital. All procedures can be reported separately, but the time spent performing these procedures needs to be subtracted from the face-to-face time.

■ 99292: Physician-provided critical care services for each 30-minute period beyond 74 minutes to a patient older than 24 months (for each additional 30 minutes of direct care with the transport patient; use in conjunction with 99291)

Note that these care codes may not be used until the physician has encountered the patient, and the times include only direct care, not preparation or transport time to the referring institution. Billing and reimbursement usually are based on the *CPT* codes and the Resource-Based Relative Value Scales offered by the federal government. Payers may have difficulty understanding the scope of these codes, and payer billing programs may not be updated frequently. As part of contract negotiations, an experienced coding expert may be useful to help all parties understand the guidelines that appear in the *CPT* codes and in *Coding for Pediatrics,* published by the

American Academy of Pediatrics. Information about the American Medical Association's *CPT* text is available at http://www.ama-assn.org/ and about *Coding for Pediatrics,* at http://www.aap.org/.

If the transport program employs nurse practitioners who will bill for their services, they may be required to receive a provider number under the specific state's Medicaid program, as the guidelines for coding and reimbursement are state-specific. Different rules may apply if the nurse practitioner is employed by a physician group. These nurse practitioners may bill for their services (under the direction of a physician) for Medicaid, managed care, and commercial insurance. If none of the nursing personnel are nurse practitioners, the hospital may bill a flat hourly fee for the nursing personnel, as well as for respiratory care personnel. In addition, supplies and equipment used during the transport may be billed according to the hospital's respective charges, individually or in prebundled sets.

Contractual Options and Vendor Relationships

Some programs find vendor services to be an efficient method of supplying essential but expensive services. Because transport vehicles are an expense that require additional certification and administrative oversight to operate, many programs find the efficiencies offered by vendors to be helpful in meeting transportation needs. Most businesses, hospitals included, use a number of outside (nonowned) service contractors to provide services. Expertise in managing service contracts should exist in the institution and should be included in all negotiations and contract management interactions. Before establishing a vendor relationship, the base facility should evaluate the availability of suppliers and the impact of the relationship on the program and the organization. A number of questions should be answered before beginning the formal search for the right supplier: Are there suppliers in the market that can provide the service? Are there suppliers in the market interested in forming a contractual relationship for services required? Will the relationship be valuable to the base facility (ie, Will the expense of the supply contract be offset by potential benefits?)? What is the base hospital willing to pay for the contracted service? What portion of the cost will be reimbursed by revenue generated as the hospital sells the contracted service to a third party? Do the suppliers in the area have expertise in managing service contracts with a health care organization? As one finds with transport in general, the benefit of the contract may reap more than financial benefits to both parties. The ability to provide efficient service to distant hospitals may promote goodwill that enhances marketing efforts to communities served.

Once the decision is made to find a vendor, a request for proposals (RFP) should be distributed to potential vendors. These are identified through an evaluation of the potential candidates and a prescreening by the transport program and/or institution. Once the RFPs are returned from interested vendors, the review and interview process begins. In essence, the base facility and transport staff must find the best value. All vendors will be eager to tout their advantages, but limitations must be presented and understood. Understanding a vendor's limitations becomes as important as understanding its strengths. Once limitations are identified, the transport program must ask, "How will limitations be overcome?" It is not acceptable to jeopardize a patient's condition, and alternatives must be developed in advance. Financial arrangements are important to evaluate in advance. How does the vendor want to be paid? Will the vendor directly bill patients for services? What is the direct avenue for dispute management and resolution? Will the base facility receive a reduced rate as a result of a guaranteed volume? It is important at this stage to identify responsible people in the vendor's organization and determine the ability of the identified people to effect change if a contract is signed.

Vendor contracts require management throughout the life of the contract. An administrative official at the base facility should be a liaison between the transport team and the hospital's administration. This person, along with the transport program manager, should monitor financial and service components of the contracts on a regular basis. A clear line of communication and frequent interaction with a responsible member of the contract service provider's staff is essential.

CHAPTER 15

Nonfinancial Components of the Transport Service (Goodwill, Exposure, and Branding)

By evaluating engineering firms in the United Kingdom, Maclaran and McGowan[1] made several observations of importance to small business that must compete in a market that includes competitors of varying sizes. Maclaran and McGowan[1] evaluated how small firms that are disadvantaged owing to size compete favorably with larger firms able to take advantage of economies of scale and major investment in research and development. They found that small firms differentiated themselves by providing better customer care and quality of service. Smaller firms maintained closer relations with clients, and, as a result, they understood the client's philosophy and approach to business. When problems arose, clients were able to approach a person at small firms directly and obtain rapid resolution. Because direct communication was possible, problems were solved quickly, and the client and the firm were more flexible. This improved customer care resulted in a positive image and significant customer loyalty.

The health care industry in general and transport services in particular could learn from these findings. Transport teams, by virtue of the fact that they are often relatively small budget subsidiaries of larger organizations, are similar to the small businesses studied by Maclaran and McGowan.[1] Because transport teams deal with a finite and usually small number of referral centers, the opportunities to use personal interaction to improve customer care and, thereby, create loyalty and a positive image are significant. By association, it is reasonable to assume that the base or sponsoring facility will make gains in loyalty and image as well. In a sense, if this pattern is followed, improved customer care will result in promotional and marketing success, leaving the transport team and its sponsoring facility with a branded image associated with quality service.

Carve-out Options

Carving out is a strategy that separates a specialty service (the carve out) from other services provided by an organization. A specialty care provider that usually assumes some financial risk to provide the service then manages the carved-out service. This strategy can result in significant cost savings and decreased financial and, potentially, legal risks for the parent organization while providing the service for its customers.

Carve-out arrangements vary significantly in form, benefit design, provider network characteristics, fee arrangements, and management techniques. The mental health care industry has used carve outs for some time to provide and manage care. Carve outs potentially could be beneficial for transport teams by allowing them to provide the service for an organization that wants to provide the service but is uncomfortable with the potential financial or other risks. The advantage of carve outs to the parent organization is the ability to share or totally mitigate financial risk for services deemed important by its customers and stakeholders. Risk sharing in this situation can take a number of forms, including a vendor contract in which the transport team that provides the service functions as a clearly separate and independent agency or an arrangement in which an agency provides the service under the name of the parent organization. Risk is minimized in either case for the parent organization because the agency providing the service agrees to manage the service and assumes responsibility for collecting reimbursable, charges and for the cost of the program.

Economies of Scale and Scope

Economies of scale and scope are defined, respectively, as follows. Reduction in cost per unit resulting from increased production achieves economies of scale through operational efficiencies. Economies of scale occur because the cost of producing an additional unit of goods falls as production increases. Economy of scope arises when the cost of performing multiple business functions simultaneously proves more efficient than performing each business function independently. Economy of scale, therefore, occurs as an organization consolidates units serving the same or similar function. Economy of scope occurs as an organization improves throughput (provides more services with the same resources).

Economies of scale reduce costs by reducing waste. The assumption is that if the same resource can be used to support 2 or more functions, it is wasteful to duplicate that resource and the functions should be merged so that all who require the resource can take advantage of it. With merger, efficiencies may occur because a single unit was too small to take advantage of economies of scale and scope. Economies of scale and scope also can be realized by merging units in a large hospital that are underutilized. In a study that reviewed a number of hospital mergers that occurred in the late 1980s, Sinay[2] compared operating efficiencies 2 years after merger occurred in 2 groups of hospitals: hospitals in one group were the result of the merger of 2 hospitals, and the other was a group of hospitals that had not merged. Mergers occurred during a 4-year period. Sinay[2] noted that merging hospitals revealed no diseconomies of scale premerger (waste), no economies of scale in the first year postmerger, and economies of scale in the second year postmerger. It seems that after the merger, hospitals needed to find and correct opportunities for saving. Differences in economies of scope were inconsistent between the control group and the merging hospital group.

This study may have some significant implications for transport services. Merging of units that provide the same function for different age groups of patients may be beneficial because it allows managerial and logistical expenses to be shared and, thus, decreases the allocated fixed cost per transport. In the classic sense, it might be difficult to appreciate how economies of scale can be realized if each transport retains an individual cost that is multiplied by simultaneous transports, although as noted, fixed costs (eg, salaried personnel, vehicles) that are allocated over more transports will indeed bring the real cost of each transport down, if within the established capacity of the current fixed assets. Economies of scope may be achieved by making transport team members more productive at the base facility when not engaged transporting a patient. Nonengaged personnel, after transport preparation and other requirements are completed, could participate in other easily transferable hospital-based activities (such as assignment to care for intensive care unit patients in stable condition, in-house transport, or phlebotomy) that could be accomplished while awaiting transport need.

References

1. Maclaran P, McGowan P. Managing service quality for competitive advantage in small engineering firms. *Int J Entrepreneurial Behav Res.* 1999;5:35–47
2. Sinay UT. Pre- and post merger investigation of hospital mergers. *East Econ J.* 1998;24:83–97

Selected Readings

Bradley JF, Salus T, eds. *Coding for Pediatrics 2006.* 11th ed. Elk Grove Village, IL: American Academy of Pediatrics; 2006

American Medical Association. *CPT 2006: Current Procedural Terminology.* Chicago, IL: AMA Press; 2005

Glaizier KL. Managing behavioral health. *J Healthc Manag.* 1998;43:393–396

Glazier KL, Eselius LL, Hu T, Shore KK, G'Sell WA. Effects of a mental health carve-out on use, costs and payers: a four-year study. *J Behav Health Serv Res.* 1999;26:381–389

Krumrey NA, Byerly GE. A step-by-step approach to identifying a partner—and making the partnership work. *Hosp Mater Manage Q.* 1995;16:10–14

Vonderabe B. Hopes and reality: a vendor's perspective on shared services in a total system. *Hosp Mater Manage Q.* 1988;10:70–75

Questions

1. Describe fixed costs that transport program management personnel should consider during the year's budgeting process.
2. Describe "economies of scale" and "economies of scope."
3. Will a responsive approach to customer service improve customer loyalty?

Answers

1. ▪ Facility costs
   ▪ Personnel costs (salaried employees)
   ▪ Equipment maintenance
   ▪ Durable equipment payments, depreciation, and replacement
   ▪ Contract requirements
2. Economies of scale occur because the cost of producing an additional unit of goods falls as production increases; economies of scale reduce cost by reducing waste. Economies of scope occur when the cost of performing multiple functions simultaneously is more efficient than performing each function independently, eg, each function requires the same infrastructure.
3. Small enterprises can distinguish themselves by providing direct and more responsive customer care and maintaining close personal relations with clients. The direct communication results in quicker problem recognition and resolution, which improves customer satisfaction and loyalty.

Database Development

Outline

- The transport database
- Development of the database
- Database architecture
- Computer database operation
- System configuration
- HIPAA and databases
- Legal discovery and databases

The transport team is often the initial recipient of patient health information. Entering referral information and data from the patient transport into a database has become increasingly important. Health care practitioners can review and evaluate data and develop critical pathways that can outline medical interventions in the care of transport patients. The data also can be used during communications with practitioners at a receiving facility for continuing care. Accessing patient databases allows the transport team to trend clinical care. As the data are monitored and reviewed, quality improvement appraisals, including analysis, study, and evaluation of patient care, will be evident. After receiving appropriate permissions and approvals, clinical research information can be derived from the database to critically evaluate present and future patient care. Quality improvement, patient outcomes, cost-effectiveness of patient care, and use of evolving transport technology are areas in which important information can be abstracted from a well-thought-out transport database.

In addition to analyzing health care issues, the transport patient database is also crucial for medical, transport, and hospital leaders and administrators to monitor and project the financial feasibility of operating a transport team and may also be used for billing purposes. Reimbursement patterns identify issues related to preauthorization, coding, and documentation. Cursory review might suggest a non-optimal financial picture but demonstrate "value added" if referring facilities find the transport team to be a valuable regional resource. Early recognition of financial challenges can result in appropriate correction of the course that minimizes their untoward effects. Furthermore, the database can help transport team management personnel define appropriate staffing patterns and requirements for supplies. Periodic review of the data allows the transport team to evaluate referral patterns and trends that can direct marketing efforts.

The Transport Database

In developing the transport database, the input data should reflect the questions and needs of people who will be accessing and using the data, such as the transport team (including the managers and directors), hospital administrators, pediatric and neonatal intensive care unit leaders, quality assurance committees, and regulators. The data should be current and relevant at the time of the patient encounter (transport), reliable, valid, legible, and comprehensible. Although the transport database does not include all elements in the medical record, there should be enough information to identify essential elements of the transport and to reconstruct the transport events (see Appendix A3).

Demographics and Other Elements

Basic demographic data positively identify each patient for the purposes of clinical care, billing, and market analysis. Each patient's name, address, date of birth, sex, and name of a responsible adult or guardian should be recorded. Because prospective forms of payment and risk sharing are becoming more prevalent, it is important to understand payment arrangements in advance. Many payers reserve the right to preauthorize a nonemergency transfer. Other inquiries in the demographic category should include patient origination (eg, facility, location within facility, contact personnel, and contact numbers within that facility), patient mix (adolescent vs pediatric vs neonatal), types of diseases, and treatment of conditions. Types of vehicles, equipment, and team composition can be ascertained from these data. An appropriately designed database can help obtain financial information as well, which can be valuable when assessing and strategizing specific or general financial issues. The database also can be useful for documenting quality management issues such as team personnel skills and experience, team composition, response time, and equipment failures.

Marketing

The transport database offers an excellent opportunity to identify potential impact of and resources for the development of marketing strategies. By identifying vital information, statistics, and trends, marketing personnel can acquire a better understanding of the health care–related needs and preferences of referring facilities and the geographic area. These specific needs can be targeted and the transport team's specialty services promoted. Data that reflect the quality of a transport team, such as excellent safety records, rapid availability of ground or air ambulances, use of experienced pediatric- and/or neonatal-trained transport personnel, and improved patient outcomes can be used to publicize a transport program.

Paper vs Electronic Databases

With the rapid advancement of computer technology, the ability to use data and information via electronic measures such as a computer database have made the transmission of patient health information more rapid and widespread. The paper record, on the other hand, has many drawbacks. Only 1 user can access the paper record at any given time; therefore, the record is restricted to 1 user at a time. As a result, communication among different health care providers is limited. Providers must rely on other practitioners' inconsistent documentation styles in terms of data organization, completeness, understandability, legibility, and chronology. Furthermore, maintenance and retrieval of thick and numerous paper records is costly and inefficient. Electronic record keeping reduces the incidence of inaccessibility and disparate information because it can serve numerous offices and organizations. The electronic record also can rapidly provide up-to-date and accurate records to people requiring their use. With the passage of the Health Insurance Portability and Accountability Act of 1996 (HIPAA), limiting access to the electronic record is required to protect patient confidentiality and security. Limited access can be achieved via a variety of methods, including operational policies and procedures and software security programs to ensure identification and accountability of all users of electronic records. Overall, as an electronic record, computer databases improve information handling, accessibility, and overall usefulness.

Development of the Database

Database users (should include the transport team medical director and representatives from the transport team, administration, admitting, medical informatics services, and communications departments, and research personnel) should collaborate with computer programmers on the development of the transport database program and interface. Other existing databases such as those from other transport programs, local emergency medical services, hospitals, and the military can serve as initial templates and can be modified to meet the specific needs of the transport team. There is not currently a universally accepted or available critical care transport database. Development of standard database application software, amendable by individual transport systems, with the ability to collect nonidentifiable data on a national level, would be useful in the quest to develop evidence-based assessments of current and future transport practices.

The database development should be done in a systematic manner in terms of objectives, design, and simplicity. By setting objectives, the users can clearly understand the function and what is expected of the data system. If this is not established early, collection of data may occur for a period before team members realize that it does not adequately address important questions posed by the users. Furthermore, buying hardware or software without outlining the objectives may result in system limitations. The design of the program must be user-friendly to ensure accuracy and to promote data entry, system use, and efficient queries.

Real-time data entry would prove advantageous to patient care. For example, if a notebook computer, tablet, or personal digital assistant (PDA) is used to record vital signs at the patient bedside during a transport, the data can be quickly analyzed for trends. Based on this analysis, critical medical interventions can be made in a timely manner. If data entry is not performed until after a transport is completed (after-the-fact entry), there is greater risk of error or omission. The data may have to be transferred from paper to an electronic record by another person or recoded for the database program. Furthermore, the additional workload and time involved in manual data entry and the potential for data loss (eg, missing chart or papers) or misrepresentation (eg, inaccurate or limited documentation) result in an inefficient process.

Data user input is essential in this process because data entry should be fluid and straightforward. For example, when accessing the various functions of the database, small details such as types of menu options (pop-up, pull-down, or radio button) need to be discussed. The data system should be kept simple, especially in the earliest phases of development. Recording every physiologic parameter on every transport patient will overwhelm the data system. Simple operational tasks such as ad hoc queries of the database to generate meaningful reports would be problematic. If the system is too complicated or inflexible, later changes may be difficult or impossible. It would be prudent for the database to be programmed to promptly produce standardized reports; therefore, the many different departments of an institution can easily access, retrieve, and have full use of the reports. These reports can be updated frequently throughout the year so that analysis of trends can be assessed rapidly. Conversely, institutional departments may also require specific and unique information. The database also should be designed to enable users to use straightforward methods to create specific reports on demand.

Understanding an organization's method of developing and maintaining its databases can prove useful to managers. Databases can communicate through programmed interfaces or function as one central database with a network of input and reading locations. Interfaced databases function as loose confederations. They are a system of individual databases designed to meet the needs of a single area. Once it becomes desirable to exchange information electronically, interfaces are created by programmers that allow the systems to exchange information. To accomplish this, programmers must examine the databases in question and create electronic links that allow communication. Even after interfaces are created, database control and maintenance may remain the responsibility of the original department. It is ideal to use a database or platform that is approved and supported by the institution's information services group. Although information and computer support 24 hours a day, 7 days a week is advantageous, departments may need contingency plans if there is a breakdown or malfunction of the data system. A person within a department who has been a part of the database development should be designated to develop a guidebook that can be used to remedy simple errors that may arise. This troubleshooting manual needs to be straightforward and easy to follow so that any qualified member of the department can address routine or simple issues and understand the appropriate response and path for resolution of more complicated concerns.

Integrated database systems develop a common database for the entire organization. This is important should a common query among departments occur. Data are made available simultaneously to the entire organization in a way that promotes networking and eliminates data duplication. Data accessibility and the ability to enter or change data, however, can (and should) be limited by user and location. These integrated data systems tend to be more efficient and improve data collection and management; however, security and confidentiality become more difficult to maintain. With more security measures (eg, passwords, data encryption, and firewalls) needed to protect the data from unauthorized viewing, accountability also becomes a factor. To restrict unauthorized access to databases, different levels of security need to be implemented. For example, a database system may be designed with 3 levels of security authorizations. The first is network security. A user is required to enter a valid password to log on to the network. The user is able to share his or her files with anyone with the same access authorization. The next level of security is database security. An additional password is required for access to the database system. The final level is administrative access, which is an exclusive right to the database file. A password is assigned to each specific person who has authorization to change, edit, add, or delete data from the database.

Once developed and functional, the transport patient database should be able to be accessed for any of the transport team's institutional and local needs. If a national database were to be developed, useful and meaningful transport data could be shared among transport teams in the United States and Canada. As a result, information exchange, care comparisons, and investigational opportunities among transport systems would be improved.

Database Architecture

It is recommended that transport services obtain data in the following categories for each patient transferred by the system:

1. **Demographic data:** Patient and referring facility identification and location within the facility and classification (can be preprogrammed for routine referral sources with prepopulated fields, although needs to be amendable if changes are needed), addresses, telephone, fax and pager numbers, Web and e-mail addresses, and referring and primary care physician identification

2. **System data:** Mode of transport, staffing levels, use of specific personnel and equipment during transport, date and time of the transport and pretransport and intratransport times, and communication attempts and successes between medical control and referring hospital with times

3. **Clinical and completion data:** Chief complaint, provisional diagnosis *(International Classification of Diseases, Ninth Revision, Clinical Modification [ICD-9-CM])*, patient acuity score, procedures *(Current Procedural Terminology [CPT])*, reason(s) for transport, clinical status (eg, intubated, pressors required), adverse events, discharge diagnoses *(ICD-9-CM)*, and disposition. Uniformity of coding will be facilitated by storing extracted lists of *ICD-9-CM* and *CPT* codes for diagnoses and procedures frequently encountered during transport and critical care. Financial data (including charges and submitted bills) also can be included in this database,

4. **Quality improvement:** Specific prospective or quality improvement monitors should be incorporated into the database. To understand the true effect of certain events or occurrences, these monitors should be capable of relating designated events to specific outcomes.

Computer Database Operation

During and on completion of a transport, data input should be accomplished by designated persons. Data input training of all transport team members increases consistency and accuracy. The medical director or transport team coordinator should supervise this process. If a hospital has an intake or communications center, pretransport data (patient name, demographics, referring hospital and physicians, telephone numbers, and initial diagnoses) should be entered before the transport team's departure. An ideal approach should be to have transport personnel input data during a patient transport. This could be accomplished via portable devices such as PDAs, graphic tablets, and notebook personal computers. The data later could be downloaded to the main database program, if not designed as a Web-based application. The download process can be done in a variety of ways: wireless (eg, infrared, Bluetooth [http://www.bluetooth.com/bluetooth/]), hardwire cable (eg, PDA cradle, USB, and serial), and a variety of storage media (eg, floppy disk, CD-ROM, memory sticks, compact flash cards, and jump drives). However, this could be a potentially expensive and troublesome venture. The data should be summarized, analyzed, and reported at periodic and routine (eg, monthly, quarterly and yearly) intervals. This report should include information about the number, ages, and diagnoses of patients transferred; methods of travel; and regions served by the team. Certifications (eg, Advanced Cardiac Life Support, Pediatric Advanced Life Support, Neonatal Resuscitation Program) and procedures performed by individual team members can be tracked and data on adverse effects on patient care and deaths identified. This information can be used as a tool during educational and quality improvement presentations at transport team staff meetings. Furthermore, reports prepared from the transport database should be distributed to appropriate management personnel, transport program administrators, transport team members, and support services.

System Configuration

System configuration will be determined by the needs of the transport team and its base facility. Individual systems may be based on a desktop platform or on a centralized mainframe and file server. Desktop database environments are characteristically single-user applications. Table size on a desktop storage system is fewer than 1 million records. Because the application resides on an individual desktop, software upgrades would have to be done for each separate computer. In contrast, mainframe systems house an entire operating system, database, and applications software. Therefore, all computers within a network can have their software upgraded at one time. Other potential advantages of mainframe computers include faster processing speeds, ultra-high storage capacities, and consistent backup and expanded levels of security.

To facilitate the exchange of data, readily available software should be used, and files should be exportable to a universal format, such as ASCII (American Standard Code for Informational Interchange). Operating systems such as Windows NT, 2000 and XP use Unicode, officially called the Unicode Worldwide Character Standard. IBM's S/390 systems use a proprietary code called EBCDIC (Extended Binary-Coded Decimal Interchange Code). Conversion programs allow different operating systems to change a file from one code to another. Technical aspects of database construction and operation should be under the direction of a qualified systems operator who confers frequently with the medical director and transport team coordinator. The system must be simple enough to provide answers to basic questions at any time, day or night.

HIPAA and Databases

The Privacy Rule

Because health-related databases are used for research purposes, they are subject to the regulations of the *Standards for Privacy of Individual Identifiable Health Information,* known as *the Privacy Rule.* As a result of HIPAA, the Department of Health and Human Services required "covered entities" such as health care providers, health plans, and health care clearinghouses to be in compliance with the Privacy Rule as of April 14, 2003. As a response to public concern about potential abuses of the privacy of health information, the Privacy Rule establishes a category of health information. This protected health information (PHI) or a person's identifiable health care information, can be used or disclosed to others in certain circumstances or under certain conditions (also see Chapter 7).

The Privacy Rule, however, allows covered entities such as hospitals, clinics, and other health care providers to continue to obtain data on their patients for treatment, payment, and health care purposes. This information can be entered into a database program without a patient's permission or "authorization." Furthermore, authorization is not needed if PHI is disclosed to government-authorized public health authorities for disease surveillance, disease prevention, and other public health purposes such as reporting disease and injury. As a result, many databases will be able to be maintained and updated and will remain available to researchers, although under new terms.

A covered entity may be permitted to use or disclose PHI for research under the following circumstances and conditions under the Privacy Rule:

- For reviews preparatory to research if certain representations are obtained from the researcher
- For research solely on a decedent's information if certain representations are obtained from the researcher
- If the subject of the PHI has granted specific written permission through an authorization
- If the covered entity receives appropriate documentation that an institutional review board (IRB) or another review body called a privacy review board has granted a waiver or an alteration of the authorization requirement
- If the PHI has been deidentified in accordance with the standards set by the Privacy Rule (in which case the health information is no longer PHI)
- If the information is released in the form of a limited data set, with certain identifiers removed and with a data use agreement between the researcher and the covered entity
- If informed consent of the individual to participate in the research, an IRB waiver of such informed consent, or other express legal permission to use or disclose the information for the research is grandfathered by the transition provisions

A waiver or alteration of authorization also provides for the databases for which no contact information is available. An IRB or a privacy review board will review criteria set forth by the Privacy

Rule to determine whether an approval of a wavier or alteration of authorization is warranted. This is based on whether PHI use or disclosure would not pose more than a minimal risk to the privacy of individuals. Criteria include the following: (1) an adequate plan presented to the IRB or privacy review board to protect PHI identifiers from improper use and disclosure; (2) an adequate plan to destroy those identifiers at the earliest opportunity; and (3) adequate written assurances that the PHI will not be reused or disclosed to any other person or entity except as required by law, for authorized oversight of the research study, or for other research for which the use of disclosure of the PHI is permitted by the Privacy Rule. Furthermore, the researcher must show that the project could not be practically conducted without the requested waiver and alteration and without access and use of the PHI.

The Limited Data Set

A limited data set refers to PHI that excludes 16 categories of direct identifiers. Certain identifiers that may include geographic information (not street addresses but city, state, and ZIP code), elements of dates (such as admission and discharge dates), and unique codes or identifiers not listed as direct identifiers defined in the Privacy Rule can be released as a limited data set to a researcher. The researcher must sign a data use agreement that describes the permitted uses and disclosures of the information received and prohibits reidentifying or using the information to contact individuals. The 16 categories of direct identifiers that must be stripped from the data set are listed in Table 16-1.

Covered entities may allow researchers to review PHI in databases for purposes preparatory for research. This allows a researcher to determine whether a sufficient number or type of records exists to conduct the research. To permit a researcher access to the PHI, the covered entity must obtain the following representations from the researcher: (1) the use of disclosure is requested solely to review PHI as necessary to prepare a research protocol or for similar purposes preparatory to research, (2) the PHI will not be removed from the covered entity in the course of review, and (3) the PHI for which use or access is requested is necessary for research. These representations can be in written or oral form.

■■■■■■■■■■■■■■■■■■■■■■■■■■■■■■■■■■■

Table 16-1: Categories of Direct Identifiers That Must Be Omitted to Create a Limited Data Set

1. Names
2. Postal address information, other than town or city, state, and ZIP code
3. Telephone numbers
4. Fax numbers
5. E-mail addresses
6. Social Security numbers
7. Medical record numbers
8. Health plan beneficiary numbers
9. Account numbers
10. Certificate and license numbers
11. Vehicle identifiers and serial numbers, including license plate numbers
12. Device identifiers and serial numbers
13. Web universal resource locators (URLs)
14. Internet protocol (IP) address numbers
15. Biometric identifiers, including finger and voice prints
16. Full face photographic images and any comparable images

The PHI of deceased persons can be disclosed for research without authorizations from the personal representative or next of kin, a waiver, or an alteration of authorization or data use agreement. The covered entity must receive the following from the researcher: (1) oral or written representations that the decedents' PHI is necessary for the research and is being sought solely for research on the PHI of decedents, (2) oral or written representations that the PHI for which use or disclosure is sought is necessary for the research purposes, and (3) at the request of the covered entity, documentation of the deaths of the study patients.

Deidentification of Health Information

Health information that has been deidentified may be used or disclosed by a covered entity without restriction under the Privacy Rule (see Chapter 7). By deleting 3 specific categories that potentially could identify the individual or the individual's relatives, employers, or household members from the limited data set, the resulting record is not PHI; therefore, it is not subject to the Privacy Rule.

The identifiers that must be removed are the following:

1. All geographic subdivisions smaller than a state, including street address, city, county, precinct, ZIP code, and their equivalent geographical codes, except for the initial 3 digits of a ZIP code if, according to the current publicly available data from the Bureau of the Census:

   a. the geographic unit formed by combining all ZIP codes with the same 3 initial digits contains more than 20 000 people and

   b. the initial 3 digits of a ZIP code for all such geographic units containing 20 000 or fewer people are changed to 000.

2. All elements of dates (except year) for dates directly related to an individual, including birth date, admission date, discharge date, and date of death; and all ages more than 89 years and all elements of dates (including year) indicative of such age, except that such ages and elements may be aggregated into a single category of age 90 years or older

3. Any other unique identifying characteristic or code

An alternative to establish deidentification of the health information, instead of removing all 18 identifiers, is to use statistical methods. Covered entities may have a qualified statistician ("a person with appropriate knowledge of and experience with generally accepted statistical and scientific principles and methods rendering information not individually identifiable"[1]) determine that there is a very small risk that the information used, alone or in combination with other reasonably available information, would be used by the anticipated recipient to identify the subject of the information.[1] The statistician also must document the methods and results of the analysis that justify such a determination.

HIPAA and Databases Before April 14, 2003

Under transition provisions, the PHI from databases that were established before the Privacy Rule's compliance date of April 14, 2003, still can be disclosed under certain conditions without an authorization. These conditions, which would have to be obtained by the covered entity by the compliance date, include the following: (1) an authorization or other express legal permission from an individual to use or disclose PHI for research, (2) the informed consent of the individual participating in the research, or (3) a waiver by an IRB of informed consent in accordance with applicable laws and regulations governing informed consent, unless informed consent is sought after the compliance date.

Legal Discovery and Databases

Because provision of health care has potential liability, databases, as a source of patient health information, are subject to legal discovery. Furthermore, existing reporting systems require disclosure of health care data to analyze errors that result in serious harm, near misses, or errors resulting in lesser harm. Protection from disclosure of submitted data, particularly in litigation, has been debated. One view holds that all information should be protected because accessed information could lead to possible litigation and interfere with quality improvement goals of reporting systems. On the other hand, another view considers that errors that are discovered in a reporting system should be disclosed because of the public's right to know.

Because databases are used for quality improvement activities, many states have quality assurance laws that protect these organizational databases from legal discovery. These laws (which vary greatly among states) do not, however, protect the databases if organizations share their data outside the organization. Federal laws seem to offer some protection to counteract the variability of 50 different states, but the laws have not been tested in court. Therefore, if a hospital shares quality improvement data about a medical error with a national reporting system such as the Patient Safety Reporting System, the data may be subpoenaed. In addition, an organization's quality improvement data also may be subpoenaed, if a specific medical error is in question.

Safeguards to decrease the risk of inadvertent discovery of errors from databases can be implemented. Private organizations may have only the option of the practice of confidentiality based on promise and practice. Organizations that have roles of quality improvement and enforcement can make data available only to those who need access for purposes of analysis and prevention. The data must be protected from unauthorized viewing within an institution. Thus, data on errors can be sequestered behind an internal curtain of confidentiality. Anonymous reporting ensures that the reporter cannot be identified from the report. This practice, however, can decrease the effectiveness of a reporting system. Because a loss of information may occur at the initial transfer of data, the recipient cannot go back to the reporter to obtain additional information. Furthermore, detailed information could be lost to a reporting system because it could identify a specific event or the reporter. Deidentified data also can be used as a practical protection against discovery. By removing specific elements from a set of identifiable health data, specific information of a reporting institution (such as type of center, size, and location) that may be crucial to a reporting system is not available.

Although these practice parameters can increase the reporting of information by providers, they do not fully protect providers from receiving a subpoena or having the data subsequently used against them. A combination of legal and practical protections enforced together provides the strongest assurance of confidentiality.

Reference

1. US Department of Health and Human Services. *Research Repositories, Databases and the HIPAA Privacy Rule.* Bethesda, MD: The National Institutes of Health; 2004. Available at: http://privacyruleandresearch.nih.gov/pdf/research_repositories_final.pdf

Selected Readings

Abdelhak M, Grostick S, Hanken MA, Jacobs, E. *Health Information: Management of a Strategic Resource.* 2nd ed. Philadelphia, PA: WB Saunders; 2001

Dorenfest SI. Health care information systems. In: Wolper LF, ed. *Health Care Administration: Principles, Practice, Structure, and Delivery.* 2nd ed. Gaithersburg, MD: Aspen Publishers, Inc; 1995:416–428

Kohn, LT, Corrigan JM, Donaldson MS, eds. *To Err is Human: Building a Safer Health System.* Washington, DC: National Academies Press; 2000

Kongstvedt PR, ed. *The Managed Health Care Handbook.* 4th ed. Gaithersburg, MD: Aspen Publishers, Inc; 2001

Pace WD, Staton EW, Higgins GS, Main DS, West DR, Harris DM. Database design to ensure anonymous study of medical errors: a report from the ASIPS Collaborative. *J Am Med Inform Assoc.* 2003;10:531–540

Roth RS. The transport data base. In: McCloskey KA, Orr RA eds. *Pediatric Transport Medicine.* St Louis, MO: Mosby–Year Book, Inc; 1995: 635–646

Questions

1. Which of the following statements regarding transport databases is *false*?
   a. Periodic review of the data allows the transport team to evaluate referral patterns and trends and can help establish risk-sharing agreements between referring and receiving facilities.
   b. Review of a transport database can show that a transport team is a financial advantage to an institution.
   c. Marketing strategies can be developed from transport databases to publicize the transport program.
   d. Quality management issues are often difficult to retrieve from a transport database.
2. Which of the following is *false* when comparing paper and electronic databases?
   a. The electronic database can rapidly provide up-to-date and accurate records.
   b. Limiting access to the electronic record is as important as limiting access to the paper record.
   c. The electronic record is restricted to 1 user at a time.
   d. Maintenance and retrieval of paper records is expensive and inefficient.
3. Which of the following is *not* one of the identifiers that must be removed from health information if the data are to qualify as a limited data set?
   a. Names
   b. Birth dates
   c. Telephone numbers
   d. Health plan beneficiary numbers

Answers

1. d. The transport database is a tool that allows transport and hospital administrators to determine the usefulness and feasibility of a transport program. Marketing a transport team in terms of safety records and improved patient outcomes can promote a transport program's record to potential referring facilities. Quality management programs are required for regulatory agencies such as the Commission on Accreditation of Medical Transport Services, Medicare, and the Joint Commission on Accreditation of Healthcare Organizations.

2. c. The electronic database allows the transmission of up-to-date and accurate patient health information rapidly to many users simultaneously. The paper record, on the other hand, is costly and inefficient. Users of the paper record are subject to legibility, organizational, and comprehensive and single-user issues. Limiting access to the electronic record to authorized users is imperative, however, especially after passage of the Health Insurance Portability and Accountability Act of 1996 (HIPAA). A combination of operational policies, procedures, and software security programs should be used to ensure accountability of all users of electronic records.

3. b. A limited data set is described as health information that excludes certain listed direct identifiers but may include city, state, ZIP code, and elements of dates. There are 16 direct identifiers listed in the Privacy Rule's limited data set provisions. These provisions apply not only to information about the individual, but also to information about the individual's relatives, employers, and household members.

Transport Research

Outline

- Medical advances studied for transport
- Potential topics for future transport research
- Funding and training in transport research

With the development of neonatal and pediatric transport medicine as a specialty during the last 70 years, there has come a need among transport providers for more evidence-based clinical practice. Although it seems logical when developing a new program to simply apply neonatal intensive care unit (NICU), pediatric intensive care unit (PICU), and emergency department clinical protocols, most transport professionals quickly discover that many techniques and therapies used in the hospital need to be adapted to the unique ground and air transport environments.

Although neonatal-pediatric transport programs are often part of children's hospitals, many teams originate from general adult and pediatric programs. Given the variability of training and experience among team members, it is of vital importance that there be more organized efforts on a national level to improve quality of care using evidence-based research. Ideally, this research will be incorporated into future evidence-based revisions of the *Transport Guidelines*.

Much neonatal-pediatric transport clinical research has focused on justification and optimal composition of specialized neonatal-pediatric transport programs. Limited investigational reports, mostly single-center studies, during the last few decades, have analyzed the benefit and efficacy of key transport equipment and therapies.

This chapter reviews some of the key pediatric advances that have been critically examined in the transport arena, lists potential areas for future research projects, and discusses funding and training opportunities to improve the quality of transport research.

Medical Advances Studied for Transport

Transport Risk Scores

Many teams have used the Pediatric Risk of Mortality (PRISM), Score for Neonatal Acute Physiology (SNAP and SNAP II), and Glasgow Coma Scale (GCS) in their clinical practice; however, except for the Glasgow Coma Scale score, these assessment tools were developed primarily for in-hospital use. In 2001, Lee et al[1] reported the development and application of the Transport Risk Index of Physiologic Stability (TRIPS) instrument. This specific infant transport assessment tool includes clinical signs such as temperature, blood pressure, respiratory status, and response to noxious stimuli. These investigators report that their scoring model was a reliable predictor of short-term mortality (<7 days), total NICU mortality, and severe intraventricular hemorrhage. Their results confirm the usefulness of risk assessment compared with arbitrary scoring methods. This method is limited, however, to neonates and infants, thereby leaving the older pediatric patients without a well-studied transport-specific risk assessment tool.

Surfactant Administration

The use of exogenous natural surfactant is the standard of care for neonates with confirmed respiratory distress syndrome (RDS). There still is debate about the benefit of administering surfactant immediately after birth (prophylactically) or within the first few hours of life (for rescue). Regardless, multiple studies have shown consistently that early administration has benefit in preventing long-term mortality and morbidity for neonates with RDS.

Although it seems logical to give surfactant to appropriate patients by the transport team at the referring hospital, there have been only a small number of abstracts and studies reporting outcomes and complications with this practice. Clinical concerns of transport team members administering surfactant include the following: (1) level and experience of personnel training, (2) sudden hypoxemia, (3) plugged or displaced endotracheal tubes, (4) air leaks due to sudden increases in lung compliance, and (5) pulmonary hemorrhage. In addition to the fact that there may be limited resources at the referring hospital should a complication occur, the need to travel with the infant can make assessment and intervention more challenging following surfactant administration. In response, many teams have arbitrarily adopted a minimum 30-minute wait time after surfactant dosing before a neonate can be moved to adjust ventilator settings, including pressure limits and the fraction of inspired oxygen.

In one small survey-based study, Costakos et al[2] found no significant differences between the neonates receiving surfactant before transport and the control group receiving surfactant after NICU admission. This study was survey data from 100 centers but was limited by lack of clear and consistent information about who gave the surfactant at the referring hospital (eg, referring team vs the transport team).

Extracorporeal Membrane Oxygenation During Transport

Extracorporeal membrane oxygenation (ECMO) is a well-established method of providing cardiopulmonary support to neonates with life-threatening cardiac and/or respiratory failure. Since the 1980s, ECMO has been used to treat more than 18,000 neonates and 4,000 pediatric patients. In general, safe performance of ECMO requires a team of medical professionals, including neonatologists, intensivists, pediatric surgeons, perfusionists, and NICU/PICU nursing and respiratory care staff. Because of the complexity of the equipment and the need for anticoagulation, only a few transport programs have developed the capability to initiate ECMO and transport patients during ECMO to tertiary centers. Wilson et al[3] recently reported a 16-year experience of transporting neonates and pediatric patients to military hospitals after cannulation for ECMO at the referring center. There are also a few case reports of smaller numbers of patients transported successfully during ECMO.

Despite the fact that several studies have demonstrated that ECMO can be performed during transport, there is no evidence that this practice is preferable to transfer of an ECMO candidate while providing critical care therapies for cardiac or respiratory failure. Most ECMO centers encourage early identification and transport of patients who may require ECMO to prevent the patient's condition from becoming too unstable for travel. If an ECMO center is considering offering ECMO services during transport, it is essential to understand the potential morbidity of ECMO transports and the added number of specialists and specialized vehicles that will be required.

Inhaled Nitric Oxide

Inhaled nitric oxide (iNO) has become the standard of care to treat severe hypoxic respiratory failure associated with pulmonary hypertension in term and near-term neonates. Nitric oxide is a selective pulmonary vasodilator with minimal systemic side effects.

After reviewing many multicenter neonatal studies, the US Food and Drug Administration approved the use of iNO in term and near-term neonates older than 34 weeks' gestation. The efficacy of iNO in preterm neonates is still being studied. Kinsella et al[4] and Jesse et al[5] have published single-center reports on the use, efficacy, and safety of iNO during ground and air transport. These studies have established the feasibility of administering iNO to critically ill neonates during transport, but they lack control groups to demonstrate improvement in patient outcome.

Commercial equipment is available to provide iNO in conjunction with many transport ventilators and manual ventilation systems. The American Academy of Pediatrics has published some key references detailing its clinical use.[6] Teams contemplating the use of iNO during transport should ensure the following: (1) training of personnel on the delivery of iNO in the NICU before transport, (2) availability of equipment for measuring dosage and monitoring for environmental exposure of personnel to gas by-products, and (3) a protocol developed with neonatal experts to determine the appropriate patients for iNO therapy.

Potential Topics for Future Transport Research

Table 17-1 details by category some potential topics for future neonatal and pediatric transport studies. The list is only a starting point and should be expanded whenever possible.

Proposed research questions should be answerable and directly relevant to clinical transport medicine. Studies must be well designed; approved by appropriate institutional review boards; performed in a compliant, ethical manner; and appropriately peer-reviewed in presentation and/or publication venues (see Chapter 18). Research

Table 17-1: Possible Topics for Neonatal and Pediatric Transport Research Studies*

A. Administration and personnel
1. Team composition (eg, nurse, neonatal nurse practitioner, registered respiratory therapist, physician): Are there optimal standards?
2. Unit-based vs stand-alone teams and their effectiveness
3. Informed consent procedures: Are they sufficient?
4. Should parents be transported with their critically ill children?
5. Telemedicine: outcomes and cost
6. Infectious disease protocols
7. Role of accreditation on quality and outcomes

B. Financial analysis
1. *Current Procedural Terminology* codes and reimbursement analysis
2. Cost justification of specialty transport teams

C. NICU medical therapies
1. Initiation of iNO during transport: Does it make a difference?
2. Thermoregulation: analysis of different incubators and techniques
3. Surfactant: analysis of effectiveness and side effects
4. Maternal transfer after neonatal transport
5. Development and testing of acuity scoring models
6. Head cooling

D. PICU and ED medical therapies
1. EMS, PICU, or ED team for pediatric and trauma transports
2. Initiation of shock treatment protocols and outcome analysis
3. Development and testing of acuity scoring models
4. Disaster management: Should transport teams be included in regional plans?

E. Outcomes
1. Morbidity and mortality comparison of critically ill neonates born at a community vs a tertiary center
2. Adult vs specialty teams for pediatric patients
3. Air vs ground: outcomes and costs
4. Reverse transport: practice, benefits, and limitations

*NICU indicates neonatal intensive care unit; iNO, inhaled nitric oxide; PICU, pediatric intensive care unit; ED, emergency department; and EMS, emergency medical services.

is needed to test new and existing equipment, therapies, and protocols for effectiveness and cost-efficacy. There is concern that some of our currently used transport equipment has not been optimally tested to determine compliance with national safety standards. Moreover, studies should be conducted to determine whether existing national safety guidelines are sufficient for neonates and children transported via specific modes of transport and with commercially available isolettes and stretchers.

Funding and Training in Transport Research

Not until 1990 did transport medicine receive section status within the American Academy of Pediatrics. The Section on Transport Medicine and other national transport organizations have recently increased their focus on efforts to improve quality of care using evidenced-based research. Because transport proposals have not constituted a large percentage of granting agency requests for research study applications through Requests for Applications, many qualified projects have not been conducted owing to lack of funds. Funding may be available through private foundations, national transport or pediatric health care organizations (Table 17-2), and some private corporations.

Table 17-2: Sources of Possible Grant Information and Support for Neonatal-Pediatric Transport Research

Name	Address
American Academy of Pediatrics	http://www.aap.org
Association of Air Medical Services	http://www.aams.org
National Association of EMS Educators	http://www.naemse.org
National Institutes of Health	http://www.nih.gov
Emergency Services for Children	http://www.ems-c.org
March of Dimes	http://www.modimes.org

In part because most transport programs have been primarily focused on the provision of clinical care, there has not been a strong emphasis on research and research funding. It is clear, however, that to improve the clinical care, quality, skilled, and funded research and researchers are required. Clinical research training (eg, study design, grant writing, biostatistics, and epidemiology) may be obtained at local medical schools or universities. In fact, many medical centers have established clinical research facilities and staff to support personnel in obtaining skills and conducting clinical studies.

References

1. Lee SK, Zupancic JA, Pendray M, et al. Transport risk index of physiologic stability: a practical system for assessing infant transport care. *J Pediatr.* 2001;139:220–226
2. Costakos D, Allen D, Krauss A, et al. Surfactant therapy prior to the interhospital transport of preterm infants. *Am J Perinatol.* 1996;13;309–316
3. Wilson BJ, Heiman HS, Butler TJ, Negaard KA, DiGeronimo R. A 16-year neonatal/pediatric extracorporeal membrane oxygenation transport experience. *Pediatrics.* 2002;109:189–193
4. Kinsella JP, Griebel J, Schmidt JM, Abman SH. Use of inhaled nitric oxide during interhospital transport of newborns with hypoxemic respiratory failure. *Pediatrics.* 2002;109:158-161
5. Jesse NM, Drury L, Weiss MD. Transporting neonates with nitric oxide: the 5-year ShandsCair experience. *Air Med J.* 2004;23:17–19
6. American Academy of Pediatrics Committee on Fetus and Newborn. Use of inhaled nitric oxide. *Pediatrics.* 2000;106:344–345

Selected Readings

American Academy of Pediatrics. *HIPAA: A How To Guide for Your Medical Practice.* Elk Grove Village, IL: American Academy of Pediatrics; 2004

Day S, McCloskey K, Orr R, Bolte R, Notterman D, Hackel A. Pediatric interhospital critical care transport: consensus of a national leadership conference. *Pediatrics.* 1991;88;696–704

Hulley SB, Cummings SR, Browner WS, et al. *Designing Clinical Research: An Epidemiologic Approach.* 2nd ed. Philadelphia, PA: Lippincott Williams & Wilkins; 2001

Woodward GA, Insoft RM, Pearson-Shaver AL, et al. The state of pediatric interfacility transport: consensus of the second National Pediatric and Neonatal Interfacility Transport Medicine Leadership Conference. *Pediatr Emerg Care.* 2002;18:38–43

Questions

1. Are most neonatal-pediatric transport medical therapies based on transport studies?
2. Which recent advances have been developed for or studied during transport?
3. Are there any topics still in need of well-organized transport studies?

Answers

1. Historically, most transport therapies and equipment were developed in the hospital setting and not studied during transport.
2. Transport risk scores, surfactant, extracorporeal membrane oxygenation, and inhaled nitric oxide have been directly studied during transport for their efficacy.
3. Yes. Topics include projects in the areas of administration, financial analysis, medical therapies, and outcomes.

Ethical Considerations

Outline

- Informed consent, parental permission, and child assent
- Refusal of care or transport: parent or guardian refusal
- Refusal of care or transport: child refusal
- Caregivers who disagree
- Respect for others and cultural and religious differences
- Do-not-resuscitate orders
- Resuscitation
- Family presence at resuscitation
- Respect for confidentiality
- Truth telling in difficult situations
- Concerns about the care given by another health care provider
- Research in the transport setting

Staff involved with the transport of critically ill or injured children regularly encounter ethical issues. These issues may include the inability to obtain parental permission to treat a child, refusal of permission to treat or transport by parents or older children, the maintenance of confidentiality, issues related to truth telling, and others. This chapter discusses some of these issues and offers strategies to assist transport team members in addressing ethical concerns.

Informed Consent, Parental Permission, and Child Assent

The requirement to obtain informed consent from a patient or legal guardian before providing medical care is a central feature of health care law and ethics. A person may not be touched, treated, or transported without his or her consent. Minors (children younger than 18 years), however, present a special problem because they do not have the legal authority to give consent. Therefore, in most states, a parent or legal guardian must give permission before a minor can be medically treated or transported. In situations in which a minor has a condition that represents a threat to life or health and a legal guardian is not readily available to provide consent, transport team members can assess the child, provide necessary medical treatment, and transport the child. The legal basis for taking action in an emergency when consent is not available is known as the *emergency exception rule*.

The emergency exception rule also is known as the *doctrine of implied consent*. For minors, this doctrine means that transport team members can presume consent and proceed with appropriate treatment and transport if the following 4 conditions are met:

1. The child has an emergency condition that places his or her life or health in danger.
2. The child's legal guardian is unavailable or unable to provide consent for treatment or transport.
3. Treatment or transport cannot be delayed safely until consent can be obtained.
4. The transport team administers only treatment for emergency conditions that pose an immediate threat to the child.

This emergency exception rule is based on the assumption that reasonable persons would consent to emergency care if able to do so and that if the legal guardian knew the severity of the emergency, he or she would consent to medical treatment of the child. Any time a minor is treated without consent, the burden of proof falls on any professional treating or transporting the child to justify that the emergency actions were necessary. The transport team must clearly document in the child's record the nature of the medical emergency and the reason the minor required immediate treatment and/or transport.

If possible, interfacility transport team members should contact online medical control for assistance when consent is unclear or unavailable. If the guardian is unavailable and cannot be notified, information about the destination emergency department should be provided to the most responsible person on scene with instructions to pass the information on to the minor's legal guardians. As a general rule, when the transport professional's authority to act is in doubt, team members should always do what they believe to be in the best interest of the minor.

Refusal of Care or Transport: Parent or Guardian Refusal

A particularly challenging situation occurs when transport team members are faced with a legal guardian who refuses to give permission for further medical treatment or transport of a child. As long as a child's legal guardian is alert, oriented, and mentally competent, he or she has the right to refuse medical care for the child. However, the guardian is required to act in the best interest of the child. When a legal guardian refuses to consent to medical care or transport that is necessary to prevent death, disability, or serious harm to the child, social service agencies and/or law enforcement officers can intervene under local and state child abuse and neglect laws.

When faced with a guardian who refuses to allow the provision of care or transport to a child whose life or health might be threatened, the transport team should first notify on-site or online medical control for guidance. The medical control physician might speak directly with the legal guardian. If the medical control physician agrees that the child's condition requires immediate treatment to prevent serious harm and the legal guardian continues to refuse consent for care, it may be necessary to notify the police and enlist their assistance in placing the child in temporary protective custody. Likewise, when a legal guardian seems to be intoxicated or otherwise impaired, involvement of law enforcement officers is necessary to place a minor in temporary protective custody. In these rare situations, the hospital attorney or legal office at the referring and receiving facilities also should be notified after the safety of the child has been assured.

Although temporary protective custody may allow the transport team to transport a minor to a medical facility for purposes of further medical evaluation and care, it does not give emergency medical professionals the right to treat a minor for medical conditions that are not serious or life threatening. A medical professional can provide medical treatment without consent only when the child has a medical condition that poses a risk of death or serious harm, when immediate treatment is necessary to prevent that harm, and when only the treatments necessary to prevent the harm are provided. The transport team should discuss these situations with medical control before initiating treatment whenever possible and clearly document these decisions in the medical record.

Transport team members should not confront a child's caregiver with accusations, moral judgments, or threats when disagreements arise over the appropriate management of the child's care. This approach aggravates the situation and will not help the child. Instead, team members should attempt to establish whether the caregiver refuses all care and transport or only certain aspects of care. For example, some caregivers may prefer that transport team members not initiate therapy or consider a different mode of transport but will permit the child to be transported to the initial or receiving hospital. If the child can be transported safely without initiating care, the caregiver's wishes concerning treatment should be respected. It may be appropriate for the caregiver of a child with a terminal illness or significant disabilities to restrict or request certain kinds of care for the child. Difficult situations involving children with chronic illness and special health care needs should be discussed with medical control when appropriate management is not clear.

Refusal of Care or Transport: Child Refusal

There are 2 situations in which a minor has the legal authority to make decisions about his or her health care. First, state law designates certain minors as emancipated and grants them the right to make decisions, including health care decisions. Children who are legally emancipated may give consent for medical treatment and transport. They may also refuse medical care and transport. Although emancipated minor laws vary from state to state, most states recognize minors to be emancipated if they are married, pregnant, a parent, economically self-supporting and not living at home, or on active-duty status in the armed services. Second, on rare occasions, transport team members might encounter a minor who has legal status to make health care decisions because a court has declared the person a mature minor. In most states, mature minors are older than 14 years and have been formally declared adults by the court. Because state laws vary, however, it is important to be familiar with the specifics of emancipated and mature minor laws in the state in which care is being provided.

If a child is not an emancipated or a mature minor, he or she has no legal authority to provide consent or refuse medical care.

Regardless of whether a child has the legal authority to provide or withhold consent, it is always prudent to try to obtain the child's agreement (assent) to treat and transport. This approach respects the personal dignity and self-determination of the child and minimizes confrontation. A willingness to provide the child with some control and some choice may allow for a compromise that allows transport personnel to achieve a safe transfer. Using force or restraint to transport a child should be reserved for the situations in which all efforts to negotiate respectfully with the child have failed and the child is at risk of serious harm if he or she is not transported. In these unusual circumstances, appropriate measures should be taken to ensure the safety of the patient and transport team members during transport.

Caregivers Who Disagree

One rare but confusing situation arises when transport team members are confronted by caregivers who disagree about whether to consent to treatment and transport of a sick or injured child. In these cases, it is important to establish whether one or both caregivers has legal decision-making authority on behalf of the child. Because state laws vary with regard to the legal authority of the father when parents are unmarried, transport team members should be familiar with state and local laws that govern this situation. If both caregivers have legal authority, transport team members may need to negotiate a plan that is acceptable to both. Focusing on the child's needs and the common desire to assist the child, while deflecting attention away from the disagreement may be successful. If the situation becomes threatening or potentially dangerous to transport team members or the child, police and legal assistance may be necessary.

Occasionally, members of the transport team may find themselves in disagreement with the referring physician about care to be provided to the child before transport. For example, the transport team may believe intubation is necessary for a safe transport, and the referring physician may disagree and not allow them to perform the procedure. In this difficult situation, transport team members should attempt to engage the individuals with whom they disagree in a respectful discussion about the differences in the transport environment that sometimes require procedures not necessary in the inpatient environment to be performed and what they consider the best management of the child. If patient condition allows, this discussion should occur away from the child and the child's family. The welfare of the child should always remain the primary focus. If an agreement cannot be reached through respectful dialogue, the transport team should contact medical control and have the medical control physician speak with the referring physician.

Respect for Others and Cultural and Religious Differences

Cultural differences and religious beliefs may place transport team members in a difficult position. Although the care of the patient is always of primary concern, transport team members should attempt to respect requests from the family or patient regarding preferences that may originate from their religious or cultural beliefs, especially when these do not interfere significantly with the provision of treatment to the child. Transport team members should always remain nonjudgmental about requests that stem from cultural or religious beliefs, acknowledge the importance of these requests to the family, and attempt to accommodate them when they do not pose a risk to the child. When the transport team cannot accommodate requests that are based on cultural or religious beliefs because they would put a child at risk of serious harm, they should respectfully explain the reasons for being unable to accommodate the requests.

Language barriers also may present a challenge as the transport team attempts to communicate with a child's caregiver. Transport team members should be familiar with the resources available locally to provide professional translation and interpretation in a timely manner. Miscommunications can have a significant impact on a child's care, especially if transport team members are unable to obtain information about a child's underlying medical conditions, allergies, current medications, and other relevant and important information. If professional interpretation services are available to transport team members, they are preferred over the use of family members or bystanders. If such services are not available, a family member or neighbor might be available to assist with a rough interpretation. Transport team members should be aware, however, that the interpretation may not be accurate when a trained interpreter is not used.

Do-Not-Resuscitate Orders

The caregivers of some children, usually in consultation with their primary physician, will have decided that limitations should be placed on the kinds of treatments and interventions provided. These decisions usually are made because of the child's underlying condition and the desire to avoid futile or burdensome interventions should a life-threatening condition develop. Transport team members, in responding to a call about a sick child, might be confronted with a do-not-resuscitate (DNR) order. A DNR order must be signed by a physician to be valid and informs the provider that cardiopulmonary resuscitation should not be initiated or should be of limited scope in a cardiopulmonary arrest. Only some jurisdictions recognize pre-hospital DNR orders as valid for children. It is very important that transport team members clarify the limits of the DNR law governing their service area and develop protocols for dealing with them. Regardless of the nature of the DNR law, a legal guardian generally may revoke a DNR order written on behalf of a child. When faced with a valid DNR order written for a child and a legal guardian requesting that the child be resuscitated, the legal guardian's wishes generally should be followed. Even in the face of a valid DNR order, it is very important to discuss with the legal guardian what kinds of interventions he or she considers acceptable and which are not considered beneficial to the child. For example, oxygen delivery, transport, and hospital admission may be acceptable and expected for some children with DNR orders written on their behalf. Discussion with on-site and online medical control and consultants may help with these potentially challenging issues.

Resuscitation

Sometimes resuscitation attempts for children in cardiopulmonary arrest are ineffective or not indicated. Resuscitation policy should define circumstances when cardiopulmonary resuscitation must be initiated, when it may be withheld, and when it may be stopped. For pediatric cases, the policy should favor resuscitation in questionable cases, but allow appropriate withholding of resuscitation to focus on grief management and family interactions.

Local resuscitation policy may allow transport team members to withhold or stop resuscitation when a child is clearly dead. This may be emotionally difficult for transport team members, and all participants should be in agreement with the decision to stop or not initiate resuscitation in these cases.

Family Presence at Resuscitation

The practice of allowing family members to be present during resuscitation remains controversial. A number of surveys of health care professionals demonstrate a reluctance of providers to consider allowing relatives during resuscitation. However, available data overwhelmingly suggest that families want to be given the opportunity to be present for the resuscitation of a child or loved one, that they do not interfere with the staff, that staff do not feel excess stress when family members are present, and that family members may deal with grief in a more healthy manner if they were present during a resuscitation in which a loved one died.

Given the absence of data that suggest the presence of relatives during transport or resuscitation is harmful and the existence of data that suggest families want to be present and that their presence is not harmful and may be helpful, offering select family members the opportunity to be present during resuscitation and transport should be considered (see Chapter 12). Having a dedicated staff person identified and available to support family members during a resuscitation will be helpful and is recommended.

Respect for Confidentiality

Medical information is considered private by most people, and carelessly or inadvertently revealing identifiable information is a risk that transport team members face because they frequently care for ill or injured people in a public environment. It is essential that transport team members remain aware of the potentially sensitive nature of identifiable information and take every possible precaution as they care for patients, including children. Sensitive discussions should, when possible, occur where bystanders cannot overhear them. The use of last names should be avoided if possible at the scene. Private information should not be shared with concerned bystanders (other than those legally responsible for the patient). Finally, because radio communication systems may be monitored by people in the community, use of names should be avoided unless absolutely essential to the receiving hospital. If use of names is important, then a telephone should be used at the scene rather than a radio.

Truth Telling in Difficult Situations

Transport team members should deal as honestly as possible with children they care for and with their caregivers. It is not unusual for caregivers to ask about the condition of a child or request information about a child's prognosis. In such situations, transport team members should refrain from speculating, but respond instead with honest reassurance. For example, "We'll take the best possible care of your child," provides an honest and reassuring statement without speculating about uncertain outcomes.

Transport team members also may face situations in which multiple injuries have occurred and parent or child requests information about someone else who may have been injured. Although a delay in providing information is often not an ideal approach, it may be appropriate for transport team members to deflect such questions, especially when the other party suffered severe injuries or died. Rather than answering dishonestly, transport members should offer an honest statement of reassurance, such as "My concern is to take care of you right now. My partners are doing their best to take care of _____." Although there is an ethical obligation to be honest, it may be appropriate to delay sharing particularly distressing information until a patient has been transported safely and other sources of emotional support can be made available to the patient.

Concerns About the Care Given by Another Health Care Provider

Occasionally, transport team members will have concerns about clinical care given to a patient before or during transport. Transport team members may have questions about their obligations to provide feedback to the person who gave the care in question or to notify

■■■■■■■■■■■■■■■■■■■■■■■■■■■■■■■■■

the patient or family that they suspect harmful or deficient care was given or that mistakes were made.

Although truthfulness about mistakes is important, transport team members also should remain aware that they rarely have a full understanding of the many factors that may have affected care given before their arrival. In most cases, transport team members should avoid making potentially premature and misinformed judgments about the care given by others. The focus initially should be on the care of the patient and stabilization of the patient's condition. Once transport has been completed, there should be a clear and direct mechanism for communicating concerns to the provider in question, collecting the necessary data to determine whether care was appropriate, and providing a formal means for review of the data and remediation, if necessary. In most situations, family members should be notified about errors or deficient care, but only after an adequate investigation of the facts has determined that this occurred.

Research in the Transport Setting

The future health of children depends on the conduct of clinical research in which children participate. As investigators design and implement research protocols, they should be aware of the ethical and legal requirements that govern research with human participants. This is especially true of research that involves children and other vulnerable groups, especially those in the midst of an emergency. Because of the inherent vulnerability of children, research must be designed carefully to ensure that the participants are not placed at excessive risk or denied potential benefits unfairly. Federal regulations governing research involving children and local institutional review boards (IRBs) exist to assure that research involving children occurs in a way that protects their welfare. For research in the transport setting to satisfy ethical and legal requirements, it must be scientifically sound and significant; subject selection must be fair; approaching families for enrollment must avoid pressure; risks to participants cannot be excessive and must be minimized; risks must be justified by the benefits of the research; informed consent, parental permission, and assent must be obtained when appropriate; enrolled subjects must be respected; and the protocol must have been approved by an

IRB. In most cases, the best source of information and guidance about research protocols will be the local IRB.

In some cases, research in the transport environment is designed to study emergency procedures that offer the prospect of direct benefit to potential participants; enrollment must take place immediately, and parents may not be available to provide permission. This presents a special situation governed by special rules. Under these circumstances, the research can proceed without permission of the parents only under restricted guidelines outlined by federal regulation: (1) The subject is facing a life-threatening or permanently disabling situation for which the only known therapy is investigational, unproven, or unsatisfactory. (2) The child is incapable or unable to provide valid consent and the parents cannot be reached for permission before the time the investigational treatment must be started. (3) There is no accepted therapy that is clearly superior to the experimental therapy. In addition, the research protocol must undergo IRB review to determine that the experimental treatment has a realistic probability of benefit that equals or exceeds that of standard care, that the risks of the experimental therapy are reasonable in comparison with the patient's condition and standard therapy, that there is minimal added risk from participation in the research protocol, that there is no possibility of obtaining prospective consent from individuals likely to need the experimental therapy, that participants and/or parents will be provided with all pertinent information about the study as soon as possible, and that alteration or waiver of consent will not adversely affect the rights and welfare of the subjects. Once the legal decision maker has been informed of the research, he or she may choose to discontinue participation at any time after being fully informed of the consequences of doing so. Finally, federal regulations require that input from community representatives be sought about the protocol before IRB approval to gain a form of "community consent" to proceed with the research and that public disclosure of the research and its risks and benefits be made to the community from which potential participants will be enrolled before initiation of the research. Public disclosure of study results also is required by law in this situation.

Selected Readings

American Academy of Pediatrics Committee on Bioethics. Informed consent, parental permission, and assent in pediatric practice. *Pediatrics*. 1995;95:314-317

American Academy of Pediatrics Committee on Bioethics. Religious objections to medical care. *Pediatrics*. 1997;99:279-281

American Academy of Pediatrics Committee on Pediatric Emergency Medicine. Consent for emergency medical services for children and adolescents. *Pediatrics*. 2003;111:703-706

American Academy of Pediatrics Committee on School Health and Committee on Bioethics. Do not resuscitate orders in schools. *Pediatrics*. 2000;105:878-879

Diekema DS. Conducting ethical research in pediatric emergency medicine. *Clin Pediatr Emerg Med*. 2003;4:273-284

Galanti GA. *Caring for Patients From Different Cultures: Case Studies From American Hospitals*. 2nd ed. Philadelphia, PA: University of Pennsylvania Press; 1997

Iserson KV, Sanders AB, Mathieu D, eds. *Ethics in Emergency Medicine*. 2nd ed. Tucson, AZ: Galen Press; 1995

Sabatino CP. Survey of state EMS-DNR laws and protocols. *J Law Med Ethics*. 1999;27:297-315

Taveras EM, Glores G. Why culture and language matter: the clinical consequences of providing culturally and linguistically appropriate services to children in the emergency department. *Clin Pediatr Emerg Med*. 2004;5:76-84

Questions

1. Under what circumstances can a child receive treatment and transport without the permission of a parent?
2. What is the best way to communicate with a family who does not speak English?
3. To maintain confidentiality, what is the best method of communication between the transport team and the receiving hospital?

Answers

1. When the provider determines that a child has an emergency condition that places his or her life or health in danger; the child's legal guardian is unavailable or unable to provide consent for treatment or transport; treatment or transport cannot be delayed safely until consent can be obtained; and the transport team members and hospital professionals administer only treatment for emergency conditions that pose an immediate threat to the child's life or health.
2. Use a certified interpreter.
3. Telephone

CHAPTER 19

Accreditation

Outline

- Accreditation for medical transport services
- CAMTS: an organization of organizations
- Mission and goals of CAMTS
- Accreditation standards
- Applying for accreditation

Accreditation for Medical Transport Services

Accreditation is a voluntary process that provides a means to demonstrate a level of quality. The Commission on Accreditation of Air Medical Services (CAAMS) was initiated in 1990 as a direct response to the unacceptable number of air-medical accidents in the 1980s. Specific standards were developed for air-medical transport to address safety and patient care issues that formed the foundation for accreditation. The Joint Commission on Accreditation of Healthcare Organizations (JCAHO) was developed out of similar circumstances. In 1915, the American College of Surgeons allocated $500.00 to establish standards for quality patient care in hospitals as a result of a study that demonstrated dismal outcomes for hospitalized patients. These *Minimum Standards for Hospitals* eventually led to voluntary accreditation for hospitals by JCAHO, chartered in 1951.

In addition to CAAMS, there are only 2 other agencies in the United States that accredit medical transport services. The Commission on Accreditation of Ambulance Services (CAAS) was initiated in 1990 to offer voluntary accreditation to advanced life support and basic life support ground transport services, mostly 911 response systems. In 1996, the Commission on Fire Accreditation International (CFAI) was initiated to offer accreditation to fire and emergency services through-

303

out the world. Neither CAAS nor CFAI addresses air-medical transport, and neither agency focuses on critical care transport. Joint Commission Resources also publishes a text regarding international accreditation standards for transport organizations (Joint Commission International Accreditation Standards for Medical Transport Organizations). These standards include focus areas of: "medical transport organizations, including those responsible for emergency treatment and transport; non-emergency transport; ambulance services; land, air, and water medical transport; and fire brigade emergency services."[1]

In 1997, the mission and scope of CAAMS expanded to meet the needs of ground critical care transport services and led to the name change to Commission on Accreditation of Medical Transport Systems (CAMTS). There were already extensive standards addressing medical direction and education of critical care teams. Many of the operational standards also could be applied to ground transport. Additional standards were developed specifically for the ground transport vehicle. This expansion was designed specifically for neo-natal-pediatric transport teams who were requesting an accreditation process that addressed the full scope of their practice. In addition, many air-medical services were adding ground transport to meet their transport needs when aircraft were not available owing to weather or maintenance.

CAMTS: An Organization of Organizations

CAMTS is a nonprofit organization supported by 16 member organizations. Each member organization is required to send a representative to serve on the board of directors. Board representatives are volunteers and are required to have previous or current experience with medical transport. They are directly responsible for accreditation decisions, policies and procedures, marketing, and budgeting. The CAMTS board meets 3 times a year.

The diversity and experience level of board representatives provide CAMTS with the integrity to offer accreditation in North America and abroad. Table 19.1 is the list of current member organizations:

Table 19.1: Current Member Organizations of CAMTS*

Aerospace Medical Association (AsMA)
Air & Surface Transport Nurses Association (ASTNA)
Air Medical Physicians Association (AMPA)
American Academy of Pediatrics (AAP)
American Association of Critical Care Nurses (AACN)
American Association of Respiratory Care (AARC)
American College of Emergency Physicians (ACEP)
Association of Air Medical Services (AAMS)
Emergency Nurses Association (ENA)
National Air Transportation Association (NATA)
National Association of Air Medical Communications Specialists (NAACS)
National Association of EMS Physicians (NAEMSP)
National Association of Neonatal Nurses (NANN)
National Association of State EMS Directors (NASEMSD)
National EMS Pilots Association (NEMSPA)
National Flight Paramedics Association (NFPA)

* CAMTS indicates Commission on Accreditation of Medical Transport Systems.

Mission and Goals of CAMTS

The following are the mission statement and goals of CAMTS:

Mission Statement

Professionals involved with air medical services and ground interfacility transport services strive to provide the highest possible quality to their constituents.

The Commission on Accreditation of Medical Transport Systems is dedicated to assisting these professionals in offering a quality service.

The Commission offers a program of voluntary evaluation of compliance with accreditation standards which demonstrates the ability to deliver service of a specific quality.

The Commission believes that the two highest priorities of an air medical or ground interfacility transport service are patient care and safety of the transport environment.

By participating in the voluntary accreditation process, services can verify their adherence to quality accreditation standards to themselves, their peers, medical professionals, and to the general public.

The goals of CAMTS include the following:

1. To provide an organized forum through which those professionals involved with air, medical and ground transport systems can participate in improving the services they provide.
2. To assist our constituents in achieving accreditation through information sharing and education programs.
3. To provide a voluntary and objective mechanism for evaluation of compliance with the accreditation standards.
4. To offer compliance with the Commission on Accreditation of Medical Transport Systems accreditation standards as a marker of excellence for federal, state and local government agencies, as well as private agencies and to the general public.
5. To maintain recognition of the accreditation standards as a measure of quality for both public and private air medical and ground transport systems.
6. To maintain currency in the accreditation standards according to medical research, ground transport and aviation developments in order to meet the dynamic needs of air medical and ground transport systems.

Accreditation Standards

The entire accreditation process is based on compliance with accreditation standards. The standards are revised every 2 to 3 years to reflect the dynamic evolution of the field of medical transport. Medical transport services that achieve accreditation must be in substantial compliance with the accreditation standards. Each standard is supported by measurable interpretations to address the general topics listed in Table 19.2.

The accreditation standards and the audit process to verify compliance with the standards are important to patients and families who

Table 19.2: Accreditation Topics

Capabilities and resources of the medical transport service
Medical director
Medical personnel: staffing, training, and continuing education
Medical configuration of the aircraft and ambulance
Operational issues
Communications
Management
Utilization review
Quality management
Infection control
Aviation certificate
Aircraft (rotor-wing and fixed-wing)
Pilots and maintenance
Refueling
Community outreach
Ambulance and maintenance of ground vehicles
Driver qualifications

rely on the quality and professionalism of the transport service. The term *specialty team* refers to an organization that provides medical transport services to a specific population, such as neonatal transport or combined neonatal-pediatric transport teams. The CAMTS accreditation process addresses issues that may pertain to a general critical care transport team that works with specialty team members under certain circumstances and issues unique to a specialty transport service. Specialty teams may contract with an aviation or ground vendor or have contracts with other medical transport programs. Whatever the arrangement for a transport vehicle, a dedicated team is eligible to apply for CAMTS accreditation.

Of note, CAMTS does not accredit brokers, who are intermediaries who arrange medical transport for a fee but who do not own or operate aircraft or manage a medical team. An accredited medical transport service may lease aircraft or outsource communications, but there must be a dedicated medical team and the medical transport service is expected to demonstrate ethical practices.

The following are some of the standards to protect patients, ensure highest quality, and promote a positive outcome. Further information can be found at http://www.camts.org.

▪ Accreditation Standard 01.01.00: "There must be written policies and procedures specifying the mission statement and scope of care to be provided by the service." (Medical section)

▪ Accreditation Standard 01.10.00: "The transport service develops and demonstrates use of a written code of ethical conduct that demonstrates ethical practice in business, marketing and professional conduct." (Medical section)

▪ Accreditation Standard 02.06.00: "A planned and structured program should be required for all regularly scheduled medical transport personnel. Competency and currency must be ensured and documented through relevant continuing education programs and certification programs." (Medical section)

▪ Accreditation Standard 01.04.00: "All patient care resources, including personnel and equipment necessary to the program's mission must be readily available in the aircraft/ground transport vehicle or available for placing in the aircraft/ground transport vehicle and operational prior to initiating the mission. This includes resources, personnel, and equipment provided by Specialty Care Providers." (Medical section)

▪ Accreditation Standard 03.06.11: "The aircraft/ambulance design and configuration must not compromise patient stability in loading, unloading or in-flight operations." (Aircraft/Ambulance section)

▪ Accreditation Standard 04.01.02: "Medical transport personnel must ensure that all medical equipment is in working order and all equipment/supplies are validated through documented checklists for both the primary and back-up aircraft/ambulance." (Aircraft/Ambulance section)

▪ Accreditation Standard 04.01.09: "A policy addresses carry-on baggage of patient or passenger that must be checked for hazardous materials before loading on the transport aircraft/ambulance." (Aircraft/Ambulance section)

▪ Accreditation Standard 03.06.12: "Patients transported by air are restrained with a minimum of three cross straps that must comply with FAA [Federal Aviation Administration] regulations. Ground ambulance patients are securely restrained in accordance with state and federal laws." (Aircraft/Ambulance section)

a. Patients under 60 pounds (27 kg) should be provided with an appropriately sized restraining device (for patient's height and weight) which is further secured by a locking device. All patients under 40 pounds must be secured in a five-point safety strap device that allows good access to the patient from all sides and permits the patient's head to be raised at least 30 degrees. Velcro straps are not encouraged for use on pediatric devices.

b. If a car seat is used, it must have an FAA approved sticker.

c. There must be some type of restraining device within the isolette to protect the infant in the event of air turbulence or poor road conditions.

■ Accreditation Standard 06.01.04: "A policy limits driver's use of cellular phones or other communication devices while driving except for vital communications."

Frequently Cited Deficiencies Regarding Specialty Teams

Most neonatal or combined neonatal-pediatric transport teams are considered specialty teams. In addition to the aforementioned standards, specialty teams may not be in compliance with certain standards and may be cited for deficiencies in areas that do not meet compliance with the standards for accreditation. For example, when transporting in helicopters, specialty teams might not wear helmets or follow the same dress standards as the regular air-medical team. Wearing only scrubs or unsuitable footwear is not appropriate in case there is an unexpected landing or survivable crash in rough terrain and weather. Safety in the environment is paramount. Of note, isolettes may be inadvertently located in the head-strike envelope of medical personnel in air and ground vehicles.

■ Accreditation Standard 02.04.01 Staffing (Medical section):

a. "Physical well-being is promoted through protective clothing and dress codes...."

■ Accreditation Standard 03.06.12: Head strike envelope (Aircraft/Ambulance section):

a. "Appropriately sized helmets are worn (by all personnel on the aircraft except for the patient) OR the interior modification of the aircraft is clear of objects/projections OR the interior of the aircraft is padded to protect the head-strike envelope of the medical personnel and patients as appropriate to the aircraft."

b. "The head strike envelope in the ambulance should be clear of hard objects that could cause injury in the event of poor road conditions or sudden stops."

■ Accreditation Standard 02.06.04: Education specific to the in-flight and ground transport environment (Medical section):

a. "Survival training/techniques/equipment...pertinent to the environment/geographic coverage area of the medical service."

■ Accreditation Standard 04.01.03: Occupant restraint devices (Aircraft/Ambulance section):

a. "Medical personnel must be in seatbelts (and shoulder harnesses if installed) that are properly worn and secured for all take-offs and landings according to FAA regulations. A policy defines when medical personnel can get out of restraints."

b. "Ambulance personnel must be seat-belted when the ambulance is in motion unless emergent patient condition precludes it."

Annual safety training is required that includes general aircraft and ambulance safety and emergency procedures unless the specialty transport team is always accompanied by a regularly scheduled crewmember, as shown in Table 19.3.

Applying for Accreditation

There currently is a pool of 32 site surveyors who are independent contractors and perform at least 2 site visits per year. Site surveyors must have at least 4 years of experience in the medical transport profession as medical, communication, or aviation professionals and must have a management background. Site surveyors are interviewed and selected based on their level of experience and positive interface with the selection committee during interviews. If selected, site surveyors are required to attend a course provided by the board of directors before being assigned to a site visit with an experienced surveyor. The site surveyor coordinator schedules site surveyors according to their experience with types of patients (eg, age groups) and modes of transport (ie, rotor-wing, fixed-wing, or ground).

To apply for CAMTS accreditation, a transport service should request an initial application and complete the following steps:

1. Complete the initial application.
2. Return it to the CAMTS office with the application fee.

Table 19.3 Annual Safety Training Requirements				
Type of Team	Verify Critical Care Education Requirements	Verify Annual Safety Training	Safety Briefing Only	Verify Dress Code
Independent specialty team: part of the transport service but flies alone	XXX	XXX		XXX
Specialty team: part of the service but always accompanied by the flight team	XXX	XXX		XXX
Specialty team that contracts for transport: not part of the service but flies alone		XXX		XXX
Specialty team that contracts for transport: not part of the service but always accompanied by flight team			XXX	XXX

3. Complete the program information form (PIF) that will be sent by e-mail or on a disk. The PIF is a self-study document that asks questions pertinent to each accreditation standard and requires certain attachments to be included with the submission. It must be completed within 1 year of receipt.
4. Submit the PIF and the attachments requested: 4 hard copies or on a CD.

After receipt of the PIF, CAMTS schedules a site visit within 4 to 6 weeks. An accreditation decision is made at the next scheduled meeting of the board of directors; meetings are held 3 times per year.

Conclusion

There are many incentives to become accredited. Voluntary participation in the accreditation process indicates a commitment to quality patient care and a safe environment for transport team personnel. The accreditation process provides a comprehensive evaluation of the transport program by experts in the transport profession and a framework for improvement to ensure safe and competent patient transport. Potential advantages also may include aviation insurance cost reduction; contracts awarded to CAMTS-accredited services by the government and industry; and reimbursement incentives from managed care organizations.

References

1. Joint Commission Resources: *Joint Commission International Accreditation Standards.* Oakbrook Terrace, IL: Joint Commission on Accreditation of Healthcare Organizations

Selected Readings

Commission on Accreditation of Medical Transport Systems. *Sixth Edition Accreditation Standards.* Anderson, SC: Commission on Accreditation of Medical Transport Systems; 2004

Duffy, M. *An Introduction to the Joint Commission: its survey and accreditation processes, standards, and services.* 3rd ed. Chicago, IL: Joint Commission on Accreditation of Healthcare Organizations; 1988

Joint Commission Resources: *Joint Commission International Accreditation Standards for Medical Transport Organizations.* Oakbrook Terrace, IL. Joint Commission of Accreditation of Healthcare Organizations; 2003.

Questions

TRUE or FALSE

1. Accreditation is a voluntary process that provides a means to demonstrate quality.
2. CAMTS does not offer accreditation to critical care ground services.
3. The American Academy of Pediatrics is a member organization of CAMTS.

Answers

1. True
2. False
3. True

■ Special Considerations for ■
Neonatal-Pediatric Transport

Outline

I.   Pediatric emergency department considerations
II. Pediatric ICU considerations
III. Neonatal ICU considerations

Neonatal-pediatric critical care transport teams serve a multitude of "customers" such as community hospitals, tertiary care centers, emergency medical services (EMS) systems, and, ultimately, patients and their families. In addition, they interact with a variety of agencies, departments, units, and practitioners, all of which have special considerations for transport team members. Transport team members must have a diverse set of skills and the flexibility to adapt to changing environments and situations, all perhaps within a single shift or day. Familiarity with the special considerations within the 3 major areas—emergency medicine, pediatric critical care, and neonatal intensive care—will contribute to the transport service's effectiveness.

Pediatric Emergency Department Considerations

Emergency Department Capabilities

It is estimated that fewer than 10% of hospitals in the United States have dedicated pediatric emergency departments (EDs). The majority of pediatric emergency care, therefore, is provided in EDs that serve adults and children. The American Academy of Pediatrics (AAP) and American College of Emergency Physicians have published joint guidelines for the care of children in the ED, addressing leadership, personnel, equipment, and policies and procedures. At present, there is no uniformly accepted method of categorizing EDs based on their capabilities with regard to pediatric emergency care. The AAP has endorsed a statement by the Society for Academic Emergency Medicine stating that although physically separate care areas for children are ideal, they are not mandatory for the provision of quality pediatric emergency care.

Trauma Centers

Trauma is the leading cause of death for children between the ages of 6 months and 14 years; consequently, the interfacility transport of critically injured children is a frequent occurrence. It is essential that pediatric transport staff be familiar with the trauma capabilities of receiving institutions. The American College of Surgeons Committee on Trauma (ACSCOT) classifies trauma center levels based on predefined criteria for staffing, facilities, and other resources and approves the designation of an individual institution through a process called verification. Guidelines for transport destination based on trauma center level typically are determined by state or regional protocols. Pediatric trauma patients may or may not be given special consideration within a state's trauma system, depending on the availability and accessibility of pediatric trauma centers in the region.

The ACSCOT criteria for trauma center levels are included in Figure 20-1. Most trauma centers undergo biannual surveys to maintain verification. Level I trauma centers may be classified as level I pediatric and/or adult trauma centers. As expected, there are additional requirements for specially trained pediatric medical and surgical specialists for facilities designated as level 1 pediatric trauma centers.

Most pediatric trauma patients have blunt injuries and are managed nonoperatively. Trauma resuscitation focuses on airway management, ventilatory support, and restoration of intravascular volume. Approximately 3% to 5% of children will undergo surgery within the first 24 hours following injury, primarily for stabilization of orthopedic injuries. An even smaller number will require emergency surgical procedures on arrival to a trauma center, such as patients with an expanding epidural hematoma or penetrating thoracic trauma. In these cases, it is important that transport programs work with receiving hospitals to develop procedures for direct admission of selected patients to the operating room (OR) or other appropriate assessment or interventional location. Components of a "direct to the OR" protocol include a communication system to notify the appropriate surgical service(s) and essential personnel (eg, anesthesia, OR nursing, blood bank, radiology). In addition, preregistration should be available so that all required materials and medications are available and consents can be obtained before or immediately on patient arrival. In most

Figure 20-1: American College of Surgeons Criteria for Trauma Centers

American College of Surgeons Committee on Trauma Classification System of Trauma Center Level

ACS Levels and Descriptions

Level I

Provides comprehensive trauma care, serves as a regional resource, and provides leadership in education, research, and system planning.

A level I center is required to have immediate availability of trauma surgeons, anesthesiologists, physician specialists, nurses, and resuscitation equipment. American College of Surgeons' volume performance criteria further stipulate that level I centers treat 1200 admissions a year or 240 major trauma patients per year or an average of 35 major trauma patients per surgeon.

Level II

Provides comprehensive trauma care either as a supplement to a level I trauma center in a large urban area or as the lead hospital in a less population-dense area.

Level II centers must meet essentially the same criteria as level I but volume performance standards are not required and may depend on the geographic area served. Centers are not expected to provide leadership in teaching and research.

Level III

Provides prompt assessment, resuscitation, emergency surgery, and stabilization with transfer to a level I or II as indicated.

Level III facilities typically serve communities that do not have immediate access to a level I or II trauma center.

Level IV & V

Provides advanced trauma life support prior to patient transfer in remote areas in which no higher level of care is available.

The key role of the level IV center is to resuscitate and stabilize patients and arrange for their transfer to the closest, most appropriate trauma center level facility.

Level V trauma centers are not formally recognized by the American College of Surgeons, but they are used by some states to further categorize hospitals providing life support prior to transfer.

Source: MacKenzie EJ, Hoyt DB, Sacra JC, et. al. National inventory of hospital trauma centers. *JAMA.* 2003;289:516. Copyright ©2003 American Medical Association. All rights reserved. Available at: http://www.amtrauma.org/tiep/reports/ACSClassification.html#. Accessed January 11, 2006. Used with permission.

cases, eligible patients already should have a secure airway, and any imaging that would be essential before surgery (eg, computed tomography scan) should have been done.

Another emergency situation that requires rapid mobilization of the receiving hospital's resources is the management of pulseless patients with severe hypothermia from exposure or cold-water drowning. Pediatric patients with core temperatures less than 30°C and no pulse are unlikely to respond to efforts at rewarming without the use of extracorporeal life support (ECLS). Referring institutions should be advised to avoid delays for efforts at less effective types of rewarming therapy in place of rapid triage to a center that can provide pediatric cardiopulmonary bypass or extracorporeal membrane oxygenation (ECMO). Receiving hospitals should individually determine whether these patients will best be resuscitated in the OR, ED, or intensive care unit (ICU).

Poisoning and Poison Centers

Toxic ingestions are a common reason for interfacility transport of pediatric patients. Regional poison centers serve as a valuable resource for the management of poisoned children and should be consulted by the transport team if not already done by the referring institution. Specific toxic ingestions may require antidotes or emergency therapies that are available only at a limited number of centers, such as fomepizole for ethylene glycol ingestion, intravenous N-acetylcysteine for acetaminophen ingestion, and hemodialysis for aspirin intoxication. In general, the ingestion of a potentially hepatotoxic substance (eg, acetaminophen or mushrooms) is not an indication for primary transport to a pediatric transplant facility, given the low frequency with which transplant actually is required in these situations.

The American Association of Poison Control Centers (AAPCC; http://www.aapcc.org) maintains a toll-free number, (800) 222-1222, through which any of the 62 poison centers in the United States, Puerto Rico, and the US Virgin Islands can be accessed.

Children With Special Health Care Needs

Children with special health care needs are those who have or are at risk for chronic physical, developmental, behavioral, or emotional conditions and who also require health and related services of a type or amount not usually required by children. This definition includes children with congenital or acquired developmental disabilities or other chronic health problems, with or without technology or device dependence. Because many children with underlying health problems have been transitioned from acute care hospitals to rehabilitation facilities or to their homes, they are frequent users of EMS, EDs, transport teams, and pediatric ICUs. Many children with complex health needs will obtain their primary medical care from a tertiary children's hospital, which may be remote from their home. As a result, critical care transport teams may be asked to transfer a patient from a community hospital to a pediatric facility at which the child's specialists or subspecialists practice.

There have been several initiatives to improve the coordination of emergency care for children with special health care needs. The Emergency Medical Services for Children Program (EMS-C), the AAP, and the American College of Emergency Physicians have all developed emergency information forms or data sets and templates for emergency care plans to be used as resources for health care providers who are unfamiliar with a child with special health care needs who has an emergency condition. Of course, this documentation must be updated and proofread by parents and health care providers on a regular basis to ensure it is current and accurate (Figure 20-2).

The transport of a child with special health care needs may be complicated by several factors, including the following:

1. Need for specialized devices or medications not typically available to critical care transport teams (eg, left ventricular assist device pumps, Huber needles, custom-designed tracheostomy tubes, and prostacyclin infusions for primary pulmonary hypertension)
2. Need for specialized equipment (eg, portable ventilators) that must be adequately secured in the transport vehicle
3. Immobility or physical limitations on positioning (eg, spica casts)
4. Importance of transporting parents or home health care providers who are familiar with the patient's usual problems and management

The AAP has issued a policy statement entitled "Transporting Children With Special Health Care Needs." This document can serve as a resource for EMS providers and transport professionals who may care for children with special needs.

Mental Health or Behavioral Emergencies

Although a patient with a primary mental health emergency is less likely to be transferred by a critical care transport team, underlying or concomitant psychological conditions may complicate an acute illness or injury. For example, an adolescent injured in a single-car vehicle accident may have intended suicide, or a patient with seizures and hyperthermia may be under the influence of mind-altering medications such as Ecstasy. Critical care transport team members, especially those who primarily transport infants and children, may be unprepared for a patient who unexpectedly becomes violent. In these situations, team safety is paramount, and consideration should be given to physical and/or pharmacologic restraint before transport. If it is not feasible to use pharmacologic methods because of the nature of the patient's condition, appropriate physical restraints are indicated. Specialized restraints such as leather wrist and ankle binders should be applied by trained law enforcement or security personnel, who should accompany the transport team in case the restraints must be removed for patient care. If referring hospital or local law enforcement policies prohibit their staff to participate in the transport process, then the team may refuse to perform the transport owing to safety concerns. When used, the description of and justification for restraints applied during transport should be entered in the medical record. Guidelines and protocols for consideration, implementation, and frequent assessment and documentation of restraints should be available and adhered to by the transport team.

Chemical, Biological, and Radiological Hazards

The concern about acts of terrorism or use of weapons of mass destruction has led many institutions to develop training programs, policies and procedures, and specialized resources for the management of potentially hazardous situations. Transport teams should be included in educational programs that address recognition and

Figure 20-2: Sample emergency information form for children with special health care needs

Emergency Information Form for Children With Special Needs

Last name:

American College of Emergency Physicians®	American Academy of Pediatrics	Date form completed	Revised	Initials
		By Whom	Revised	Initials

Name:	Birth date:	Nickname:
Home Address:	Home/Work Phone:	
Parent/Guardian:	Emergency Contact Names & Relationship:	
Signature/Consent*:		
Primary Language:	Phone Number(s):	

Physicians:

Primary care physician:	Emergency Phone:
	Fax:
Current Specialty physician: Specialty:	Emergency Phone:
	Fax:
Current Specialty physician: Specialty:	Emergency Phone:
	Fax:
Anticipated Primary ED:	Pharmacy:
Anticipated Tertiary Care Center:	

Diagnoses/Past Procedures/Physical Exam:

1.	Baseline physical findings:
2.	
3.	Baseline vital signs:
4.	
Synopsis:	Baseline neurological status:

*Consent for release of this form to health care providers

Figure 20-2: Sample emergency information form for children with special health care needs, *continued*

Diagnoses/Past Procedures/Physical Exam continued:

Medications:

1.
2.
3.
4.
5.
6.

Significant baseline ancillary findings (lab, x-ray, ECG):

Prostheses/Appliances/Advanced Technology Devices:

Last name:

Management Data:

Allergies: Medications/Foods to be avoided   and why:

1.
2.
3.

Procedures to be avoided   and why:

1.
2.
3.

Immunizations

Dates						Dates					
DPT						Hep B					
OPV						Varicella					
MMR						TB status					
HIB						Other					

Antibiotic prophylaxis: Indication: Medication and dose:

Common Presenting Problems/Findings With Specific Suggested Managements

Problem	Suggested Diagnostic Studies	Treatment Considerations

Comments on child, family, or other specific medical issues:

Physician/Provider Signature: **Print Name:**

Reproduced with permission from *Pediatrics,* Vol. 104, Page. e53, © October 1999 by the AAP management of patients who may require special handling or decontamination. To protect transport team members, communications and medical personnel who participate in the intake process should notify the team members of any possible concern for hazardous conditions. Likewise, to protect the receiving hospital staff and patients, the transport team must take the necessary precautions when transferring the patient and coordinate with the medical control physician and hospital officials about patient disposition, especially the need for isolation or decontamination.

The Occupational Safety and Health Administration (OSHA) develops standards for workplaces and worker training with which transport program administrators should be familiar. OSHA standard 29 CFR 1910.120, referred to as the hazardous waste operations and emergency response (HAZWOPER) standard, describes training requirements for employees who may be involved in emergency response operations that include the potential release of hazardous substances. These include the following:

- Names of personnel and alternates responsible for site safety and health
- Safety, health, and other hazards present on the site
- Use of personal protective equipment (PPE)
- Work practices by which the employee can minimize risks from hazards
- Medical surveillance requirements, including recognition of symptoms and signs that might indicate exposure to hazards
- Specific contents of the site safety and health plan, including decontamination procedures, PPE, confined space entry procedures, and spill containment program

The requirements for emergency providers are much less stringent than for personnel involved in clean-up operations and include an "initial briefing at the site prior to their participation in any emergency response. The initial briefing shall include instruction in the wearing of appropriate personal protective equipment (PPE), what chemical hazards are involved, and what duties are to be performed." Additional information can be found on the OSHA Web site at http://www.osha.gov.

The AAP (http://www.aap.org) also has published guidelines for the isolation and treatment of children exposed to bioterrorism or chemical hazards.

Infection Control

Similar to other health care providers, transport team members may be exposed to patients or family members with contagious diseases. In general, transport personnel always should use standard precautions, including gloves and frequent hand washing, as their primary means to avoid disease transmission. The availability of alcohol-based hand washes and gels eliminates the need for a source of running water, making it more practical for transport team members to maintain hand hygiene in a mobile environment. When transporting a patient with a suspected contagious disease, the transport team should communicate with the receiving facility so that the patient can be triaged to an appropriate point of entry and/or an isolation area, as indicated.

Certain patient conditions require additional measures to protect health care providers and/or prevent disease transmission to other patients. For example, when treating patients who are colonized or infected with multiresistant organisms such as MRSA (methicillin-resistant *Staphylococcus aureus*) or VRE (vancomycin-resistant *Enterococcus*), transport team members should wear disposable gowns over their clothes or uniforms to avoid contact. Patients may have known or suspected infectious conditions that are transmitted by respiratory secretions or droplets, such as meningococcal disease and varicella, necessitating the use of masks to prevent transmission. When highly virulent diseases are suspected, such as severe acute respiratory syndrome, or SARS, the use of disposable high-filtration respirators is indicated. Information on specific diseases and recommendations for health care providers can be found on the Centers for Disease Control and Prevention Web site at http://www.cdc.gov.

Transport team members should consider obtaining available immunizations for certain contagious diseases to which they may be exposed. Vaccinations are available against hepatitis A, hepatitis B, influenza, mumps, measles, rubella, meningococcus (certain strains), varicella, polio, tetanus, diphtheria, and pertussis. Persons who are not vaccinated or naturally immune also can receive postexposure passive immunization for hepatitis A, hepatitis B, tetanus, and vari-cella. Antibiotic prophylaxis may be indicated following a significant exposure to a patient with meningococcal disease. Transport team members should undergo OSHA-approved training regarding preven-tion and management of exposure to blood and body fluids. Health care workers should be familiar with institutional procedures in the event of an accidental needle stick or blood or body fluid exposure owing to the potential indication for passive immunization against tetanus or hepatitis B or postexposure prophylaxis against human immunodeficiency virus.

Pediatric ICU Considerations

Pediatric ICU Levels

As with trauma centers and neonatal ICUs, pediatric ICUs may be classified by level based on their resources and capabilities. Guidelines for pediatric ICUs have been updated by the AAP and the Society of Critical Care Medicine (Figure 20-3). Level I facilities provide a full range of pediatric subspecialty services and meet specific require-ments for availability of personnel, equipment, and support services on a 24-hour basis. For level II facilities, some of these resources are considered optional, although there are still minimum requirements for staffing and other services. In most states, the classification of pediatric ICUs is an informal practice that does not have any bearing on patient triage or transfer or any impact on the type or complexity of care that is permitted at a particular institution. The availability of certain services, however, may be regulated by a state agency such as the department of public health, which may have the authority to license ICU beds, approve expansion of services and physical facilities, and control expenditures for capital resources. For example, these types of regulations may specify that hospital-based transport pro-grams must demonstrate sufficient need in the region or state to expand physical facilities or enact major purchases such as aircraft.

It has been demonstrated that critically ill or injured children admitted to a pediatric ICU, with its concentration of specialized personnel and resources, have an improved outcome compared with pediatric patients admitted to an adult ICU. Despite this, approxi-mately 7% of hospitals in the United States report that they routinely

Figure 20-3: Levels of Pediatric Intensive Care Units (PICUs)

Minimum guidelines and levels of care for PICUs (abridged) are given. E indicates essential; D, desired; O, optional; NA, not applicable. Guideline designations are given for Level 1, Level 2.

I. Organization and administrative structure
  A. Category I facility: E, E
  B. Organization
    1. PICU committee: E, E
    2. Distinct administrative unit: E, E
    3. Delineation of physician and nonphysician privilege: E, E
  C. Policies
    1. Admission and discharge: E, E
    2. Patient monitoring: E, E
    3. Safety: E, E
    4. Nosocomial infection: E, E
    5. Patient isolation: E, E
    6. Family-centered care: E, E
    7. Traffic control: E, E
    8. Equipment maintenance: E, E
    9. Essential equipment breakdown: E, E
    10. System of record keeping: E, E
    11. Periodic review
      a. Morbidity and mortality: E, E
      b. Quality of care: E, E
      c. Safety: E, E
      d. Critical care consultation: E, E
      e. Long-term outcomes: D, D
      f. Supportive care: D, D
  D. Physical facility—external
    1. Distinct, separate unit: E, D
    2. Distinct unit (not necessarily physically separate) with auditory and visual separation: E, E
    3. Controlled access (no through traffic): E, E
  E. Physical facility—internal
    1. Patient isolation capacity: E, E
    2. Patient privacy provision: E, E
    3. Satellite pharmacy: D, O
    4. Medication station with drug refrigerator and locked narcotics cabinet: E, E
    5. Emergency equipment storage: E, E

II. Personnel
  A. Medical director
    1. Appointed by appropriate hospital authority and acknowledged in writing: E, E
    2. Qualifications
      a. Board-certified or actively pursuing certification in 1 of the following:
        i. Pediatric critical care medicine: E, E
          • Initial board certification in pediatrics: E, E
          • Codirector if director is not a pediatrician: E, D
        ii. Anesthesiology with practice limited to infants and children and special qualifications in critical care medicine: E, E
        iii. Pediatric surgery with added qualification in surgical critical care medicine: E, E
    3. Responsibilities documented in writing: E, E
      a. Acts as primary attending physician: D, D
      b. Has authority to provide consultation when physician is not available: E, E
      c. Assumes patient care if primary attending physician is not available: E, E
      d. Participates in development, review, and implementation of PICU policies*: E, E
      e. Maintenance of database and/or vital statistics*: E, E
      f. Supervises quality-control and quality-assessment activities (including morbidity and mortality reviews)*: E, E
      g. Supervises resuscitation techniques (including educational component)*: E, E
      h. Ensures policy implementation*: E, E

Figure 20-3: Levels of Pediatric Intensive Care Units (PICUs), *continued*

Minimum guidelines and levels of care for PICUs (abridged) are given. E indicates essential; D, desired; O, optional; NA, not applicable. Guideline designations are given for Level 1, Level 2.

B. Physician staff
  1. A physician in-house 24 h/d: E, E
    a. A physician at the postgraduate year 2 level or higher assigned to the PICU: E, D
    b. A physician at the postgraduate year 2 level or higher available to the PICU (advanced practice nurse or physician assistant may be used): E, E
    c. A physician at the postgraduate year 3 level or higher (in pediatrics or anesthesiology) in-house 24 h/d: E, O
  2. Available in 30 min or less (24 h/d)
    a. Pediatric intensivist or equivalent: E, D
  3. Available in 1 h or less
    a. Anesthesiologist: E, E
      i. Pediatric anesthesiologist: E, D
    b. General surgeon: E, E
    c. Surgical subspecialists
      i. Pediatric surgeon: E, D
      ii. Cardiovascular surgeon: E, O
        • Pediatric cardiovascular surgeon: D, O
      iii. Neurosurgeon: E, E
        • Pediatric neurosurgeon: E, O
      iv. Otolaryngologist: E, D
        • Pediatric otolaryngologist: D, O
      v. Orthopedic surgeon: E, D
        • Pediatric orthopedic surgeon: D, O
      vi. Craniofacial, oral surgeon: D, O
  4. Pediatric subspecialists
    a. Intensivist: E, E
    b. Cardiologist: E, D
    c. Nephrologist: E, D
    d. Hematologist/oncologist: D, D
    e. Pulmonologist: D, D
    f. Endocrinologist: D, D
    g. Gastroenterologist: D, D
    h. Allergist: D, D
    i. Neonatologist: E, E
    j. Neurologist: E, D
    k. Geneticist: D, D
  5. Radiologist: E, E
    a. Pediatric radiologist: E, O
  6. Psychiatrist or psychologist: E, D
C. Nursing staff
  1. Manager/director: E, E
    a. Training and clinical experience in pediatric critical care: E, E
    b. Master's degree in pediatric nursing or nursing administration: D, D
  2. Nurse/patient ratio based on patient need: E, E
  3. Nursing policies and procedures in place: E, E
  4. Orientation to PICU: E, E
  5. Completion of clinical and didactic critical care course: E, E
  6. Address psychosocial needs of patient and family: E, E
  7. Participate in continuing education: E, E
  8. Completion of critical care registered nurse (pediatric) certification: D, D
  9. Completion of PALS or an equivalent course: D, D
  10. Nurse educator on staff (clinical nurse specialist): E, D
    a. Responsible for pediatric critical care in-service education: E, D
  11. Nurse coordinator for regional continuing education: O, O
D. Respiratory therapy staff
  1. Supervisor responsible for training registered respiratory therapy staff: E, E
  2. Maintenance of equipment and quality control and review: E, E
  3. Respiratory therapist in-house 24 h/d assigned primarily to PICU: E, D

Figure 20-3: Levels of Pediatric Intensive Care Units (PICUs), *continued*

Minimum guidelines and levels of care for PICUs (abridged) are given. E indicates essential; D, desired; O, optional; NA, not applicable. Guideline designations are given for Level 1, Level 2.

4. Respiratory therapist in-house 24 h/d: E, E
5. Respiratory therapists familiar with management of pediatric patients with respiratory failure: E, E
6. Respiratory therapists competent with pediatric mechanical ventilators: E, E
7. Completion of PALS or an equivalent course: D, D

E. Other team members
1. Biomedical technician (in-hospital or available within 1 h, 24 h/d): E, E
2. Unit clerk on staff 24 h/d with a written job description: E, D
3. Child life specialist: E, D
4. Clergy: E, E
5. Social worker: E, E
6. Nutritionist or clinical dietitian: E, E
7. Physical therapist: E, E
8. Occupational therapist: E, E
9. Pharmacist (24 h/d): E, E
10. Pediatric clinical pharmacist: D, D
11. Radiology technician: E, E
12. Bereavement coordinator: D, D

III. Hospital facilities and services
A. Emergency department
B. Intermediate care unit or step-down unit separate from PICU and pediatric acute care unit: D, D
C. Pediatric rehabilitation unit: D, D
D. Blood bank
1. Comprehensive (all blood components): E, E
2. Type and crossmatch within 1 h: E, E
E. Radiology services and nuclear medicine
1. Portable radiograph: E, E
2. Fluoroscopy: E, D
3. Computed tomography scan: E, E
4. Magnetic resonance imaging: E, D
5. Ultrasound: E, E
6. Angiography: E, O
7. Nuclear scanning: E, O
8. Radiation therapy: D, O
F. Laboratory with microspecimen capability
1. Available within 15 min
   a. Blood gases: E, E
2. Available within 1 h
   a. Complete blood cell, platelet, and differential counts: E, E
   b. Urinalysis: E, E
   c. Chemistry profile (electrolytes, serum urea nitrogen, glucose, calcium, and creatinine): E, E
   d. Clotting studies: E, E
   e. Cerebrospinal fluid analysis: E, E
3. Available within 3 h
   a. Ammonia concentration: E, E
   b. Drug screening: E, E
   c. Osmolality: E, E
   d. Magnesium and phosphorus concentrations: E, E
   e. Toxicology screen: E, D
4. Preparation available 24 h/d
   a. Bacteriology (culture and Gram stain): E, E
5. Point-of-care diagnostic testing: D, D
G. Department of surgery
1. Operating room available within 30 min, 24 h/d: E, E
2. Second operating room available within 45 min, 24 h/d: E, D
3. Capabilities
   a. Cardiopulmonary bypass: E, D
   b. Bronchoscopy (pediatric): E, D
   c. Endoscopy (pediatric): E, D
   d. Radiograph in operating room: E, E
H. Cardiology department with pediatric capability
1. Electrocardiography: E, E

Figure 20-3: Levels of Pediatric Intensive Care Units (PICUs), *continued*

Minimum guidelines and levels of care for PICUs (abridged) are given. E indicates essential; D, desired; O, optional; NA, not applicable. Guideline designations are given for Level 1, Level 2.

2. Echocardiography
   a. Two-dimensional echocardiography with Doppler: E, E
3. Catheterization laboratory (pediatric): D, O
I. Neurodiagnostic laboratory
   1. EEG: E, E
   2. Evoked potentials: D, D
   3. Transcranial Doppler flow: D, O
J. Hemodialysis: E, O
K. Peritoneal dialysis or continuous renal replacement therapy: E, O
L. Pharmacy with pediatric capability: E, E
   1. Available 24 h/d for all requests: E, E
   2. Located near PICU and pediatric acute care unit: D, O
   3. Urgent drug-dosage form at bedside: E, E
   4. Satellite pharmacy located in PICU: D, O
   5. Pediatric pharmacist available for medical rounds: D, O
M. Rehabilitation department with pediatric capability
   1. Physical therapy: E, E
   2. Speech therapy: E, E
   3. Occupational therapy: E, E
IV. Drugs and equipment
   A. Emergency drugs: E, E
   B. Portable equipment
      1. Emergency cart: E, E
      2. Procedure lamp: E, E
      3. Doppler ultrasonography device: E, E
      4. Infusion pumps (with micro-infusion capability): E, E
      5. Defibrillator and cardioverter: E, E
      6. Electrocardiography machine: E, E
      7. Suction machine (in addition to bedside): E, E
      8. Thermometers: E, E
      9. Expanded scale electronic thermometer: E, E
      10. Automated blood pressure apparatus: E, E

11. Otoscope and ophthalmoscope: E, E
12. Automatic bed scale: E, D
13. Patient scales: E, E
14. Cribs (with head access): E, E
15. Beds (with head access): E, E
16. Infant warmers, incubators: E, E
17. Heating and cooling blankets: E, E
18. Bilirubin lights: E, E
19. Transport monitor: E, D
20. EEG machine: E, E
21. Isolation cart: E, E
22. Blood warmer: E, E
23. Pacer (transthoracic or transvenous): E, E
C. Small equipment
   1. Tracheal intubation equipment: E, E
   2. Endotracheal tubes (all pediatric sizes): E, E
   3. Oropharyngeal and nasopharyngeal airways: E, E
   4. Vascular access equipment: E, E
   5. Cut-down trays: E, E
   6. Tracheostomy tray: E, E
   7. Flexible bronchoscope: E, D
   8. Cricothyroidotomy tray: E, E
D. Respiratory support equipment
   1. Bag-valve-mask resuscitation devices: E, E
   2. Oxygen tanks: E, E
   3. Respiratory gas humidifiers: E, E
   4. Air compressor: E, E
   5. Air-oxygen blenders: E, E
   6. Ventilators of all sizes for pediatric patients: E, E
   7. Inhalation therapy equipment: E, E
   8. Chest physiotherapy and suctioning: E, E
   9. Spirometers: E, E
   10. Continuous oxygen analyzers with alarms: E, E
E. Monitoring equipment
   1. Capability of continuous monitoring of:
      a. Electrocardiography, heart rate: E, E
      b. Respiration: E, E

■■■■■■■■■■■■■■■■■■■■■■■■■■■■■■■■■

Figure 20-3: Levels of Pediatric Intensive Care Units (PICUs), *continued*

Minimum guidelines and levels of care for PICUs (abridged) are given. E indicates essential; D, desired; O, optional; NA, not applicable. Guideline designations are given for Level 1, Level 2.

c. Temperature: E, E
d. Systemic arterial pressure: E, E
e. Central venous pressure: E, E
f. Pulmonary arterial pressure: E, D
g. Intracranial pressure: E, D
h. Esophageal pressure: D, O
i. Capability to measure 4 pressures simultaneously: E, D
j. Capability to measure 5 pressures simultaneously: D, D
k. Arrhythmia detection and alarm: E, E
l. Pulse oximetry: E, E
m. End-tidal CO_2: E, E

2. Monitor characteristics
   a. Visible and audible high and low alarms for heart rate, respiratory rate, and all pressures: E, E
   b. Hard-copy capability: E, E
   c. Routine testing and maintenance: E, E
   d. Patient isolation: E, E
   e. Central station: E, E

V. Prehospital care
   A. Integration and communication with EMS system: E, E
   B. Transfer arrangements with referral hospital: E, E
   C. Transfer arrangement with level I PICU: NA, E
   D. Educational programs in stabilization and transportation for EMS personnel: E, D
   E. Transport system (including transport team): E, O
   F. Emergency communication into PICU and pediatric acute care unit (eg, phone, radio) 24 h/d: E, E
   G. Communication link to poison control center: E, E

VI. Quality improvement

VII. Training and continuing education
   A. Physician training
      1. Unit in facility with accredited pediatric residency program D, O
      2. Unit provides clinical rotation for pediatric residents in pediatric critical care: D, O
      3. Fellowship program in pediatric critical care: D, O
      4. Cardiopulmonary resuscitation certification: E, E
      5. PALS or advanced pediatric life support: E, E
      6. Ongoing continuing medical education for physicians specific to pediatric critical care: E, E
      7. Staff physicians to attend and participate in pediatric critical care: E, E
   B. Unit personnel
      1. Cardiopulmonary resuscitation certification for nurses and respiratory therapists: E, E
      2. Resuscitation practice sessions: E, E
      3. Ongoing continuing education (on-site and/or off-site workshops and programs for nurses respiratory therapists, clinical pharmacists): E, E
      4. Certified by the American Association of Critical Care Nurses: D, D
      5. PALS or advanced pediatric life support certification: E, E
      6. Critical care registered nurse certification: D, D
   C. Regional education
      1. Participation in regional pediatric critical care education: E, O
      2. Service as educational resource center for public education in pediatric critical care: D, D
      3. Prehospital care and interhospital transport: D, O

*In conjunction with nurse manager. PALS indicates Pediatric Advanced Life Support.

Reproduced with permission from *Pediatrics*, Vol. 114, Page(s) 1114-1125, © October 2004 by the AAP admit children requiring intensive care to an adult unit rather than transferring them to a pediatric facility. The practice seems to be more common with trauma, in which up to 10% of hospitals have reported a practice of admitting critically injured children to an adult ICU.

Burn Centers

The management of pediatric burn patients may require specific resources because serious burns are uncommon and highly complex. Although adult burn units commonly are found at major medical centers, specialized care for pediatric burn patients is concentrated among a small number of facilities, such as the nationwide Shriner's Hospital system. Transfer to a pediatric burn center is often a secondary or even tertiary transport following resuscitation and/or stabilization at a community hospital or pediatric institution without a burn unit.

For the most part, pediatric burn centers are accustomed to receiving patients in transfer from other institutions, although some may be prepared to accept patients directly from the field under certain circumstances. Critical care transport programs should work with the closest regional pediatric burn center to develop procedures for the triage of seriously burned children directly to the burn center or in secondary transfer following resuscitation and stabilization at another facility. The American Burn Association has developed guidelines for transfer of pediatric patients to a pediatric burn center, as shown in Figure 20-4 (http://www.ameriburn.org).

Burn patients are often transported by helicopter but, in many cases, air transport may be unnecessary owing to an observed practice of "overtriage." Studies have shown that referring physicians regularly overestimate burn size, favoring the use of air transport and increasing the costs of acute burn care.

Hyperbaric Oxygen Therapy

Treatment in a hyperbaric oxygen chamber is available at selected centers in the United States. The most common indications for emergency use of hyperbaric oxygen therapy are acute carbon monoxide (CO) poisoning and cerebral air embolism or "the bends" from decompression accidents as occur with scuba diving. For patients with CO poisoning, oxygen content is reduced by the very high affinity of

■ ■

Figure 20-4: American Burn Association Burn Unit Referral Criteria

1. Partial-thickness burns greater than 10% total body surface area (TBSA)

2. Burns that involve the face, hands, feet, genitalia, perineum, or major joints

3. Third-degree burns in any age group

4. Electrical burns, including lightning injuries

5. Chemical burns

6. Inhalation injury

7. Burn injury in patients with preexisting medical disorders that could complicate management, prolong recovery, or affect mortality

8. Any patients with burns and concomitant trauma (eg, fractures) in which the burn injury poses the greatest risk of morbidity or mortality. In such cases, the patient's condition may be initially stabilized in a trauma center before transfer to a burn unit. Physician judgment will be necessary in such situations and should be in concert with the regional medical control plan and triage protocols.

9. Burned children in hospitals without qualified personnel or equipment for the care of children

10. Burn injury in patients who will require special social, emotional, or long-term rehabilitative intervention

---

Adapted from *Guidelines for the Operations Burn Units* (pp. 55–62), Resources for Optimal Care of the Injured Patient: 1999, Committee on Trauma, American College of Surgeons, Chicago, IL.

CO for hemoglobin. Administration of 100% oxygen at atmospheric pressure will reduce the level of carboxyhemoglobin in the blood over several hours' time. Hyperbaric oxygen therapy (HBOT) has the theoretical additional benefits of accelerating the reduction in carboxyhemoglobin and increasing the concentration of dissolved oxygen in the blood, thus improving oxygen delivery to the tissues, especially the brain. In decompression sickness, patients who breathe pressurized gas mixtures and return to atmospheric pressure too quickly may be harmed by the formation of gas bubbles in the tissues as the solubility of the gas in the blood decreases. In these cases, treatment of the patient under hyperbaric conditions will permit the gas to redissolve in the blood, after which the rate of decompression can be carefully controlled.

As with all emergency care, standard resuscitation and stabilization measures take priority over adjunctive therapies such as HBOT. For example, a patient with CO exposure from a house fire also might have thermal burns, inhalation injury, and/or cyanide toxicity and should be treated first for problems with the airway, breathing, and circulation. After the immediate life-threatening problems have been identified and treated, the risks and benefits of additional therapies such as HBOT should be considered, based on the patient's condition and the severity of the suspected CO intoxication.

In general, patients who are unconscious after exposure to CO or those with a carboxyhemoglobin level of more than 40%, are considered candidates for HBOT. However, a patient with acute lung injury may be served best by admission to an ICU for expert management of mechanical ventilation. Given that controversy exists about the efficacy of HBOT in preventing or ameliorating the neuropsychiatric sequelae of CO intoxication, especially in pediatric patients, the transport destination should not routinely be determined by the availability of a hyperbaric oxygen chamber. Guidelines should be developed, in concert with the HBOT medical director and personnel, regarding when direct transport to HBOT should be considered, with an emphasis on ensuring optimal pediatric assessment and monitoring in the HBOT location. This should include expectations for which physicians, nurses, and technicians will attend to the patient during the prolonged exposures, at the bedside and outside the chamber.

Implantable Pacemakers and Automated Internal Cardiac Defibrillators

Although primary cardiac disease is encountered less frequently in children than in adults, there is a population of children with congenital or acquired heart disease for whom there may be special considerations during critical care transport. Children with conduction system abnormalities often require placement of an implantable pacemaker, even during the neonatal period. These devices typically are placed subcutaneously in the abdomen owing to the limited size and expandability of the chest wall. Automated internal cardiac defibrillators (AICDs) may be placed in children at high risk for developing life-threatening ventricular arrhythmias. These larger devices also are placed in the abdominal region; to date, the youngest recipient weighed 10 kg. Malfunction of an implanted pacemaker or AICD can lead to serious complications in children, as in adults. Device failure can be managed by externally providing any therapy that is being inadequately performed, such as use of transthoracic pacing. Device mishaps, such as inappropriate discharges, may require that the device be disabled for the patient's safety. This can be accomplished by placing a specialized magnet over the device. Fortunately, most hospital EDs have access to magnets because of the more widespread use of pacemakers and AICDs in adult patients.

Organ Procurement and Transplantation

Solid organ transplantation is a highly specialized area of medicine that requires the close cooperation of multiple agencies, programs, and personnel. In most states, there is a mandatory requirement to notify the regional organ procurement organization (OPO) when a diagnosis of brain death is likely or when a patient dies. The success of an organ transplant procedure is determined by many factors, among which are time to harvest and time to transplant following harvest (ischemic time). Most patients who are evaluated and listed for organ transplantation are required to relocate to the vicinity of the transplant center so that they can respond rapidly for surgery in case an organ becomes available. More often than not, however, it is necessary for the transplant team to travel to harvest the organ and transport it back to the transplant center. In certain cases, transport teams may be requested to facilitate the transport of medical personnel or of the organs themselves because of the time-sensitive nature of the process. The United Network for Organ Sharing has published guidelines for the transport of organs for transplantation within the United States. In general, it is the responsibility of the "host" OPO (ie, the organization that makes the organ available) to make arrangements to transport the organ to the receiving facility. Interestingly, the costs of transporting a kidney are borne by the host OPO, whereas the costs associated with the transport of other organs are the responsibility of the recipient facility. Transport team members should not be expected to package, label, or handle the organ for transplantation, which is the responsibility of the host OPO.

Neonatal ICU Considerations

Neonatal ICU Levels

Unlike trauma centers or pediatric ICUs, neonatal ICUs typically are licensed by the individual state to provide a specific level of services for neonatal patients. The level of neonatal ICU care usually is designated by the state's hospital regulatory agency, such as the department of public health, whose definitions may vary from state to state. The AAP recommends a uniform classification and subclassification of neonatal ICUs based on their capabilities (Figure 20-5).

Level I (basic): neonatal resuscitation, postnatal care of healthy neonates, care of infants born at 35 to 37 weeks' gestation who are physiologically stable, and stabilization of the condition of sick neonates or those who are less than 35 weeks' gestational age before transfer to a higher level facility

Level II (specialty): neonatal resuscitation, postnatal care of infants born at more than 32 weeks' gestation and birth weight more than 1500 g, care of neonates who are moderately ill and do not require urgent subspecialty services, and care of premature infants who are convalescing after a course in a level III nursery

Level III (subspecialty): neonatal resuscitation and postnatal care that includes advanced life support and/or comprehensive care for high-risk or critically ill neonates

ECMO and Inhaled Nitric Oxide

There are approximately 115 ECMO centers in the United States, a number that has decreased during the past 10 years. This reflects the decreased demand for ECLS owing to the use of therapies such as high-frequency oscillatory ventilation, inhaled nitric oxide (iNO), and surfactant replacement.

In 2000, the US Food and Drug Administration (FDA) approved the use of iNO for the treatment of hypoxic respiratory failure in term and near-term neonates with clinical or echocardiographic evidence of pulmonary hypertension. As a result, many neonatal ICUs have begun to provide iNO therapy, including facilities that do not have ECMO capabilities. The initiation of iNO therapy in a non-ECMO center is controversial because it may delay transfer to a facility with ECMO capability.

Figure 20-5; Levels of Neonatal Intensive Care Units (NICUs). Proposed Uniform Definitions for Capabilities Associated With the Highest Level of Neonatal Care Within an Institution

Level I neonatal care (basic)
- Well-neonatal nursery: has the capabilities to
  - Provide neonatal resuscitation at every delivery
  - Evaluate and provide postnatal care to healthy neonates
  - Stabilize and provide care for infants born at 35 to 37 weeks' gestation who remain physiologically stable
  - Stabilize the condition of neonates who are ill and those born at <35 weeks' gestation until transfer to a facility that can provide the appropriate level of neonatal care

Level II neonatal care (specialty)
- Special care nursery: level II units are subdivided into 2 categories on the basis of their ability to provide assisted ventilation including continuous positive airway pressure
- Level IIA has the capabilities to:
  - Resuscitate and stabilize preterm and/or ill infants before transfer to a facility at which neonatal intensive care is provided
  - Provide care for infants born at >32 weeks' gestation and weighing ≥1500 g (1) who have physiologic immaturity such as apnea of prematurity, inability to maintain body temperature, or inability to take oral feedings or (2) who are moderately ill with problems that are anticipated to resolve rapidly and are not anticipated to need subspecialty services on an urgent basis
  - Provide care for infants who are convalescing after intensive care
- Level IIB has the capabilities of a level IIA nursery and the additional capability to provide mechanical ventilation for brief durations (<24 hours) or continuous positive airway pressure

Level III (subspecialty) NICU: level III NICUs are subdivided into 3 categories
- Level IIIA has the capabilities to:
  - Provide comprehensive care for infants born at >28 weeks' gestation and weighing >1000 g
  - Provide sustained life support limited to conventional mechanical ventilation
  - Perform minor surgical procedures such as placement of central venous catheter or inguinal hernia repair
- Level IIIB NICU has the capabilities to provide:
  - Comprehensive care for extremely low birth weight infants (≤1000 g and ≤28 weeks' gestation)
  - Advanced respiratory support such as high-frequency ventilation and inhaled nitric oxide for as long as required
  - Prompt and on-site access to a full range of pediatric medical subspecialists
  - Advanced imaging, with interpretation on an urgent basis, including computed tomography, magnetic resonance imaging, and echocardiography
  - Pediatric surgical specialists and pediatric anesthesiologists on site or at a closely related institution to perform major surgery such as ligation of patent ductus arteriosus and repair of abdominal wall defects, necrotizing enterocolitis with bowel perforation, tracheoesophageal fistula and/or esophageal atresia, and myelomeningocele
- Level IIIC NICU has the capabilities of a level IIIB NICU and also is located in an institution that has the capability to provide extracorporeal membrane oxygenation and surgical repair of complex congenital cardiac malformations that require cardiopulmonary bypass

Reproduced with permission from *Pediatrics*, Vol. 114, Page(s) 1341-1347, © November 2004 by the AAP

This practice has major implications for critical care transport teams who may be asked to urgently transfer a critically ill neonate who is already receiving maximal medical therapy, short of ECMO. In these situations the transport team is unlikely to have any additional therapies that may offset the instability precipitated by transitioning from high-frequency oscillatory ventilation to conventional ventilation or by the stress of a mobile or air-medical environment.

For these reasons, it is essential that non-ECMO centers that provide iNO therapy for neonatal respiratory failure work closely with an ECMO center to develop criteria for transfer to ensure that there is a "window of opportunity" during which the transport can be accomplished safely. These guidelines should be evaluated regularly by reviewing the outcome of infants transported for ECMO. A certain incidence of "unnecessary" transports (ie, neonates who are referred for but do not require ECMO) may be necessary if the transfer criteria are adequately conservative. Furthermore, any transport team that may be asked to transport a neonate who is already receiving iNO therapy must have the capability of providing iNO during transport because abrupt discontinuation may result in serious deleterious effects.

Because iNO is an FDA-approved therapy, transport teams also may choose to *initiate* iNO on transport under appropriate circumstances. Infants with hypoxic respiratory failure and clinical or echocardiographic evidence of pulmonary hypertension are candidates for iNO therapy. Of note, there is controversy about the administration of iNO without echocardiographic confirmation of the absence of structural heart disease. The source of the concern is the fact that iNO therapy may be harmful to neonates whose systemic blood flow is dependent on right-to-left flow through the ductus arteriosus, because the subsequent reduction in pulmonary vascular resistance may compromise systemic blood flow. Examples include left-sided obstructive lesions such as critical aortic stenosis, hypoplastic left heart syndrome, and interrupted aortic arch. At a minimum, protocols regarding the initiation of iNO during transport should specifically address the possibility of congenital heart disease and the appropriate steps to take if the patient's condition worsens while receiving iNO. The decision to initiate iNO during transport should reflect consideration of the potential risks and benefits of its use outside of the ICU, including the severity of illness and distance or time to the receiving facility. The practice of empirically initiating iNO during transport to facilitate the transition from high-frequency oscillatory ventilation to conventional mechanical ventilation has been reported, but there is no evidence that it improves patient safety or outcome.

Ideally, a neonate with hypoxic respiratory failure whose trajectory predicts the need for ECMO will be transferred to an ECMO center before meeting criteria for cannulation or his or her condition becoming too unstable to transport. When this is not possible, a few select programs have the capability to respond to requests for transport by mobilizing an ECMO team that is capable of cannulating at the referring facility and then transporting the patient while receiving ECMO to the base institution. This practice, although labor-intensive, expensive, and high risk, has been carried out safely and successfully in civilian and military programs.

The Extracorporeal Life Support Organization (ELSO), based at the University of Michigan, promulgates guidelines for ECLS and maintains a registry of patients who have been treated with ECMO (http://www.elso.med.umich.edu). Neonates represent the largest treatment group to date. ELSO's materials indicate that the decision to transfer a neonate to an ECMO center should be influenced by a number of factors and states that there are no standard criteria. In general, ELSO recommends that a neonate whose condition is deteriorating be transferred at a time when the conversion to conventional ventilation still can be tolerated and suggests that an infant whose condition has not improved after 6 hours of high-frequency oscillatory ventilation be considered a candidate for expedient transfer. Individual institutions may use the alveolar-arterial oxygen difference, the oxygenation index, or the persistence of a PaO_2 of less than 50 torr as predictors of the need for ECMO. Unfortunately, published experience indicates that the transfer of neonates for ECMO often occurs after the patient has reached commonly agreed on criteria for cannulation.

The staff at the ECMO center who accept a neonate in transfer should clearly indicate to the referring physician that the patient is being transported as an ECMO candidate, without a guarantee that ECMO will be provided. This practice may diminish the likelihood that the referring hospital or the family will question the decision to transport in case ECMO is not required. Furthermore, it communicates the fact that the ECMO center will be evaluating the patient and determining whether the infant is an appropriate candidate for ECMO after arrival.

The decision to cannulate for ECMO may be facilitated by requesting that the referring facility perform certain diagnostic studies while the transport team is mobilizing and responding. These include a cardiac ECHO to evaluate for noncorrectable conditions or cyanotic heart disease that might have been misdiagnosed as pulmonary hypertension. In addition, a recent cranial ultrasound to assess for the presence of intracranial hemorrhage is helpful. Because the patient will need to undergo type and cross-matching for blood at the receiving facility, it is unnecessary to perform this at the referring hospital unless there is an anticipated need for transfusion of blood products during transport.

Extreme Prematurity

The threshold for viability of premature infants has decreased progressively with improvements in perinatal care. Although survival rates for infants born between 22 and 25 weeks' gestation have improved progressively, there remains a significant incidence of neurodevelopmental disability and other chronic health problems. Parental counseling and decision making around the birth of an extremely premature infant have medical, legal, and ethical considerations. A published survey of neonatologists in the New England region indicated that the decision to resuscitate at the lower limits of viability is based on gestational age and parental wishes. For example, the majority of neonatologists surveyed indicated that they would consider resuscitation for infants born at less than $23^{0}/_{7}$ weeks to be futile, but one third would attempt resuscitation at the parents' request. For infants born at $25^{1}/_{7}$ weeks' gestation and later, most neonatologists reported that they would consider treatment clearly beneficial, and 91 % would provide resuscitation, even if the parents requested to withhold treatment. Between $24^{1}/_{7}$ and $24^{6}/_{7}$ weeks' gestation, neonatologists were divided on the benefit of treatment, but the majority reported that they would defer to parental wishes with regard to resuscitation.

The AAP and the American College of Obstetricians and Gynecologists have published guidelines for decision making at the threshold of viability. The guidelines acknowledge that delivery room management is made more challenging by the narrow range of gestations during which prognosis can vary significantly. The most reliable indicator of estimated gestational age is the date of the mother's last menstrual period, followed by a first trimester ultrasonographic evaluation. The approximation of gestational age based on estimated fetal weight at the time of presentation in preterm labor has a significant error rate of 15% to 20%. Furthermore, gestational age is a better marker of outcome than birth weight, as demonstrated by the outcome of infants who are growth-restricted but more mature than their birth weight suggests. In situations in which there has been inadequate prenatal care or when there is uncertainty about actual gestational age, it may be necessary to postpone decisions about resuscitation until the time of birth when the infant's physical appearance, weight, and condition can be assessed directly. The AAP's Neonatal Resuscitation Program states that it is appropriate to consider noninitiation of delivery room resuscitation when an infant is born at less than 23 weeks' gestation or a birth weight of less than 400 g. When there is doubt on the part of the clinician, most experts would recommend an initial trial of therapy, followed by reassessment and discussion with the parents about the risks and benefits of further life-sustaining care.

Transport teams are faced with several dilemmas when the birth of an extremely preterm infant is imminent. Whenever feasible, it is preferable for the referring institution to transfer the mother with the fetus in utero, so that delivery can occur in a facility with experience in the care of premature neonates. If delivery is imminent or maternal transfer is judged to be an unacceptably high risk to the mother or the fetus, delivery should occur in the referring institution. Neonatal transport teams may be requested to "stand by" to assist in the delivery room resuscitation of an extremely premature infant who then will require transport after birth. The decision to mobilize a transport team for anticipated problems with a premature neonate should be made in consultation with the referring providers, the medical control physician, and the transport team leadership. If the timing of delivery can be predicted with reasonable certainty (ie, decision to perform a cesarean section), the infant's estimated gestational age and weight indicate the potential for viability, and the referring facility has inadequate resources to manage the initial resuscitation and stabilization of an extremely preterm infant, it may be appropriate to dispatch the transport team before the infant's birth. The transport team may need to be augmented with additional personnel if expectations of assessments and/or interventions could exceed the standard team's level of expertise or scope of practice. Issues surrounding level of involvement and credentialing should be anticipated and agreed on before need. On the other hand, it is usually not appropriate to dispatch the team if there will be an unpredictable period of waiting for a vaginal delivery, if there is a high likelihood that the infant is previable, or if there are providers who can perform initial resuscitation and stabilization before the transport team's arrival.

Selected Readings

American Academy of Pediatrics Committee on Environmental Health and Committee on Infectious Diseases. Chemical-biological terrorism and its impact on children: a subject review. *Pediatrics*. 2000;105:662–670

American Academy of Pediatrics Committee on Fetus and Newborn. Levels of neonatal care. *Pediatrics*. 2004;114:1341–1347

American Academy of Pediatrics Committee on Fetus and Newborn. Perinatal care at the threshold of viability. *Pediatrics*. 2002;110:1024–1027

American Academy of Pediatrics Committee on Fetus and Newborn. Use of inhaled nitric oxide. *Pediatrics*. 2000;106:344–345

American Academy of Pediatrics Committee on Injury and Poison Prevention. Transporting children with special health care needs. *Pediatrics*. 1999;104:988–992

American Academy of Pediatrics Committee on Pediatric Emergency Medicine. Emergency preparedness for children with special health care needs. *Pediatrics*. 1999;104:e53 Available at: http://pediatrics.aappublications.org/cgi/content/full/104/4/e53. Accessed January 11, 2006

American Academy of Pediatrics Committee on Pediatric Emergency Medicine and American College of Emergency Physicians. Care of children in the emergency department: guidelines for preparedness. *Pediatrics*. 2001;107:777–781

American Academy of Pediatrics Section on Critical Care and Committee on Hospital Care. Guidelines and levels of care for pediatric intensive care units. *Pediatrics*. 2004;114:1114–1125

American Academy of Pediatrics. Statement of endorsement. Pediatric care in the emergency department. *Pediatrics*. 2004;113:420

American Academy of Pediatrics. *Textbook of Neonatal Resuscitation*. 4th ed. Elk Grove Village, IL: American Academy of Pediatrics; 2000

Athey J, Dean JM, Ball J, Wiebe R, Melese-d'Hospital I. Ability of hospitals to care for pediatric emergency patients. *Pediatr Emerg Care*. 2001;17:170–174

■ ■

DeWing MD, Curry T, Stephenson E, Palmieri T, Greenhalgh DG. Cost-effective use of helicopters for the transportation of patients with burn injuries. *J Burn Care Rehabil.* 2000:21;535–540

Foley DS, Pranikoff T, Younger JG, et. al. A review of 100 patients transported on extracorporeal life support. *ASAIO J.* 2002:48;612–619

McPherson M, Arango P, Fox H, et al. A new definition of children with special health care needs. *Pediatrics.* 1998;102:137–140

Mitchell CS, Doyle ML, Moran JB, et al. Worker training for new threats: a proposed framework. *Am J Ind Med.* 2004;46:423–431

Peerzada JM, Richardson DK, Burns JP. Delivery room decision-making at the threshold of viability. *J Pediatr.* 2004;145:492–498

Rosenberg DI, Moss MM, and the American College of Critical Care Medicine of the Society of Critical Care Medicine. Guidelines and levels of care for pediatric intensive care units. *Crit Care Med.* 2004;32:2117–2127

Sacchetti A, Gerardi M, Barkin R, et al. Emergency data set for children with special needs. *Ann Emerg Med.* 1996;28:324–327

Saffle JR, Edelman L, Morris SE. Regional air transport of burn patients: a case for telemedicine? *J Trauma.* 2004;57:57–64

Slater H, O'Mara MS, Goldfarb IW. Helicopter transportation of burn patients. *Burns.* 2002;28:70–72

Weaver LK, Hopkins RO, Chan KJ, et al. Hyperbaric oxygen for acute carbon monoxide poisoning. *N Engl J Med.* 2002;347:1057–1067

Westrope C, Roberts N, Nichani S, Hunt C, Peek GJ, Firmin R. Experience with mobile inhaled nitric oxide during transport of neonates and children with respiratory insufficiency to an extracorporeal membrane oxygenation center. *Pediatr Crit Care Med.* 2004;5:542–546

Wilson BJ, Heiman HS, Butler TJ, Negaard KA, DiGeronimo R. A 16-year neonatal/ pediatric extracorporeal membrane oxygenation transport experience. *Pediatrics.* 2002;109:189–193

Questions

1. Which of the following services may be affected by regulatory agencies based on the level of services provided?
   a. Pediatric emergency departments, trauma centers
   b. Trauma centers, pediatric intensive care units
   c. Pediatric intensive care units, neonatal intensive care units
   d. Neonatal intensive care units, trauma centers
2. Examples of children with special health care needs include those with all of the following conditions *except:*
   a. Chronic lung disease
   b. Diabetes
   c. Respiratory distress syndrome
   d. Congenital heart disease
3. Which of the following is true regarding newborns with pulmonary hypertension?
   a. Inhaled nitric oxide should be initiated only in extracorporeal membrane oxygenation (ECMO) centers.
   b. Mobile ECMO is widely available for use during transport in the United States.
   c. Abrupt discontinuation of nitric oxide can result in acute worsening of pulmonary hypertension.
   d. High-frequency oscillatory ventilation is the preferred mode of ventilation during transport.

Answers

1. d
2. c
3. c

International Transport

Outline

- General considerations for international transport
- Team configuration and medical control
- Legal and regulatory issues
- Communications
- Medications and equipment
- Personnel considerations
- Logistical issues
- Financial considerations

General Considerations for International Transport

Increasing globalization and international travel are eliminating geographic boundaries in the health care environment. The demands and requirements for international transport of pediatric and neonatal patients are, therefore, increasing. Despite the growth of this practice, most transport programs have limited opportunity or demand to participate in international transports, unless they are located in a border community.

If planning to participate in international transports, the service should develop specific guidelines in advance to avoid significant delays in or failure to complete the transport. There are certain issues to consider that would generally not be of concern within the confines of the US borders. These include the legitimacy of the referral request, equipment compatibility, and limitations of local and international communications. Additional factors that need to be considered are pharmaceutical issues, legal and custody issues, language barriers and need for interpretation services, customs (immigration) protocols, patient and family citizenship, currency availability, contingency planning, and personnel health and safety issues.

■■■■■■■■■■■■■■■■■■■■■■■■■■■■■■■■■■■

Neonatal-pediatric transport services in proximity to bordering countries may have the opportunity to use a ground ambulance for patient transfer. More commonly, international transports will be accomplished using fixed-wing transportation. Pediatric transport programs operating a fixed-wing program must determine whether the aircraft is adequately equipped for international travel, including the potential for travel over open water. If not, just as for programs without direct access to fixed-wing aircraft, a third-party operator needs to be secured. There should be a minimum standard for the medical configuration of aircraft for international neonatal-pediatric transport supplied by the carrier. The transport program should be aware that these services are costly and, unless a previous relationship has been developed, often require payment in advance. The success of the transport can depend on the communication with each party involved. Expectations must be well defined before departure to avoid complications that could jeopardize the mission or patient, transport team, or flight crew safety.

Before leaving the United States, familiarity with the destination country should be established. The legitimacy of the referral must be investigated thoroughly by the medical and administrative representatives of the accepting hospital. Opportunity for putting the transport team and flight crew at risk abounds in many parts of the world. Standard societal and legal expectations do not apply in all countries. Countries with civil or political unrest should be avoided if possible, especially if there might be risks to the transport team. Turmoil in certain regions does not necessarily mean, however, that the transport cannot be accomplished or that the entire country is off limits. The location of the patient within the country (and alternative pick-up locations if necessary), will influence the decision in such cases. Updated information for every country is available on the US State Department's Web site at http://travel.state.gov. Detailed research before transport will provide information that will help avoid complications. Direct communication with staff in the State Department with regard to international transport planning may be advisable. This should be the responsibility of the aircraft owner or vendor but also may require input from the transport team.

International patients often have similar medical needs to the patients transported on a daily basis by teams around the United

States, although issues (medical and care) may be encountered that are less common than in the receiving center's routine transport or inpatient population. Timing of the referral may be delayed, and the type of health care and available and provided resources may vary, however, owing to local or other circumstances. The international transport standards published by the Joint Commission may help to standardize local care and transport options and improve the uncertainty and complexity surrounding transfer of patients between international locations. Therefore, the condition of the internationally transported patient may be less predictable or at a more advanced stage of illness than would be predicted or optimally desirable. Alterations and accommodations may need to be made depending on the length of the transport, the amount and sophistication of care given before transport, the acuity and medical needs of the patient during long-distance travel, and any accompanying nonmedical participants. Considerations include additional staff to relieve primary medical and logistical staff on long flights, professional interpretation services, and equipment redundancy and increased supplies.

Team Configuration and Medical Control

The initiation of an international neonatal-pediatric transport should be by direct physician-to-physician communication. Direct contact between physicians may help prevent miscommunications and false expectations by all parties. Consideration should be given to adding a physician to the team configuration for international transports because it may help overcome certain obstacles and potentially minimize medical or legal issues in the referring or receiving country. Some countries may even require that a physician be present for the patient to be released from the country. A physician may be particularly helpful in case the patient's condition deteriorates or the patient dies before or during transport.

Before departure, it is imperative that as much information as possible about the patient be obtained. This should include pertinent medical history, diagnosis, medical management and therapy with responses, and all medications the patient is receiving. This information should be used to develop a plan of care with medical control. If a physician will not be accompanying the transport team, it will be important to address all scenarios and actions to be taken in various possible situations. The plan for medical management must be comprehensive in case communication with medical control is not available during transport. These scenarios should be discussed in detail between the medical control physician and the transport team before departure. Alternative care plans, hospitals, and/or facilities should be identified in case of overnight delays, unanticipated deterioration of the patient's condition, or equipment failure.

Legal and Regulatory Issues

Although countries bordering the United States currently do not require passports for visiting US citizens,* it is highly recommended that all staff participating in international transport carry a passport and another form of identification. It is also important to predetermine which documents will be required for the *patient* to exit the country of origin and enter the United States. Often a passport and a visa are required and may take time to obtain. If the parent(s) or legal guardian(s) will not be traveling with the patient, the team may need notarized legal documents authorizing the removal of the patient from the particular country. In case both parents are not living, a copy of their death certificates may need to be presented as evidence of such. Neonates are treated no differently from adults for the purpose of transport in or out of a foreign country; however, it can take several days to acquire these documents for the child. All documents should be in order before the team is dispatched.

Enlisting the assistance of the Office of the Consulate or the embassy for the country is recommended in difficult cases. Establishing these contacts before their need in an emergency can help streamline the process.

Communications

Communication with the base facility often is difficult, if not impossible, from many foreign countries. Many cell phones and calling cards do not work outside the United States, and the toll-free numbers for many facilities do not accept international calls. Programs that will be servicing many international patients per year may want to purchase a satellite phone or GSM (Global System for Mobile communications)

*Law will change on January 1, 2007.

cell phones. This service will provide direct communication via phone from almost anywhere in the world. However, such phones and programs are expensive. An alternative would be to contact a provider for a limited lease agreement if the program will not have an extended need for such equipment. Before departure, it should be determined whether the referring facility will allow international calls to the United States for communication with medical control. Calls initiated from the United States to foreign countries can use the AT&T language line, (888) 419-0167, for interpretation services. When anticipating a significant language barrier, it may be beneficial to use the service of a professional interpreter for the transport. If accommodations cannot be made for this person to accompany the transport team, a mechanism for accessing interpretation services should be established. Whenever possible, all consent forms and other documentation should be translated before departure.

Medications and Equipment

Medications

Medications in other parts of the world are not regulated as strictly as they are in the United States, and strengths, dosages, and availability may vary. Some drugs may even be manufactured under different names than in the United States. Nontraditional therapies and medications also may be encountered in some parts of the world. Before departure, the transport team should make every effort to identify any and all medications or therapies the patient is or has been receiving. The transport team should be equipped with adequate amounts of medications for the duration of the trip and should factor in potential delays. One should not expect to be able to obtain preferred or additional medications or supplies at the referring location, a practice that many teams rely on in the United States. Examination of laws pertaining to narcotics also must be reviewed before entering another country. Certain countries may not allow narcotics to enter with the transport team, meaning these drugs would have to remain with the aircraft. By knowing this in advance, medical control can direct the transport team and referring facility accordingly.

Equipment

Electrical outlets and voltages are different in other parts of the world. As a result, it is essential to ensure that aircraft or ground vehicles that will be involved in international transport are equipped with a medical inverter and that before departure, batteries are fully charged with spares available for all equipment. Electrical adapters also should accompany each piece of equipment. Referral centers in other countries may not have high-pressure connections for oxygen. Programs using oxygen-powered ventilators must take this into account, as well as the fact that connectors vary throughout the world, and prepare accordingly. Critical noninvasive and invasive physiologic and blood monitoring systems may not be compatible owing to climate (heat or cold effects) or electrical power source. Table 21-1 can be used as a minimal equipment checklist for international transport and should be modified at the time of a transport to meet the needs of an individual patient's disease process.

Personnel Considerations

Health Issues

Transport team members may need immunizations before traveling to certain countries. Recommendations for pretravel immunizations and prophylaxis for diseases such as malaria may be obtained from the Centers for Disease Control and Prevention (http://www.cdc.gov/travel). An ample supply of bottled water should be available, and medication for various anticipated indigenous communicable diseases should accompany the transport team. Staff who require personal medication(s) should be reminded to bring an adequate supply for the anticipated duration of the transport and for potential unplanned delays.

Currency and Personal Belongings

Many areas of the world do not have the facilities or technology to accept credit cards. The transport team should be provided cash, in small denominations, to pay for unexpected expenses while traveling. Airports in remote locations may require cash payment for fees and taxes. Distribute the money among the team members so as not to display large amounts of cash when paying for expenses. Incidents

Table 21-1: International Transport Equipment List*

Equipment

_____ Transport bag stocked with usual supplies and equipment
_____ Monitor with multiple outlet charger
_____ Defibrillator
_____ Syringe pumps with power cords
_____ A/C plug adapters
_____ Spare batteries for all equipment

Airway

_____ Ventilator with extra battery packs, power cord, and extra circuits
_____ Oxygen tanks and regulators
_____ O$_2$ adapter connections
_____ Airway adjuncts (ETT, LMA) and self-inflating bag
_____ Manual backup suction

Medications and IV fluids

_____ IV fluids (multiple bags and solutions)
_____ Narcotic pack
_____ Additional medications (depends on duration of the transport, patient's diagnosis, and condition)

Standard precautions supplies

_____ Gowns, gloves, and masks
_____ Bedpan and urinal
_____ Emesis basin
_____ Biohazard bags
_____ Germicidal cloths and antiseptic foam

Miscellaneous

_____ Petty cash, credit cards
_____ Mobile phone and international phone card
_____ Linens, blankets, and towels
_____ Chart packet: transport records, patient information, and consent form
_____ Passports and/or visas, birth certificates, or other proof of citizenship
_____ Notarized statement (or other validation) from family giving permission to transport and care for the minor child
_____ Personal items

* ETT indicates endotracheal tube; LMA, laryngeal mask airway; and IV, intravenous.

of price gouging may occur if it is known that large amounts of cash are readily available. Overnight accommodations and meals usually are arranged by the fixed-wing vendor and included in the price quote but should be verified before departure. The best policy for personal items, such as jewelry and cameras, is not to take them. A good quality disposable camera is an acceptable alternative. This eliminates the problem of robbery or need for bartering with these items. Space limitations also should be considered when packing baggage for the trip.

Logistical Issues

Vendors and Liaisons

The selection of an appropriate vendor for a particular international transport can be confusing, and guidelines for selection are listed in Table 21-2. A sample of vendors is noted in Appendix E, although individual listings should not be interpreted as implying endorsement. Commission on Accreditation of Medical Transport Systems accreditation indicates a commitment to a defined set of standards for trans-

---

Table 21-2: Vendor and Equipment Analysis

I. Choosing a vendor
   a. Check AAMS (Association of Air Medical Services) resource guide for vendors that provide international transport services.
   b. Do an Internet search. This is a good way to find a variety of vendors and narrow the search to the specifics needs of the transport.
   c. History
      i. How often does the vendor do international transports?
      ii. Has the vendor been to the country that this transport will be done in?
      iii. If so, how familiar are the vendor and the pilots with the country?
      iv. Does the vendor have a handler for that country, or will one be employed?
         1. If one is to be employed, where from?
         2. Will the handler provide set up of all services such as ground transportation, hotels, and interpretation and translation services if required and will the vendor cover all expenses incurred while out of the United States (eg, customs fees)?
      v. Will the vendor handle all outbound and inbound customs regulations?
      vi. Does the vendor have references?
II. Equipment
   a. What type of plane will the vendor use for this transport?
   b. Is the program providing the plane and crew accredited by Commission on Accreditation of Medical Transport Systems (CAMTS)?
      i. This is not necessarily a requirement if it is a reputable organization with a proven record in the international community.
         1. Check the references from above.
   c. What are the billing options?
      i. Before transport
      ii. Payable on completion of transport

---

port but does not specifically address issues related to international transports. When traveling to other countries, it is recommended that a "handler" be secured to assist with the incidentals of entering and exiting the foreign country. The vendor should employ a handler who is skilled in assisting with customs, scheduling interpreters, and arranging for ground transportation, security, and other services that may be necessary for a successful mission. Depending on the duration of the mission, it may be necessary for the transport team and flight crew to schedule departure at the beginning of a duty shift or stay overnight in the foreign country to have an adequate period of rest before the return segment of the trip. Before departing, such details should be verified with the fixed-wing vendor. Fees vary widely for such services and should be included in the fixed-wing vendor's quote. Pilots, as always, should be expected and prepared to provide documentation of ownership and insurance for the aircraft, as well as appropriate pilot licensure and current Federal Aviation Administration flight physical certificate.

Ground Transportation

Repositioning the crew and the patient requires ground transportation, which may be limited and often requires cash payment. To avoid complications at the time of transport, this should be set up by the handler before departure. Ambulances and emergency medical services in foreign countries can be very different, often with a significantly lower standard of technology, from those operated in the United States. Adequately charged equipment, electrical adapters, and ample supplies should accompany the team for this portion of the transport.

Family Members

Family members planning to travel with the patient also will need a current passport and/or visa. In case the size of the aircraft and crew configuration will not allow for transport of a parent, this should be addressed when setting up the transport to provide the family adequate time to secure another form of transportation.

Financial Considerations

International transports can be costly. Securing payment or guarantee of payment in advance for such transports should be a priority. This prevents the potential for the transport team to be placed in an awkward or potentially dangerous situation. If the patient has insurance, prior authorization should be obtained for the transport and the inpatient treatment at the receiving facility. Most often, patients coming into the United States will not be eligible for state Medicaid programs at the time of transport; thus, the inbound trip may not be reimbursable by state insurance. Administrators for the transport team and the accepting facility should work in conjunction with one another to determine the best arrangements for payment. Be aware that many foreign hospitals require full payment of medical expenses before releasing the patient for transfer. Before departing for transport, ensure that the patient's guarantor has settled all debts with the referring foreign health care system.

Medical transport on commercial airlines usually is limited to patients in extremely stable condition who require little ongoing treatment. Commercial airlines differ in how they accommodate the medical needs of an infant and child and usually require that any specialized equipment be inspected before travel. Oxygen sources may or may not be available, and access to a source of electricity is variable. All commercial carriers have an affiliated medical director, who may be a valuable source of information and assistance.

Selected Readings

Association of Air Medical Services. *Association of Air Medical Services Resource Guide.* Available at: http://www.aams.org. Accessed January 13, 2006

Centers for Disease Control and Prevention. Travelers' Health. Available at: http://www.cdc.gov. Accessed January 13, 2006

Commission on Accreditation of Medical Transport Systems web site. Available at: http://www.CAMTS.org. Accessed January 13, 2006

Joint Commission Resources: *Joint Commission International Accreditation Standards for Medical Transport Organizations.* Oakbrook Terrace, IL: Joint Commission on Accreditation of Healthcare Organizations; 2003

US Department of State. Travel.State.Gov. Available at: http://travel.state.gov/travel. Accessed January 13, 2006

Veldman A, Diefenbach M, Fischer D, Benton A, Bloch R. Long-distance transport of ventilated patients: advantages and limitations of air medical repatriation on commercial airlines. *Air Med J.* 2004;23:24-28

Woodward GA, Insoft RM, Pearson-Shaver AL, et al. The state of pediatric interfacility transport: consensus of the second national pediatric and neonatal interfacility transport medicine leadership conference. *Pediatr Emerg Care.* 2002;18:38-43

Questions

1. International transport is becoming less frequent with the improvement in medical care throughout the world.
   a. True
   b. False
2. Logistical challenges with international transport include which of the following?
   a. Prolonged travel time
   b. Language issues
   c. Medication restrictions
   d. Staff rest requirements
3. Including a physician in international transport is recommended.
   a. True
   b. False

Answers

1. b, false. Requests for international transport are increasing. Each transport system should decide at what level it will participate in international transport before a request is made.
2. All of the above
3. a, true. A physician who accompanies an international transport team may help minimize legal or medical issues that may arise, especially with a patient whose condition deteriorates before or during transport.

■ Stress Management, Debriefing, ■ and Team Health

Outline

■ Sources of stress for members of a transport team
■ Effects of stress on team function and morale
■ Critical incident stress management and its role in transport team stress management
■ Methods for relieving stress and maintaining team health

Sources of Stress for Members of a Transport Team

"If a scientist were to create a stressful environment, it might look like our jobs."[1] So says an experienced flight nurse in a review of literature describing the transport environment.

Monitoring and managing a transport team's physical health and stress level is an important component in ensuring that the team is able to provide a safe and appropriate level of clinical care. Maintaining team health and recognizing and dealing with deficits proactively may help team members to deal more effectively with the effects of cumulative stress (burnout) and traumatic (critical incident) stress. Transport team members have many stressors that, although not individually unique to transport, probably *are* unique in the combination in which they occur in the transport setting. The amount of stress generated on a routine basis in the transport setting may not be recognized or acknowledged until it reaches a critical level. Stresses of flight are summarized in Table 22.1 (see also Chapter 11).

Some emphasis must be placed on the fatigue factor. One of the biggest challenges faced by transport programs is maintaining an adequate balance between rest and duty time. This is addressed with

Table 22-1: Stresses of Flight

Stressor	Effects
Decreased partial pressure of oxygen	Hypoxia
Barometric pressure changes	Barotitis media, barosinusitis, barodontalgia, gastrointestinal changes
Thermal changes	Hypothermia, hyperthermia
Decreased humidity	Dehydration
Noise	Degradation of communication, fatigue, temporary or permanent hearing loss
Vibration	Motion sickness, fatigue, shortness of breath, abdominal or chest pain, increased metabolic rate, increased respirations, orthopedic problems
Fatigue	Impaired judgment, difficulty maintaining attention to details and tasks, lessened ability to communicate effectively; increased risk of error; diminished critical thinking skills
Gravitational forces	Exposure to positive and negative acceleration forces, decompression sickness
Spatial disorientation	Cannot interpret or process information being given by the senses
Flicker vertigo	Nausea, vomiting
Fuel vapors	Altered mental status, nausea, eye inflammation

respect to the pilot component of the team via the Federal Aviation Regulations requirement under Part 135, which requires that a pilot must have a minimum of 10 hours of uninterrupted rest within every 24-hour period. (On-call time, when the pilot is required to carry and respond to a pager, is counted as "duty time" and cannot be included in the minimum 10 hours of required rest.) However, duty time is not similarly regulated for other transport team members, unless the team is using residents, who are governed by the Accreditation Council on Graduate Medical Education work rules.

In its position paper, Flight Nurse Safety in the Air Medical Environment, the Air and Surface Transport Nurses Association states: "Lengthy duty time associated with 24-hour shifts creates an environment that promotes conditions of fatigue and compromised judgment abilities unless the necessary 10-hour rest period can be ensured. Scheduling shorter shift duration does not guarantee that crew members will receive sufficient rest or be free from fatigue and compromised performance."[2] According to the National EMS Pilot's Association Safety Guidelines, "...fatigue cannot always be self-determined, and in most cases...may not be apparent until serious errors are made."

In addition to functioning in an environment where they are subject to multiple physical and physiologic variables, transport team members are expected to attain and maintain a high level of proficiency in their roles as critical thinkers, in their ability to be autonomous practitioners for complex patient care issues, and in their performance of advanced invasive procedures. All of this is accomplished in an environment with limited resources: a small, enclosed work space; few to no additional personnel to provide assistance; limited definitive diagnostic capabilities; potential equipment limitations; less than optimal lighting; and limited access to the patient.

The transport environment demands excellence in communication and teamwork to be successful. Yet, effective communication, in itself, requires significant thought and effort and adds to the workload. Transport team members depend on one another's knowledge, expertise, and skill and a collaborative use of those assets in the highly variable and ever-changing transport environment. If interpersonal dynamics between team members are less than optimal, communication can quickly deteriorate.

Communication with referral health care providers is another essential, yet stress-producing component of the transport environment. The team may walk into a situation that is chaotic and find a patient in a much different condition from that originally described. The team members need to integrate themselves immediately with a referral team that is already "in the thick of things." This includes gathering pertinent information, assisting in and eventually assuming the provision of care, and documenting patient status and treatments. Team members also may be placed in the role of teacher as referral staff question them about the treatment they are providing and ask for feedback on their performance.

In addition, there is an important need to communicate with family members, who can run the gamut from detached, to stoic, to emotionally needy, to highly volatile. They may look to transport team members for information and reassurance, and the team's response may necessarily be bad news. Team members who are already stressed with the accountability for provision of autonomous and advanced care now are taxed with the demand for sophisticated and sensitive communication skills.

Psychological factors add to the cumulative effect. There is often a strong emotional impetus to rescue a critically ill infant or child despite an adverse environment. The team may feel the need to attempt the mission, even in the face of poor and/or deteriorating weather conditions. In other cases, fear for personal safety may occur as the team is asked to respond to situations in which there is potential for harm due to fire, hazardous materials, or even volatile family members.

The final group of stressors are those that are self-imposed by team members and are represented by the acronym "DEATH": **D**rugs, **E**xhaustion (fatigue), **A**lcohol, **T**obacco, and **H**ypoglycemia.

■ Prescription and nonprescription medications and the conditions for which they are taken may interfere with performance, perception, decision making, and motor skills. Team members must be aware of the adverse and toxic effects, allergic responses, and synergistic effects of the medications they are taking.

■ Exhaustion and fatigue must be avoided to prevent errors in judgment, poor attention span, and decreased work capacity and performance.

■ The effects of alcohol ingestion tend to be exacerbated by altitude. Ingesting 1 alcoholic beverage at 10 000 ft is equivalent to ingesting 2 or 3 times as much at sea level.

■ Similarly, the effects of tobacco are magnified during flight. The carbon monoxide by-product of smoking at sea level may result in mild hypoxia similar to that seen at an altitude of 8000 ft. This may occur with smoking as few as 3 cigarettes in rapid succession.

■ An inadequate or improper diet can result in nausea, headache, dizziness, errors in judgment, and loss of consciousness. Many air transport programs have a weight limitation based on aircraft weight and balance restrictions, and care must be taken to ensure that compliance does not lead to hypoglycemia and dehydration.

Effects of Stress on Transport Team Function and Morale

The aforementioned stressors can have immediate and dramatic physical and psychological effects on individual team members and on their ability to function within the team in any given situation.

Maintaining individual physical health, mental hardiness, and team health can help to mitigate or alleviate stress. If the symptoms of stress are unrecognized or ignored, the effects will progress relentlessly. "Working in an emotionally charged milieu with stakes as high as they can get, however rewarding, must have fallout."[1]

Burnout, the concept of literally being consumed (and/or depleted) by work, is the inevitable end of cumulative, unmitigated stress. The onset of burnout is usually insidious and closely resembles depression. As burnout progresses, team members will have less and less emotional reserve and, thus, less physical and emotional energy to expend in the care of patients and in interpersonal relationships with coworkers. There is a loss of satisfaction once received from interaction with patients and a loss of connections with peers. Symptoms of burnout are many and varied and include those in Table 22-2.

The incidence of traumatic or critical incident stress is of additional significance to transport team members. A *critical incident* is any event that can exert an impact so stressful that it overwhelms an individual's usual coping mechanisms. They are generally events that are unexpected, out-of-the-ordinary, and emotionally distressing. They have an overwhelming impact on even the most highly trained and experienced personnel. Some examples are line-of-duty death, serious line-of-duty injury, coworker suicide, multicasualty incidents, police-involved shooting, injury or death of a civilian as a result of operational procedures (eg, fire engine vs private car), failed mission after extensive effort, or any event that has personal significance for the team member (which may be different for different people). Of special significance to transport teams who care for children are injury to or death of a child, especially if caused by an adult. In critical incidents in the United States in which a debriefing for involved personnel was conducted, 95% involved children.[3,4]

Table 22-2: Symptoms of Burnout

- Anxiety
- Negativity
- Cynicism
- Increased physical and emotional fatigue
- Loss of motivation or enthusiasm for the job
- Frequent absenteeism
- Apathy
- Sleep disturbances
- Memory loss
- Head, neck, back, or muscle aches
- Withdrawal from social contacts
- Irritability
- Sexual dysfunction
- Persistent or frequent infections
- Gastrointestinal problems
- Self-medication with alcohol or nonprescription or prescription drugs
- Overeating or undereating or a gain or loss in weight not related to dieting
- Inability to concentrate
- Inability to make decisions
- Short attention span
- Forgetfulness
- Elevated blood pressure
- Cardiac problems
- Irrational, impulsive behavior
- Self-destructive behavior
- Inability to do the job (substandard patient care)
- Inability to manage life in general
- Paranoia
- Overreaction to events
- Frequent accidents

Posttraumatic stress disorder (PTSD), previously most often seen in combat survivors, now is recognized as a potential response to any form of traumatic event. Acute PTSD generally occurs within 4 weeks of the event and lasts from 2 days to 4 weeks. Symptoms include a sense of detachment or absence of emotional responsiveness, decreased awareness of surroundings, depersonalization, associative amnesia, persistent reenactment of the traumatic event in dreams, flashbacks, distress when reminded of the event, anxiety or hypersensitivity, and impairment in performing usual tasks in social, work, or personal situations.

Chronic PTSD is a life-changing dysfunctional state. Mitchell and Everly[3] quote the 10th edition of the *World Health Organization: International Classification of Disease:* "PTSD may be so chronic as to transition into an enduring personality change as a direct result of the traumatic stressor." Chronic PTSD is characterized by a month or more of the following: recurrent and distressing recollections of the event, avoidance of anything associated with the traumatic event, an overall decrease in the ability to respond to and interact with others, and a persistent increased state of arousal (difficulty falling or staying asleep, irritability, hypervigilance, difficulty concentrating, or an exaggerated startle response).

Critical Incident Stress Management and Its Role in Transport Team Stress Management

Everly and Mitchell[4] state that "the ultimate goal of critical incident stress management (CISM) is the prevention of acute, disabling psychological discord and the rapid restoration of adaptive functioning in the wake of a critical (crisis) incident." Critical incident stress management is a comprehensive concept that includes the following:

- Primary prevention: Identification and mitigation of pathogenic stressors. This part of the program emphasizes preincident education and includes introduction of team members to the stressors of the job in a realistic manner, education about stress responses they may experience, and appropriate coping skills and survival techniques.
- Secondary prevention: Identification and mitigation of acute distress and dysfunctional symptom patterns. This phase includes defusing and debriefings.
  - Defusing takes place 8 to 12 hours following the incident, is informal, and is facilitated by peers trained in CISM. It provides an opportunity for participants to talk about their role and what happened from their perspective. They may discuss any stress-related responses they are experiencing. Peers provide information about other symptoms team members may experience in the next few hours or days and teach positive coping skills.

❖ Debriefing is a more formal and structured intervention and takes place between 24 and 72 hours after the event. This session is facilitated by a mental health professional. Participants are encouraged, within the confines of a safe and confidential environment, to express their thoughts, feelings, fears, and recollections. If possible, the debriefing process should include involvement of family members of transport team personnel. These family members will almost certainly have fears (some perhaps long unexpressed) about their loved one's involvement in such a high-risk profession. Spouses and adult children may benefit by participation in a debriefing session, separate from the session held for transport team members, which also is conducted by a mental health professional and is not attended by their spouse or parent who is a transport team member. Teenagers and younger children may be divided by age groups and also have an opportunity to express their fears and other feelings through play and talk.

▪ Tertiary prevention: Follow-up mental health treatment. Participants are offered ongoing, formal, and more advanced mental health intervention.

In its position paper Flight Nurse Safety in the Air Medical Environment, the Air and Surface Transport Nurses Association states that its recommendation is that each (air) medical transport program develop CISM programs, both informal and formal.[2] Peer support and debriefings on an informal basis could be used more frequently when a small number of team members are affected. Formal CISM should be used when multiple team members and/or the surrounding community, other emergency medical services providers, coworkers, and others are affected by a major event. Formal CISM requires involvement of an outside group of trained professionals who are not members of the affected groups.

Methods for Relieving Stress and Maintaining Team Health

Acknowledging and identifying stressors in the transport environment and a willingness to deal with them in a positive and proactive manner are essential steps in relieving stress and maintaining individual and team health. Transport team members can be adept at using their exceptional critical thinking skills to identify problems and solutions for their patients but not for themselves.

The physiologic stressors of transport cannot realistically be eliminated, but they may be mitigated with education and planning. Some examples include the following:

- Preemployment and annual physical screening examinations (including hearing) to identify areas of concern
- A general physical fitness program, including resources to assist with exercise and nutrition counseling
- Provision of hearing protection to staff working in and around aircraft
- Provision of adequate fluids and nutrition, even during the busiest service periods
- Weather-appropriate clothing and footwear required and, to the extent possible, provided by the employer

Maintaining a balance between adequate rest and duty time is a priority that must be attended to vigilantly by every transport program. The Air and Surface Transport Nurses' position paper, Flight Nurse Safety in the Air Medical Environment, recommends the following for flight nurses[2] (similar suggestions seem appropriate for all transport personnel who are not already subject to stricter rules or regulations regarding duty availability and participation):

- Structured scheduling that ensures that each medical crew member receives a minimum of 10 hours of uninterrupted rest in any 24-hour period
- A written policy acknowledging the crew member's responsibility to request relief from duty when feeling excessively fatigued or inadequately rested should be established. The policy should include a process for identification and activation of backup personnel to relieve excessively fatigued crew members.
- Structured scheduling of crew members to provide for infrequent changes between night, evening, and day shifts and with shift changes made in a forward rotation. Scheduling of days off should allow for maximum quality rest and transition between shifts.

Active training in and cultivation of communication skills should be an acknowledged, formal, and ongoing part of annual training requirements. This may be conducted by trained facilitators from the facility's employee assistance program or others with the necessary background and skill. In any case, individual communication skills should be monitored by team leaders and administrators just as closely as clinical skills. Additional resources for stress management are included in Table 22-3.

Table 22-3: Resources for Transport Teams Interested in Exploring Stress Management Options

- Employee assistance program: hardiness training, communication, teamwork, individual counseling
- Employee physical fitness programs and nutrition counseling
- Occupational health professionals: physical screenings, hearing examinations
- Critical incident stress management programs: preincident education, defusing, debriefings

---

When effective interpersonal communication skills are combined with medical and administrative support, formal and informal debriefing sessions provide a safe and nurturing environment that is crucial to the health of the team. A review of care provided, along with a discussion of other stressful variables that occurred during the transport, allows team members to express their questions, fears, self-doubts, and concerns and, in turn, receive social support from their peers and supervisors. High levels of social support are associated with low levels of occupational stress. On the other hand, griping and negative sessions prove to be ineffective in reducing stress and may, conversely, increase it. Formal, comprehensive, system-wide safety and quality programs also provide a forum for identification and resolution of a wide variety of issues. Prompt follow-up of issues and reporting of resolution to team members can significantly reduce stress and instill confidence that concerns are being addressed in an effective and timely way.

Regular training in survival techniques and emergency equipment and procedures is mandatory for every team, regardless of the mode of transport or the type of terrain routinely encountered. Practicing these procedures in and around their usual transport vehicles and environment instills not only knowledge, but also confidence. All team members should be encouraged to carry personal survival gear appropriate to their transport environment.

Regardless of their comfort level with emergency procedures and survival skills, each and every transport team and crew member has not only the right, but also the responsibility to refuse to participate in a transport when there is a legitimate concern for personal safety. A transport team member, when voicing concerns for his or her own safety, as well as that of the patient(s) and other team members, should be supported and protected by written policy of the program so that refusal to participate in and/or complete a transport does not lead to disciplinary or other negative action against the individual. This is true not only for air transport, but also for transport by ground ambulance when road conditions may be just as or more hazardous than those in the air.

It is essential that personnel who provide medical and administrative support to transport teams are highly aware of the potential and real stressors of transport. Transport team members, as a rule, tend to be hyperaccountable and hold themselves to an almost impossibly high standard of performance. If patient outcome is less than ideal, even in the face of overwhelming injury or disease, transport team members may assume unreasonable levels of personal accountability and guilt. Every effort must be made by medical advisors and administrators to set and reaffirm reasonable levels of performance; to provide adequate resources, education, and training; and to provide positive feedback. Team members must be actively monitored for symptoms of stress, burnout, and cumulative stress and appropriate counseling and referrals made promptly and proactively when symptoms first appear.

References

1. Prag PW. Stress, burnout, and social support: a review and call for research. *Air Med J.* 2003;22:18–22
2. Air and Surface Transport Nurses Association Position Paper. Flight Nurse Safety in the Air Medical Environment. October 2001:3,10, 11, 13. Available at: http://www.astna.org/Position-papers/Safety1.pdf. Accessed March 3, 2006
3. Mitchell JT, Everly GS. *Critical Incident Stress Debriefing: An Operations Manual for CISD, Defusing and Other Group Crisis Intervention Services.* 3rd ed. Ellicott City, MD: Chevron; 2001:10
4. Everly GS, Mitchell JT. *Critical Incident Stress Management-CISM: A New Era and Standard of Care in Crisis Intervention.* 2nd ed. Ellicott City, MD: Chevron; 1999:12

Selected Readings

Hickman BJ, Mehrer R. Stress and the effects of air transport on flight crews. *Air Med J.* 2001;20:6–9

Holleran RS, ed. Critical care transport: stress and stress management in the workplace. In: *Air & Surface Patient Transport Principles and Practice.* 3rd ed. St Louis, MO: Mosby; 2003:671–688

Holleran RS, ed. Transport physiology. In: *Air & Surface Patient Transport Principles and Practice.* 3rd ed. St Louis, MO: Mosby; 2003:41–66

Mitchell JT, Everly GS. *Critical Incident Stress Debriefing: An Operations Manual for Defusing and Other Group Crisis Intervention Services.* 3rd ed. Ellicott City, MD: Chevron; 2001

Sherman DW. Nurses' stress and burnout. How to care for yourself when caring for patients and their families experiencing life-threatening illness. *Am J Nurs.* 2004;104:48–57

Singh RG. Relationship between occupational stress and social support in flight nurses. *Aviat Space Environ Med.* 1990;61:349–352

US Department of Transportation. Federal Aviation Regulations. Part 135. Washington, DC: Federal Aviation Administration; 2001. Available at: http://www.access.gpo.gov/nara/cfr/waisidx_06/14cfr135_06.html. Accessed August 11, 2006

Questions

1. What are the physiologic stressors that transport team members can expect to face during their usual practice and what symptoms may be associated with the stressors?
2. What is burnout, and how may it be manifested in transport team members?
3. What are some ways in which individual and team mental and physical health may be maintained?

Answers

1. Depending on the environment and mode of transport, team members can expect to be affected by some or all of the following: a decrease in the partial pressure of oxygen (hypoxia), barometric pressure changes (barotitis media, barosinusitis, barodontalgia [pain in teeth associated with pressure change], gastrointestinal changes), thermal changes in the environment (hypothermia or hyperthermia), decreased humidity (dehydration), noise (degradation of communication, fatigue, temporary or permanent hearing loss), vibration (motion sickness, fatigue, shortness of breath, abdominal or chest pain, increased metabolic rate, increased respiratory rate, orthopedic problems), fatigue (decreased ability to process information and make decisions), gravitational forces, spatial disorientation (cannot interpret or process information being given by senses), flicker vertigo (nausea, vomiting), and fuel vapors (altered mental status, nausea, eye inflammation).
2. Burnout resembles depression and is the end point of cumulative, unmitigated stress. Team members experiencing burnout often will have noticeably less physical and emotional energy to expend in the care of their patients and in their relationships with coworkers. Job satisfaction declines significantly. See Table 22-2 for additional manifestations.
3. a. Acknowledgement and mitigation of physiologic stressors
   b. Adequate rest
   c. Training in communication skills
   d. Formal and informal debriefing sessions
   e. Training in survival skills and emergency procedures
   f. A formal mechanism to express concern for personal safety
   g. Medical and administrative support

Involvement and Integration With EMS

Outline

- Overview
- Integrating CCITTs with EMS
  - Long-term entrapment
  - Triage
  - Unexpected medical encounters
  - Disasters
- Training opportunities

Overview

Because of the nature of their employment, nurses, physicians, respiratory therapists, and technicians with pediatric critical care interfacility transport teams (CCITTs) may have little involvement or integration (cooperative training or practice) with the local emergency medical services (EMS) system, although to the public eye, they often are considered components of the same emergency transport system. Each has a tremendous amount to gain from the expertise of the other. This chapter discusses how sharing some of these perspectives and skills can be an advantage to EMS and CCITTs as they perform their mission of providing mobile patient care.

If one takes a closer look at both disciplines, the similarities in the way they provide care are striking. The CCITT performs telephone triage and evaluation and management of the patient, which in many ways is the interfacility transport version of 911. If the decision to accept the transfer is made, the CCITT is dispatched and on arrival at the referring hospital (or on scene for EMS) performs on-site triage and evaluation, management, and stabilization of the patient's condition. It then is the responsibility of the CCITT, like EMS, to successfully transport the patient to the receiving facility while continuing ongoing efforts at stabilization.

There are also differences. For example, in most cases, patients referred to the CCITT have been triaged, assessed, and often treated by advanced medical providers, usually physicians. This is rarely the case when EMS is involved. EMS providers are often the first and only responders on scene, and, depending on the availability of online medical direction, they provide the highest level of care the patient is likely to receive before hospital arrival.

Integrating CCITTs With EMS

There often is a casual integration with EMS as the CCITT performs its job. This integration may range from using the same parking spaces outside of the emergency department to the use of EMS providers or vehicles as a core component of the CCITT. Further efforts and development of this relationship can be mutually beneficial. There are many areas of expertise in the EMS system, which can be invaluable for the CCITT, including the following:

- Emergency vehicle operations
- Communications
- Use of the incident command (IC) system (Figure 23-1)
- Continuing education specific to the prehospital environment
- Triage of multiple patients
- Rapid and efficient on-scene triage, evaluation, and management of patients
- Consistent, effective, and outcome-driven phone triage algorithms
- Mass casualty preparedness

There also are many areas of expertise within the critical care transport environment that could be shared with EMS providers, such as the following:

- Phone direction of advanced care
- Advanced and thorough medical assessments and care provision
- Integration with hospital personnel
- Anticipation of next steps in critical care patient management
- Provision of thorough care with complete written and verbal patient care reports
- Ability to use hospital-based resources and educational opportunities

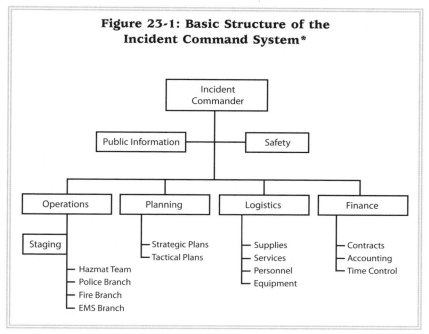

Figure 23-1: Basic Structure of the Incident Command System*

*EMS indicates emergency medical services.
Available at: http://www.training.fema.gov/EMIWeb/IS/is100.asp. Accessed January 23, 2006.

■ Access to the academic and tertiary medical settings and the opportunity to work with students, residents, and fellows

■ Nationally standardized education, training, licensing, and certification of providers

■ Consistent advanced medical control

■ Implementation and use of research protocols

■ Successful integration of effective quality assurance programs into medical practice

Integration between groups requires an understanding of educational backgrounds and care capabilities. The standard levels of EMS training and personnel in the prehospital environment are as follows:

■ First responders: can assist with basic first aid, use an automated external defibrillator, and perform cardiopulmonary resuscitation and very basic airway support; typically have approximately 40 hours of training

■ Emergency medical technician-basic (EMT-B): can perform the preceding skills and immobilization, extrication, oxygen support, and patient transport in an ambulance; typically have approximately 100 hours of training

■ Emergency medical technician-intermediate (EMT-I): can perform preceding skills and may have advanced airway skills such as intubation and the ability to obtain intravenous access; relatively few EMT-Is trained and have wide variability in skills performed; training time, approximately 200 hours

■ Emergency medical technician-paramedic (EMT-P): have advanced skills and can perform advanced airway support and administer medications in the field; training of more than 1000 hours (often closer to 2000 hours) with extensive field internships that are integral to the certification process

■ "Critical care transport" EMS provider: available in some areas; training builds on the skills of an EMT-B, EMT-I, or EMT-P; courses usually presented in a modular format over several months and include didactic and clinical instruction

The different levels of EMT's can be confusing. When teaming with an EMS provider, it is important to clarify professional capabilities and personal comfort level with expected involvement.

Whether it is through day-to-day casual encounter, ride-alongs (strongly encouraged as a learning opportunity), or an integrated educational and training program, the importance of sharing expertise between EMS and CCITTs cannot be overstated. This sharing should start with a better understanding of one another's mode of operations. For example, hospital transport and other medical professionals may not be aware of the education, capabilities, or scope of practice of prehospital providers. The converse is often true for EMS providers who typically work in the field and may not regularly interact with CCITT members. Understanding one another's roles and responsibilities is especially important during high-volume and high-acuity situations or in the case of limited care availability (such as a mass casualty or evacuation with use of both resources), when the distinctions between EMS and CCITT may blur. Situations such as mass casualty incidents or disasters of any kind may demand that the CCITT move into a role to which it is unaccustomed. Issues such as definitions of words used can add to confusion and communication difficulties for teams working together without previous training. For example, "casualty" may mean something different to an EMS-trained provider than to a transport team member (death vs an injured patient). Operational training in the aspects of EMS will be of a great benefit to the CCITT if it is needed to integrate into EMS-level care. In addition, it is always in the best interests of the CCITT and the EMS to have predesignated plans of action for these types of situations. Examples where this may be useful include the following:

Long-term Entrapment

It is possible that a CCITT may be asked to bring specialty care to the scene of a prolonged entrapment that requires ongoing medical management or a critical intervention, such as an amputation. Under these circumstances, the CCITT must know how to function under the IC system for safety and accountability. Every team member should understand the basic concepts of IC and understand that scene work or evaluation of multiple patients demands a level of personal and team awareness and communication that may not be realized in routine daily single-patient or transfer operations. Some states require that CCITT members have EMT-B certification (or higher), which helps to prepare the interfacility participant for EMS activities. Some CCITTs will require nursing or other members to obtain EMT-B, EMT-I, or EMT-P certification in addition to their primary academic preparation to help prepare for potential EMS activities. In Pennsylvania, for example, a critical care transport nurse is required to have additional EMS certification, which leads to a recognized designation as a prehospital registered nurse (PHRN). This helps ensure that these nurses possess the necessary skills to function in the prehospital environment on a routine and an emergency basis.

Triage

During the first phases of an ongoing emergency, especially involving large numbers of children, the neonatal-pediatric CCITT may be asked to assume a role in triage and stabilization of patients' conditions in the field. The CCITT members are often the highest medically trained participants in mobile medical care who are available on an emergency basis, and unusual (eg, EMS participation and triage) requests may be made of them in a crisis, such as a local disaster or mass casualty situation. Basic awareness and training in a triage protocol such as JumpSTART or other mass casualty triage tools greatly increases the efficiency by which CCITT members can assess and treat patients (Figure 23-2). The specific tool recommended or used by the local EMS and emergency preparedness groups should be the triage tool used for training. Introductory training in triage enables CCITT members to provide better assistance to EMS personnel who are trained to triage in the most effective manner during a mass casualty. Drills with local EMS agencies and classroom training that typically is reserved for EMS providers are excellent opportunities to become exposed to and practice these skills.

Unexpected Medical Encounters

It is likely that the CCITT eventually will be the first to arrive at a vehicle accident or medical emergency in the field. It is in the best interests of the CCITT to have a predesignated plan of action for these situations. Policies should be developed for when the ambulance has a patient in transit, is on the way to pick up a patient, and is returning from a transport without another commitment. These policies should be made with legal input and combine the employment and other jurisdictional requirements of the specific transport personnel and other participants in the process (eg, EMT driver).

Because CCITT members might not have prehospital credentials such as EMT, they should know whether their state's Good Samaritan laws protect on-duty health care professionals and whether they are required to stop and provide care. Many teams stop and provide emergency care as needed and simultaneously contact 911. The decision to do so when transporting a patient or en route to pick up a patient depends on multiple factors, including the status of the patient, the condition of the accident scene and victims, team policy, and the opinion of medical control, if applicable. The condition of the patient the CCITT has agreed to transport must be continuously monitored and care maintained regardless of any external situation and must remain the team's top priority. A poor outcome possibly linked to a delay in care or transport may be grounds for legal action (see Chapter 7).

Figure 23-2: JumpSTART Pediatric Triage Algorithm*†

JumpSTART Pediatric MCI Triage©

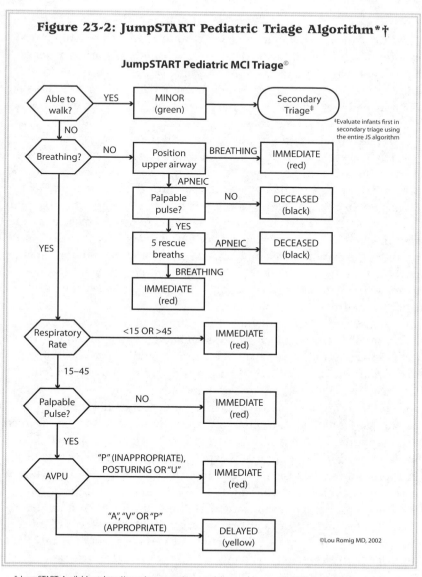

‡Evaluate infants first in secondary triage using the entire JS algorithm

©Lou Romig MD, 2002

* JumpSTART. Available at: http://www.jumpstarttriage.com/. Accessed January 20, 2006. Used with permission: Lou E. Romig, MD, FAAP, FACEP.

† AVPU indicates **A**lert, responds to **V**erbal stimuli, responds to **P**ainful stimuli, **U**nresponsive.

Disasters

The CCITT may be asked to take a critical or even a leadership role in internal or external hospital disasters or events requiring patient movement within, to, or from the hospital. Depending on the scale and scope of the incident, outside fire and EMS agencies and personnel may be involved and in charge. A working knowledge of the IC system will be useful for assisting in maintaining command and control of the situation and for integration with the outside agencies.

The Federal Emergency Management Agency became part of the new Department of Homeland Security in March 2003 and has championed a new disaster management structure. The National Incident Management System (NIMS), developed by the Secretary of Homeland Security, integrates effective practices in emergency preparedness and response into a comprehensive national framework for incident management (http://www.fema.gov/nims/). Understanding and participating in NIMS training should enable CCITT and EMS personnel to work together more effectively to manage domestic incidents no matter what the cause, size, or complexity.

The Hospital Emergency Incident Command System (HEICS) is a version of IC that is specific to hospital emergency planning and operations (Figure 23-3). CCITT members should be trained in how to operate within the HEICS system to function optimally and maintain accountability and safety when operating within the hospital system. If an incident involves special medical considerations, such as one with a biological or chemical agent, the CCITT may be involved as an important participant in providing organized and optimal care for large numbers of potentially exposed children. In such cases, it is important for the CCITT to rely on current training and have clear access to specific medical and logistical information and personnel for the appropriate and safe care of children in this environment. It is in the best interest of CCITT members to hold themselves to the highest standard in terms of operational awareness and medical knowledge in situations involving weapons of mass destruction. Even if CCITT members do not serve as a resource in this role on a day-to-day basis, they likely will be considered experts if a crisis develops. Hospitals may be so overwhelmed that they cease to be a resource for EMS, so CCITT members may need to provide care in

Figure 23-3: Basic Structure of the Hospital Emergency Incident Command System*

HOSPITAL EMERGENCY INCIDENT COMMAND SYSTEM

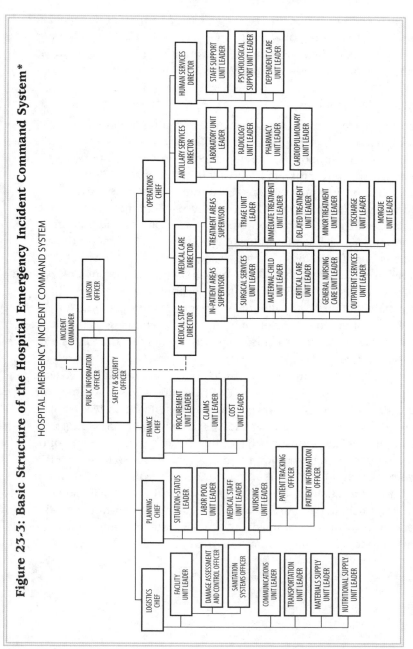

* Available at: http://www.emsa.ca.gov/Dms2/heics3.htm. Accessed January 20, 2006. Adapted from the San Mateo County Emergency Services Agency's Hospital Emergency Incident Command System Update Project.

the field and perform primary triage, care, and transport, especially during the first hours of a crisis. An excellent resource for disaster preparedness is the AAP Web site on Children, Terrorism, and Disaster Management (http://www.aap.org/terrorism/index.html).

Training Opportunities

Many opportunities exist to overlap the training of EMS and CCITT personnel. Routine standardized certification classes such as Pediatric Advanced Life Support (PALS), Advanced Cardiac Life Support (ACLS), Pediatric Education for the Prehospital Professional (PEPP), and Advanced, Basic, and Prehospital Trauma Life Support (ATLS, BTLS, and PHTLS) help integrate CCITT and EMS personnel toward the goals of standardizing and improving patient assessment and emergency treatment. The principles, knowledge, and skills learned in these courses apply seamlessly across the prehospital and hospital environments. Neonatal-pediatric CCITT members must be proficient in these skills and must be flexible enough to respond to unexpected circumstances such as an adult or pregnant pediatric patient. When they have attained this level, members can participate as instructors and reinforce their own skills while forging new relationships with EMS providers.

Specialized training in EMS and emergency operations is also an important consideration for CCITT members. By developing a relationship with EMS providers, it may be possible for CCITT members to participate in EMS training such as teaching EMT classes, participating in IC classes, and participating in community first responder classes such as the community emergency response teams (CERTs). Prehospital and CCITT personnel can benefit from participation in organizations such as federal disaster medical assistance teams (DMATs) or the local CERT. In these specialized environments, all levels of providers from inside and outside the hospital environment can serve together with a common goal.

Selected Readings

2005 American Heart Association Guidelines for Cardiopulmonary Resuscitation and Emergency Cardiovascular Care. Available at: http://circ.ahajournals.org/content/vol112/24_suppl/. Accessed January 20, 2006

Advanced Trauma Life Support. Available at: http://www.facs.org/trauma/atls/index.html. Accessed January 20, 2006

American Academy of Pediatrics. Children, Terrorism and Disasters. Available at: http://www.aap.org/terrorism/index.html. Accessed January 20, 2006

Basic Trauma Life Support. Available at: http://www.itrauma.org/. Accessed January 20, 2006

Community emergency response teams. Available at: http://www.fema.gov/kids/02cert_table.pdf. Accessed January 20, 2006

Hospital Emergency Incident Command System. Available at: http://www.emsa.ca.gov/Dms2/heics3.htm. Accessed January 20, 2006

JumpSTART. Available at: http://www.jumpstarttriage.com/. Accessed January 20, 2006

National Disaster Medical System. Available at: http://ndms.dhhs.gov/dmat.html. Accessed January 20, 2006

National Incident Management System. Available at: http://www.fema.gov/nims/index.shtm. Accessed January 20, 2006

Pediatric Advanced Life Support. Available at: http://www.americanheart.org. Accessed January 20, 2006

Pediatric Education for Prehospital Professionals: Available at: http://www.peppsite.com. Accessed January 20, 2006

Questions

1. Outline the transport ream member's role at your sponsoring institution when an external disaster is declared.

2. You are transporting a 10-year-old child with severe asthma who is receiving continuous albuterol when your contracted emergency medical services (EMS) crew pulls over to assist at the scene of a serious motor vehicle crash. How do you proceed at this time?

3. What are the likely benefits of using a pediatric-specific triage tool such as JumpSTART?

Answers

1. This answer depends on individual hospitals and polices. All transport team members should have a working knowledge of their potential role in an internal or external disaster.

2. It is important to have an established transport team policy for this situation. Your first priority is your on-board patient. Delaying transport could increase your patient's risk and the team's liability. The critical care transport crew should call 911 to ensure that help is dispatched to the scene and then continue to the receiving facility. If the on-board patient is in stable condition and there are extra care providers in the transport ambulance, stopping to offer assistance until EMS arrives could be considered. An ambulance engaged as a transport vehicle with a patient in unstable condition or limited providers should not be considered available for primary EMS response.

3. Triage can be difficult to perform objectively, especially when children are involved. Using a triage algorithm is a means of using nonarbitrary information to effectively and rapidly identify victims who will benefit from the use of limited resources.

Sample Position Descriptions*

1. Critical Care Transport Transport Nurse
2. Critical Care Transport Respiratory Therapist
3. Critical Care Transport Emergency Medical Technician-Paramedic
4. Transport Emergency Medical Technician-Basic
5. Critical Care Transport Physician
6. Critical Care Transport Medical Control Physician

The following are provided as examples of position descriptions from neonatal and pediatric transport programs. Licensing and practice regulations vary considerably from state to state. Transport programs should take into consideration local regulatory and licensure requirements and individual program policies when configuring their team composition, defining practice parameters, and developing position descriptions.

1. Sample Position Description—Critical Care Transport Nurse

Position Description

■ Practices in accordance with philosophy, policies, procedures, and standards of the hospital; functions within the guidelines of the protocols for the transport program that are reviewed and agreed on by medical and nursing directors.

■ Functions include the identification, planning, implementation, and evaluation of emergency care for acutely ill neonates, infants, children, and/or adolescents in collaboration with the medical control physician (MCP; sometimes called medical control officer, or MCO). This person is responsible for obtaining pertinent maternal,

---

*NICU indicates neonatal intensive care unit; PICU, pediatric intensive care unit; NRP, Neonatal Resuscitation Program; TNCC, Trauma Nursing Core Course; ATLS, Advanced Trauma Life Support; IV, intravenous; EMS, emergency medical services; and CPR, cardiopulmonary resuscitation.

neonatal, and childhood histories, performing physical examinations (neonates through adolescents), and formulating differential diagnoses and care management plans. Responsibilities include performing necessary diagnostic and therapeutic procedures as indicated for identification and management of problems, including, but not limited to, umbilical line placement, peripheral or central venous access, endotracheal tube placement, needle aspiration, chest tube placement, and interpretation of laboratory and radiographic data.

- Also important is the need to provide family-centered care, including psychosocial support, education, and transfer planning in conjunction with referral staff.
- Represents the hospital to health care professionals in referring hospitals.
- Maintains effective communication with referral staff and families.
- Educates referral staff through informal teaching and planned educational conferences.
- Initiates and participates in educational, research, professional, and organizational activities that contribute to improving patient care, the transport program operation, and the individual's own professional development.

Reporting Relationship

Reports to:
- Medical director of the transport program for supervision and guidance in expanded role function.
- MCP as designated for medical supervision concerning the management of individual neonatal and pediatric patients during transport.
- Nursing (or program) director, or designee, for care and administrative aspects of practice.

Requirements

1. Requires a minimum of 3 years of NICU or PICU or pediatric emergency department experience within the last 5 years. Critical care transport experience preferred.

2. Current in Basic Life Support for the Health Care Provider, Advanced Cardiac Life Support, and Pediatric Advanced Life Support. Certification in NRP and TNCC or ATLS preferred.
3. BSN-prepared at a minimum.
4. State licensure as a registered nurse.
5. Computer literacy.
6. Holds current passport or is eligible to apply for one if program will be doing international transports.
7. Demonstrates strong written and verbal communication skills at staff, patient, and family levels.

Major Responsibilities and Duties

I. Patient care activities
   A. Obtains pertinent maternal, neonatal, and pediatric histories with emphasis on risk factors and their implications for problems.
   B. Performs pertinent physical examination using techniques of observation, inspection, auscultation, palpation, and percussion.
   C. Assesses patient weight for use in calibration of medication and fluid management.
   D. Formulates differential diagnosis and a plan for management of existing and potential problems in collaboration with the MCP.
   E. Performs necessary diagnostic and therapeutic procedures as indicated for identification and management for problems as indicated by protocol, including (but not limited to):
      1. Peripheral percutaneous arterial sampling and line placement
      2. Umbilical venous and arterial catheterization
      3. Airway management, including assessment, stabilization, bag-mask oxygenation and ventilation, endotracheal intubation, tracheostomy management, and rescue airways
      4. Needle aspiration of pleural space and chest tube placement
      5. Interpretation of routine laboratory and radiographic data
      6. Insertion of central venous catheters (femoral vein only)

7. Insertion of intraosseous needle for emergency vascular access
8. Spinal immobilization
9. Trauma triage care
10. Blood drawing (venous and arterial) and insertion of peripheral IVs

F. Provides clinical management for resuscitation of the neonatal, pediatric, and/or adolescent patient, including necessary pharmacological support.

G. Performs in accordance with standing orders, and accurately documents delivery of care.

H. Communicates information about the patient's "working" diagnosis, plan of management, and prognosis to the referring physician, parents, and other members of the health care team.

I. Assesses parents' psychosocial needs, and initiates referral to appropriate consultants.

J. Obtains informed consent from parent(s)/guardian(s).

K. Provides ongoing monitoring, assessment, and appropriate interventions in transit.

L. Ensures patient safety in the transport process.

M. Completes documentation in an accurate and timely manner, and transfers care of the patient to the receiving hospital staff.

II. Education
A. Contributes to community outreach and education.
B. Assists in the assessment of staff developmental needs, and participates actively in plans to meet those needs.
C. Participates in teaching or coordination of in-service classes or workshops for the transport staff.
D. Serves as a preceptor in the training of future transport team members.

III. Operation of transport equipment
A. Demonstrates knowledge of operation and troubleshooting of all transport equipment. Ensures proper functioning and availability of equipment before transport.
B. Participates in the ongoing evaluation of transport equipment needs. Reports and documents transport equipment repairs as needed to biomedical engineering.

   C. Demonstrates knowledge of aircraft and ambulance operating procedures and safety practices.

IV. Special assignments/project responsibilities

   A. Assists with medical procedures in the NICU/PICU or emergency department on request.

   B. Performs the following transport quality improvement activities:

      1. Maintains, supports, and documents evidence of a planned, systematic quality improvement program that includes effective mechanisms for monitoring and evaluating the patient care provided by the transport service.

      2. Ensures appropriate and adequate response to findings from quality improvement activities.

      3. Maximizes the efficient use of resources available to provide neonatal-pediatric transports.

      4. Identifies opportunities to improve care.

V. Leadership

   A. Initiates and participates in the implementation of change in transport nursing policy, procedures, and/or practice to enhance the quality of patient care.

   B. Participates with transport staff in problem identification, goal setting, and transport care delivery evaluation.

   C. Uses previous clinical experience and knowledge to identify potential patient care problems related to transport.

   D. Serves as a resource or consultant to nursing and medical staff regarding neonatal and pediatric transport.

VI. Professional accountability

   A. Demonstrates continued professional growth through continuing education and review of current literature pertaining to neonatal-pediatric transport.

   B. Maintains licensure, certifications, and competency through required training and/or education.

   C. Maintains professional relationships with community physicians, nurses, and other health care professionals.

   D. Participates in peer review of the transport team members and case reviews with the medical director.

VII. Research
    A. Identifies researchable patient and nursing care problems related to transport.
    B. Uses evidence-based research findings in patient care.
    C. Cooperates and/or collaborates with other health care team members in the conduct of research studies.

VIII. Physical capabilities
    A. Frequently requires sitting, standing, and walking for long periods. Requires bending, crouching, and kneeling. Requires use of hands, keyboarding, fine motor skills, frequent lifting up to 50 lb, occasional moving up to 250 lb. Must be able to work in small confined spaces and be able to work in a mobile environment, either ground or air.
    B. There is a potential for regular exposure to patients with infectious diseases requiring observance of appropriate precautions.
    C. Flexible working hours required to provide 24 hour/day, 7 day/week coverage, including rotating shifts, weekends, holidays, and on call.
    D. Dependability in regard to attendance at work, team meetings, nursing meetings, committee meetings, etc.

IX. Environmental conditions
Indoor and outdoor environment with possible exposure to infectious, biological, and chemical agents. Occasionally requires working in proximity to sources of radiation. Work area includes riding in enclosed spaces such as ambulances, helicopters, and airplanes. Work environment commonly provides exposure to high noise levels.

2. Sample Position Description—Critical Care Transport Respiratory Therapist

Position Description

■ Practices in accordance with philosophy, policies, procedures, and standards of the hospital; functions within the guidelines of the protocols for the transport program that are reviewed and agreed on by medical, nursing, and respiratory care directors.

■ Evaluates and maintains respiratory care services for all critically ill patients. Establishes patient care plans and collaborates with team members and medical control physician (MCP).

■ Provides family-centered care to meet family needs, including psychosocial support, education, and transfer planning in conjunction with referral staff.

■ Participates in the educational and professional development of transport team members.

■ Represents the hospital to health care professionals in referring hospitals.

■ Maintains effective communication with referral staff and families.

■ Educates referral staff through informal teaching and planned educational conferences.

■ Initiates and participates in educational, research, professional, and organizational activities that contribute to improving patient care, the transport program operation, and the individual's own professional development.

Reporting Relationship

Reports to:

■ Medical director of the transport program for supervision and guidance in expanded role function.

■ The MCP as designated for medical supervision concerning the management of individual neonatal and pediatric patients during transport.

■ Transport program manager for administrative and care aspects of transport.

■ Respiratory care director, or designee, for respiratory therapy and administrative aspects of practice. This designee is usually but not exclusively within the transport program.

Requirements

1. Requires a minimum of 3 years of NICU/PICU or pediatric emergency department experience within the last 5 years. Critical care transport experience preferred.

2. Current in Basic Life Support for the Health Care Provider, Advanced Cardiac Life Support, and Pediatric Advanced Life Support. Certification in NRP and ATLS preferred.

3. Requires National Board for Respiratory Care (N.B.R.C.) Registered Respiratory Therapist.

4. Requires degree from a Committee on Accreditation for Respiratory Care (CoARC)-accredited respiratory care program.

5. Requires N.B.R.C. neonatal-pediatric specialist examination.

6. State licensure (if required) as a registered respiratory therapist.

7. Computer literacy.

8. Holds current passport or is eligible to apply for one, if program participates in international transports.

9. Demonstrates strong written and verbal communication skills at staff, patient, and family levels.

Major Responsibilities and Duties

I. Patient care activities

  A. Assists in obtaining pertinent maternal, neonatal, and pediatric histories with emphasis on risk factors and their implications for problems.

  B. Performs and/or assists with as appropriate pertinent physical examination of the respiratory system using techniques of observation, inspection, auscultation, and percussion.

  C. Formulates a plan for management of existing and potential respiratory system problems in collaboration with the team leader and the MCP.

  D. Performs necessary diagnostic and therapeutic procedures as indicated for identification and management of problems indicated in the program's protocols, including (but not limited to):

    1. Peripheral percutaneous arterial sampling
    2. Assist in umbilical venous and arterial catheterization
    3. Airway management, including assessment, stabilization, bag-mask oxygenation and ventilation, endotracheal intubation, tracheostomy management, and rescue airways
    4. Needle aspiration of pleural space
    5. Interpretation of routine laboratory and radiographic data
    6. Assist in spinal immobilization
    7. Assist in trauma triage care

E. Provides clinical management for resuscitation of neonatal, pediatric, and adolescent patients, including assisting in necessary pharmacological support.

F. Performs in accordance with standing orders, and accurately documents delivery of care.

G. Provides ongoing monitoring, assessment, and appropriate respiratory care interventions in transit.

H. Ensures patient safety in the transport process.

I. Completes documentation in an accurate and timely manner, and transfers care of the patient to the receiving hospital staff.

II. Education

A. Contributes to community outreach and education.

B. Assists in the assessment of staff developmental needs, and participates actively in plans to meet those needs.

C. Participates in teaching or coordination of in-service classes or workshops for the transport staff.

D. Serves as a preceptor in the training of future transport team members.

III. Operation of transport equipment

A. Demonstrates knowledge of operation and troubleshooting of all transport equipment, and ensures proper functioning before transport. Is primarily responsible for the respiratory care equipment, including ventilators, pulse oximeters, gas cylinders, and oxygen and other medical gas delivery devices.

B. Participates in the ongoing evaluation of transport equipment needs. Reports and documents transport equipment repairs as needed to biomedical engineering.

C. Demonstrates knowledge of aircraft and ambulance operating procedures and safety practices.

IV. Special assignments/project responsibilities

A. Assists with medical procedures in the NICU/PICU or emergency department on request.

B. Performs the following transport quality improvement activities:

1. Maintains, supports, and documents evidence of a planned, systematic quality improvement program that includes effective mechanisms for monitoring and evaluating the patient care provided by the transport service.

2. Ensures appropriate and adequate response to findings from quality improvement activities.
3. Maximizes the efficient use of resources available to provide neonatal-pediatric transports.
4. Identifies opportunities to improve care.

V. Leadership
   A. Initiates and participates in the implementation of change in transport respiratory therapy policies, procedures, and/or practice to enhance the quality of patient care.
   B. Participates with transport staff in problem identification, goal setting, and transport care delivery evaluation.
   C. Uses previous clinical experience and knowledge to identify potential patient care problems related to transport.
   D. Serves as a resource or consultant to nursing and medical staff regarding respiratory care aspects of neonatal and pediatric transport.

VI. Professional accountability
   A. Demonstrates continued professional growth through continuing education and review of current literature pertaining to neonatal-pediatric transport.
   B. Maintains licensure, certifications, and competency through required training and/or education.
   C. Maintains professional relationships with community physicians, nurses, respiratory therapists, and other health care professionals.
   D. Participates in peer review of the transport team members and case reviews with the medical director.

VII. Research
   A. Identifies researchable patient and respiratory care problems related to transport.
   B. Uses evidence-based research findings in patient care.
   C. Cooperates and/or collaborates with other health care team members in the conduct of research studies.

VIII. Physical capabilities

A. Frequently requires sitting, standing, and walking for long periods. Requires bending, crouching, and kneeling. Requires use of hands, keyboarding, fine motor skills, frequent lifting up to 50 lb, occasional moving up to 250 lb. Must be able to work in small confined spaces and be able to work in a mobile environment, either ground or air.

B. There is a potential for regular exposure to patients with infectious diseases requiring observance of appropriate precautions.

C. Flexible working hours required to provide 24 hour/day, 7 day/week coverage, including rotating shifts, weekends, holidays, and on call.

D. Dependability in regard to attendance at work, team meetings, respiratory care meetings, committee meetings, etc.

IX. Environmental conditions

A. Indoor and outdoor environment with possible exposure to infectious, biological, and chemical agents. Occasionally requires working in proximity to sources of radiation. Work area includes riding in enclosed spaces such as ambulances, helicopters, and airplanes. Work environment commonly provides exposure to high noise levels.

3. Sample Position Description—Critical Care Transport Emergency Medical Technician-Paramedic

Position Description

- Practices in accordance with philosophy, policies, procedures, and standards of the hospital; functions within the guidelines of the protocols for the transport program that are reviewed and agreed on by medical and nursing directors.

- As a team member during transport, functions to identify, plan, implement, and evaluate the stabilization and emergency care of the acutely ill neonates, infants, children, and/or adolescents in collaboration with the team leader and medical control physician. The transport paramedic is responsible for assisting the team leader in obtaining pertinent maternal, neonatal, and childhood histories, performing physical assessments (neonates through adolescents), and formulating and implementing care management plans. Responsible for performing necessary diagnostic and therapeutic procedures within the scope of practice of a paramedic.

■ With expertise in the prehospital setting, the paramedic is responsible for ensuring that while in the out-of-hospital setting, the transport team is working in a safe and secure environment. Provides family-centered care to meet family needs, including psychosocial support, education, and transfer planning in conjunction with referral staff.

■ Participates in educational and professional development of transport and other team members.

■ Represents the hospital to health care professionals in referring hospitals.

■ Maintains effective communication with referral staff, families, and the EMS system.

■ Participates in the education of referral staff and prehospital care providers through informal teaching and planned educational conferences.

■ Initiates and participates in educational, research, professional, and organizational activities that contribute to improving patient care, the transport program operation, and the individual's own professional development.

Reporting Relationship

Reports to:

■ Medical director of the transport program for the supervision and guidance in expanded role function.

■ Medical control physician (MCP) as designated for medical supervision concerning the management of individual neonatal and pediatric patients during transport.

■ Transport program director or designee for clinical and administrative aspects of practice. If EMS services are outsourced, may report to EMS director of contracted service.

Requirements

1. Requires a minimum of 3 years of practice as a paramedic. Pediatric and critical care transport experience preferred.
2. Current in Basic Life Support for the Health Care Provider, Advanced Cardiac Life Support, and Pediatric Advanced Life Support. Certification in NRP and ATLS preferred. Critical care EMT-P certification preferred.
3. State licensure as a paramedic.
4. Computer literacy.
5. Holds current passport or is eligible to apply for one, if the program intends to perform international transports.
6. Demonstrates strong written and verbal communication skills at EMS, staff, patient, and family levels.

Major Responsibilities and Duties

I. Patient care activities
   A. Obtains pertinent maternal, neonatal, and pediatric histories with emphasis on risk factors and their implications for problems.
   B. Performs pertinent physical assessment.
   C. Assists in assessing patient weight for use in calibration of medication and fluid management.
   D. Formulates a plan for management of existing and potential problems in collaboration with the team leader and MCP.
   E. Performs (or assists with, as per team protocol) necessary diagnostic and therapeutic procedures as indicated for identification and management of problems including (but not limited to):
      1. Airway management, including assessment, stabilization, bag-mask oxygenation and ventilation, endotracheal intubation, tracheostomy management, and rescue airways
      2. Needle aspiration of pleural space
      3. Insertion of intraosseous needle for emergency vascular access
      4. Spinal immobilization
      5. Trauma triage care
      6. Blood drawing and insertion of peripheral IVs

F. Provides clinical management for resuscitation of the newborn, pediatric, and adolescent patients, including necessary pharmacological support.

G. Performs in accordance with standing orders, and accurately documents delivery of care.

H. Communicates information about the patient's diagnosis, plan of management, and prognosis to the referring physician, parents, and other members of the health care team.

I. Assesses parents' psychosocial needs, and initiates referral to appropriate consultants.

J. Obtains informed consent from parents or guardians.

K. Provides ongoing monitoring, assessment, and appropriate interventions in transit.

L. Ensures patient safety in the transport process.

M. Completes documentation in an accurate and timely manner, and transfers care of the patient to the receiving hospital staff.

II. Education

A. Contributes to community outreach and education.

B. Assists in the assessment of staff developmental needs, discusses the assessment with the transport team coordinator and medical director, and participates actively in plans to meet those needs.

C. Participates in teaching or coordination of in-service classes or workshops for the transport staff.

D. Serves as a preceptor in the training of future transport paramedics.

III. Operation of transport equipment

A. Demonstrates knowledge of operation of all transport equipment, and ensures proper functioning before transport.

B. Participates in the ongoing evaluation of transport equipment needs. Reports and documents transport equipment repairs as needed to biomedical engineering.

C. Demonstrates knowledge of aircraft and ambulance operating procedures and safety practices.

IV. Special assignments/project responsibilities
   A. Assists with medical procedures in the NICU/PICU and emergency department on request.
   B. Performs the following transport quality improvement activities:
      1. Maintains, supports, and documents evidence of a planned, systematic quality improvement program that includes effective mechanisms for monitoring and evaluating the patient care provided by the transport service.
      2. Ensures appropriate and adequate response to findings from quality improvement activities.
      3. Maximizes the efficient use of resources available to provide neonatal-pediatric transports.
      4. Identifies opportunities to improve care.

V. Leadership
   A. Initiates and participates in the implementation of change in transport paramedic policies, procedures, and/or practice to enhance the quality of patient care.
   B. Participates with transport staff in problem identification, goal setting, and transport care delivery evaluation.
   C. Uses previous clinical experience and knowledge to identify potential patient care problems related to transport.
   D. Serves as a resource or consultant to nursing and medical staff regarding prehospital and triage in neonatal and pediatric transport.

VI. Professional accountability
   A. Demonstrates continued professional growth through continuing education and review of current literature pertaining to neonatal-pediatric transport.
   B. Maintains licensure, certifications, and competency through required training and/or education.
   C. Maintains professional relationships with the EMS system, community physicians, nurses, and other health care professionals.
   D. Participates in peer review of the transport team members and case reviews with the medical director.

VII. Research
    A. Identifies researchable patient care problems related to transport.
    B. Uses evidence-based research findings in patient care.
    C. Cooperates and/or collaborates with other health care team members in the conduct of research studies.

VIII. Physical capabilities
    A. Frequently requires sitting, standing, and walking for long periods. Requires bending, crouching, and kneeling. Requires use of hands, keyboarding, fine motor skills, frequent lifting up to 50 lb, occasional moving up to 250 lb. Must be able to work in small confined spaces and be able to work in a mobile environment, either ground or air.
    B. There is a potential for regular exposure to patients with infectious diseases requiring observance of appropriate precautions.
    C. Flexible working hours required to provide 24 hour/day, 7 day/week coverage, including rotating shifts, weekends, holidays, and on call.
    D. Dependability in regard to attendance at work, team meetings, paramedic meetings, committee meetings, etc.

IX. Environmental conditions
Indoor and outdoor environment with possible exposure to infectious, biological, and chemical agents. Occasionally requires working in proximity to sources of radiation. Work area includes riding in enclosed spaces such as ambulances, helicopters, and airplanes. Work environment commonly provides exposure to high noise levels.

4. Sample Position Description—Transport Emergency Medical Technician-Basic

Position Description

■ Practices in accordance with philosophy, policies, procedures, and standards of the hospital; functions within the guidelines of the protocols for the transport program that are reviewed and agreed on by medical and nursing directors.

- Provides family-centered care to meet family needs including psychosocial support, education, and transfer planning in conjunction with referral staff.
- Participates in the educational and professional development of transport team members.
- Represents the hospital to health care professionals in referring hospitals.
- Maintains effective communication with community EMS system, referral staff, and families.
- Initiates and participates in educational, research, professional, and organizational activities that contribute to improving patient care, the transport program operation, and the individual's own professional development.

Reporting Relationship

Reports to:
- Medical director of the transport program for supervision and guidance in expanded role function.
- Medical control physician (MCP) as designated for medical supervision concerning the management of individual neonatal and pediatric patients during transport.
- Transport director, or designee, for clinical and administrative aspects of practice. In cases in which EMS services are outsourced, the emergency medical technician (EMT) may report to the EMS director of the contracted service.

Requirements

1. Requires knowledge of state and regional EMS codes and regulations.
2. Emergency vehicle operator certification.
3. State licensure as an EMT.
4. Computer literacy.
5. Demonstrates strong written and verbal communication skills at EMS, staff, patient, and family levels.

Major Responsibilities and Duties

I. Patient care activities
   A. Assists in obtaining pertinent maternal, neonatal, and pediatric histories, if required.
   B. Handles multiple tasks, and is self-directed.
   C. Speaks clearly and concisely over the radio and telephone.
   D. Performs in accordance with regional and program standing orders, and accurately documents delivery of care.
      1. Ensures patient and transport team safety in the transport process.
      2. Completes documentation in an accurate and timely manner, and transfers care of the patient to the receiving hospital staff.
      3. Assists with patient care activities within scope of practice, such as spinal immobilization, oxygen therapy, and CPR.
II. Education
   A. Contributes to community outreach and education.
   B. Assists in the assessment of staff developmental needs, and participates actively in plans to meet those needs.
   C. Participates in teaching or coordination of in-service classes or workshops for the transport staff.
   D. Serves as a preceptor in the training of future transport team members.
III. Operation of transport equipment
   A. Demonstrates knowledge of operation of all ambulance equipment, and ensures proper functioning before transport.
   B. Participates in the ongoing evaluation of transport equipment needs. Reports and documents transport equipment repairs as needed to biomedical engineering.
   C. Demonstrates knowledge of ambulance operating procedures and safety practices.

IV. Special assignments/project responsibilities
   A. Assists in the emergency department or other clinical areas on request within scope of practice and employment.
   B. Performs the following transport quality improvement activities:
      1. Maintains, supports, and documents evidence of a planned, systematic quality improvement program that includes effective mechanisms for monitoring and evaluating patient care.
      2. Ensures appropriate and adequate response to findings from quality improvement activities.
      3. Maximizes the efficient use of resources available to provide neonatal-pediatric transports.
      4. Identifies opportunities to improve care.
V. Leadership
   1. Initiates and participates in the implementation of change in transport EMT policies, procedures, and/or practice to enhance the quality of patient care.
   2. Participates with transport staff in problem identification, goal setting, and transport care delivery evaluation.
   3. Uses previous clinical experience and knowledge to identify potential patient care problems related to transport.
   4. Serves as a resource or consultant to nursing and medical staff regarding prehospital and EMS aspects of neonatal and pediatric transport.
VI. Professional accountability
   1. Demonstrates continued professional growth through continuing education and review of current literature pertaining to neonatal-pediatric transport.
   2. Maintains licensure, certifications, and competency through required training and/or education.
   3. Maintains professional relationships with other health care professionals and the EMS community.
   4. Participates in peer review of the transport team members and case reviews with the medical director.

VII. Research
    A. Cooperates and/or collaborates with other health care team members in the conduct of research studies.
VIII. Physical capabilities
    1. Frequently requires sitting, standing, and walking for long periods. Requires bending, crouching, and kneeling. Requires use of hands, keyboarding, fine motor skills, frequent lifting up to 50 lb, occasional moving up to 250 lb. Must be able to work in small confined spaces and be able to work in a mobile environment.
    2. There is a potential for regular exposure to patients with infectious diseases requiring observance of appropriate precautions.
    3. Flexible working hours required to provide 24 hour/day, 7 day/week coverage, including rotating shifts, weekends, holidays, and on call.
    4. Dependability in regard to attendance at work, team meetings, EMT meetings, committee meetings, etc.
IX. Environmental conditions
    A. Indoor and outdoor environment with possible exposure to infectious, biological, and chemical agents. Occasionally requires working in proximity to sources of radiation. Work area includes enclosed spaces such as ambulances, helicopters, and airplanes. Work environment commonly provides exposure to high noise levels.

5. Sample Position Description—Critical Care Transport Physician

Position Description

- Practices in accordance with philosophy, policies, procedures, and standards of the hospital; functions within the guidelines of the protocols for the transport program that are reviewed and agreed on by medical and nursing directors.
- As team leader/member during transport, functions to identify, plan, implement, and evaluate the stabilization and emergency care of acutely ill neonates, infants, children, and adolescents in collaboration with the medical control physician. The transport

team physician is responsible for obtaining pertinent maternal, neonatal, and childhood histories, performing physical examinations (neonates through adolescents), and formulating differential diagnoses and care management plans. He or she is responsible for performing necessary diagnostic and therapeutic procedures as indicated for identification and management of problems, including but not limited to, umbilical line placement, airway management, needle aspiration of the chest, chest tube placement, and interpretation of laboratory and radiographic data.

- Provides family-centered care to meet such family needs as psychosocial support, education, and transfer planning in conjunction with referral staff.
- Participates in educational and professional development of transport and other team members.
- Represents the hospital to health care professionals in referring hospitals.
- Maintains effective communication with transport team members, referral staff, and families.
- Educates referral staff through informal teaching and planned educational conferences.
- Initiates and participates in educational, research, professional, and organizational activities that contribute to improving patient care, the transport program operation, and the individual's own professional development.

Reporting Relationship

Reports to:
- Medical director of the transport program for the supervision and guidance in expanded role function.
- Medical control physician (MCP) as designated for medical supervision concerning the management of individual neonatal and pediatric patients during transport.

Requirements

1. Must be board-certified or eligible in pediatrics (and have additional formal training or certification in transport and acute care medicine).

2. Current in Basic Life Support for the Health Care Provider, Advanced Cardiac Life Support, and Pediatric Advanced Life Support. Certification in NRP and ATLS.
3. Computer literacy.
4. Holds current passport or is eligible to apply for one, if program intends to perform international transports.
5. Holds active, unrestricted state medical license and Drug Enforcement Agency (DEA) certificate.

Major Responsibilities and Duties

I. Patient care activities

A. Obtains pertinent maternal, neonatal, and pediatric histories with emphasis on risk factors and their implications for problems.

B. Performs pertinent physical examination using techniques of observation, inspection, auscultation, palpation, and percussion.

C. Formulates differential diagnosis and a plan for management of existing and potential problems in collaboration with the MCP.

D. Performs necessary diagnostic and therapeutic procedures as indicated for identification and management for problems including (but not limited to):

1. Peripheral percutaneous arterial sampling and line placement
2. Umbilical venous and arterial catheterization
3. Airway management, including assessment, stabilization, bag-mask oxygenation and ventilation, endotracheal intubation, tracheostomy management, and rescue airways
4. Needle aspiration of pleural space and chest tube placement
5. Interpretation of laboratory and radiographic data
6. Insertion of central venous line for central venous access
7. Insertion of intraosseous needle for emergency vascular access
8. Spinal immobilization
9. Trauma care

10. Blood drawing and insertion of peripheral IVs
11. Clinical management for resuscitation of neonatal, pediatric, and adolescent patients, including necessary pharmacological support.

E. Performs in accordance with standards of care and accurately documents delivery of care.

F. Communicates information about the patient's diagnosis, plan of management, and prognosis to the referring and receiving physicians, parents, and other members of the health care team.

G. Assesses parents' psychosocial needs, and initiates referral to appropriate consultants.

H. Obtains informed consent from parents or guardians.

I. Provides ongoing monitoring, assessment, and appropriate interventions in transit.

J. Ensures patient safety in the transport process.

K. Completes documentation in an accurate and timely manner, and transfers care of the patient to the receiving hospital staff.

II. Education
A. Contributes to community outreach and education.
B. Assists in the assessment of staff developmental needs, and participates actively in plans to meet those needs.
C. Participates in teaching or coordination of in-service classes or workshops for the transport staff.
D. Serves as a preceptor in the training of future transport team members.

III. Operation of transport equipment
A. Participates in the ongoing evaluation of transport equipment needs. Reports and documents transport equipment repairs as needed to biomedical engineering.
B. Demonstrates knowledge of aircraft and ambulance operating procedures and safety practices.

IV. Special assignments/project responsibilities
A. Assists with medical procedures in the NICU/PICU and emergency department on request.

B. Performs the following transport quality improvement activities:
1. Participates in, supports, and documents evidence of a systematic quality improvement program that includes effective mechanisms for monitoring and evaluating the patient care provided by the transport service.
2. Helps to ensure appropriate and adequate response to findings from quality improvement activities.
3. Maximizes the efficient use of resources available to provide neonatal-pediatric transports.
4. Identifies opportunities to improve care.

V. Leadership
A. Initiates and participates in the implementation of change in transport policies, procedures, and/or practice to enhance the quality of patient care.
B. Participates with transport staff in problem identification, goal setting, and transport care delivery evaluation.
C. Uses previous clinical experience and knowledge to identify potential patient care problems related to transport.
D. Serves as a resource or consultant to nursing and medical staff regarding neonatal and pediatric transport.

VI. Professional accountability
A. Demonstrates continued professional growth through continuing education and review of current literature pertaining to neonatal-pediatric transport.
B. Maintains licensure, certifications, and competency through required training and/or education.
C. Maintains professional relationships with community physicians, nurses, and other health care professionals.
D. Participates in peer review of the transport team members and case reviews with the medical director.

VII. Research
A. Identifies researchable patient care problems related to transport.
B. Uses evidence-based research findings in patient care.
C. Cooperates and/or collaborates with other health care team members in the conduct of research studies.

VIII. Physical capabilities
   A. Frequently requires sitting, standing, and walking for long periods. Requires bending, crouching, and kneeling. Requires use of hands, keyboarding, fine motor skills, frequent lifting up to 50 lb, occasional moving up to 250 lb. Must be able to work in small confined spaces and be able to work in a mobile environment, either ground or air.
   B. There is a potential for regular exposure to patients with infectious diseases requiring observance of appropriate precautions.
   C. Flexible working hours required to provide 24 hour/day, 7 day/week coverage, including rotating shifts, weekends, holidays, and on call.
   D. Dependability in regard to attendance at work, team meetings, transport meetings, committee meetings, etc.
IX. Environmental conditions
   Indoor and outdoor environment with possible exposure to infectious, biological, and chemical agents. Occasionally requires working in proximity to sources of radiation. Work area includes riding in enclosed spaces such as ambulances, helicopters, and airplanes. Work environment commonly provides exposure to high noise levels.

6. Sample Position Description—Critical Care Transport Medical Control Physician (MCP) (also known as Medical Control or Command Officer, or MCO)

Position Description

■ Practices in accordance with philosophy, policies, procedures, and standards of the hospital and transport service; functions within the guidelines of the protocols for the transport program that are reviewed and agreed on by medical and nursing directors. Adds online critical care expertise and direction to transport team members. Participates in knowledge and skill preparation of team members.

- As senior medical consultant for each transport, functions to identify, plan, implement, and evaluate the stabilization and emergency care of acutely ill neonates, infants, children, and adolescents in collaboration with the referring and transport teams.
- Represents the hospital to health care professionals in referring hospitals.
- Maintains effective communication with transport team members and referral staff.
- Educates referral staff through informal teaching and planned educational conferences.
- May initiate and participate in educational, research, professional, and organizational activities that contribute to improving patient care, the transport program operation, and the individual's own professional development.

Reporting Relationship

Reports to:
- Medical director of the transport program

Requirements

1. Board-certified or eligible in pediatrics and specialty trained in a critical care specialty (intensive care medicine, emergency medicine, neonatology, cardiac intensive care medicine, or pediatric/trauma surgery) and additional formal training or certification in transport medicine
2. Current in Basic Life Support for the Health Care Provider, Advanced Cardiac Life Support, and Pediatric Advanced Life Support. Certification in NRP and ATLS as appropriate.
3. Holds active, unrestricted state medical license and Drug Enforcement Agency (DEA) certificate.
4. Is oriented to and knowledgeable regarding critical care transport.
5. Ideally has background that includes actual transport experience.

Major Responsibilities and Duties

I. Patient care activities

    A. Supervises and directs transport-related patient care activities Availability within scope of team guidelines (immediate for most teams). Ensures optimal, consistent, correct advice and seamless transition from referring team to transport team to definitive care location. Documents involvement, information, and advice.

    B. Formulates differential diagnosis and a plan for management of existing and potential problems in collaboration with the transport team.

    C. Performs in accordance with standards of care, and accurately documents information, communication, and direction of care.

II. Education

    A. Contributes to community outreach and education.

    B. Assists in the assessment of staff developmental needs, and participates actively in plans to meet those needs.

    C. Participates in teaching or coordination of in-service classes or workshops for the transport staff.

III. Transport capabilities

    A. Understands and is literate with transport equipment and team and personnel capabilities.

    B. Demonstrates knowledge of aircraft and ambulance limitations, standard operating procedures, and safety practices.

IV. Special assignments/project responsibilities

    A. Participates in transport quality improvement activities:

        1. Participates in, supports, and documents evidence of a systematic quality improvement program that includes effective mechanisms for monitoring and evaluating the patient care provided by the transport service.

        2. Helps to ensure appropriate and adequate response to findings from quality improvement activities.

        3. Maximizes the efficient use of resources available to provide neonatal-pediatric transports.

        4. Identifies opportunities to improve care.

V. Leadership
   A. Initiates and participates in the implementation of change in transport policies, procedures, and/or practice to enhance the quality of patient care.
   B. Participates with transport staff in problem identification, goal setting, and transport care delivery evaluation.
   C. Uses clinical experience and knowledge to identify potential patient care problems related to transport.
   D. Serves as a resource or consultant to nursing and medical staff regarding neonatal and pediatric transport.

VI. Professional Accountability
   A. Demonstrates continued professional growth through continuing education and review of current literature pertaining to neonatal-pediatric transport and specific specialty.
   B. Maintains licensure, certifications, and competency through required training and/or education.
   C. Maintains professional relationships with community physicians, nurses, and other health care professionals.
   D. Participates in peer review of the transport team members and case reviews with the medical director.

VII. Research
   A. Identifies researchable patient care problems related to transport.
   B. Uses evidence-based research findings in patient care.
   C. Cooperates and/or collaborates with other health care team members in the conduct of research studies.

VIII. Specific Capabilities
   A. Requires rapid phone or in-person availability when in role as MCP.
   B. Requires knowledge and use of appropriate phone etiquette and terminology.
   C. Flexible working hours required to provide 24 hour/day, 7 day/week coverage, including rotating shifts, weekends, holidays, and on call.

■ Sample Pediatric Transport Intake Record* ■

Sample Transport Intake Record

Date/time of Request _____

Name of Patient _____

_____

Age of Patient _____

Birth Date _____

Referring Physician _____

_____

Referral Hospital _____

Referring Unit _____

Phone Number _____

Team Composition

1. _____

2. _____

3. _____

	NAME	TIME
Referral Call Received _____		
Command Center Notified _____		
Transport Nurse Notified _____		
Transport Physician Notified _____		
Referring Physician Callback _____		
Other Notification _____		
Accepting Physician/Unit _____		

Mode of Transport/Time Notified

Ground Ambulance _____

Helicopter _____

Fixed-wing Airplane _____

Expected Availability _____

Anticipated ETA _____

Medical Database

Chief Complaint/Working Diagnosis _____

History
History of Present Illness _____

Medical History/Neonatal History/Maternal History _____

Allergies _____

Exposures _____

Physical
Vital Signs: (include most recent)

Time	Temperature	HR	RR	BP	Pulse Oximetry

*HR indicates heart rate; RR, respiratory rate; BP, blood pressure; GI, gastrointestinal; CSF, cerebrospinal fluid; Hgb, hemoglobin; Hct, hematocrit; WBC, white blood cell count; Na, sodium; K, potassium; Cl, chloride; BUN, blood urea nitrogen; Cr, creatinine, Ca, calcium; BE, base excess; sat, saturation. This is not meant to be an all inclusive intake record but to present a potential data collection and organization example.

General Appearance _____ Patient's weight (kg) _____ Actual/Estimated

Respiratory

    Exam _____

    Supplemental Oxygen (% and mode) _____

    Artificial Ventilation (mode and settings) _____

    Tracheal Tube Size and Location _____

Cardiovascular

    Exam _____

    Vascular Access _____

GI _____

Neurologic _____

Other _____

Labs Cultures obtained—blood, urine, CSF, other

Time	Hgb	Hct	WBC	Differential	Platelets	Coagulation Profile				
Time	Na	K	Cl	CO_2	BUN	Cr	Ca	Glucose	Other Labs	
Blood Gases		Type	Time	pH	Pco_2	Po_2	BE	HCO_2	o_2 sat	Fio^2	Ventilator Settings
		Type	Time	pH	Pco_2	Po_2	BE	HCO_2	o_2 sat	Fio^2	Ventilator Settings

Radiographs/Other studies _____

	Therapeutic Interventions Completed	Interventions Recommended
Fluids		
Medications		
Medications		
Other		

Signature of Transport Intake Coordinator(s) _____

■ Sample Transport Database Collection Fields* ■

I. **Demographic data**
   Unique transport identifier
   Medical record number
   Date of birth (and time of birth for neonates)
   Age (gestational age for neonates)
   Sex
   Weight (kg)
   Race/ethnicity
   Patient address
   Referring physician/medical professional with telephone/
     fax number
   Date of transport
   Name of parents (responsible for consent)
   Name of guarantor (responsible for bill)
   Primary physician (with contact information)
   Religious preference if stated
   Special family circumstances (eg, sick mother from birth, deaf
     family member, need for translator)

II. **System data**
   Community code (community, city, county, region, or state name)
   Transport system type (public, private, hospital, volunteer)
   Type of team (neonatal, pediatric, trauma, ECMO, burn)
   Mode of vehicle (ground, fixed-wing, helicopter, combination,
     other)
   Type of transport (acute vs return)
   Team configuration (personnel dispatched with names, identifiers,
     eg, physician, RN, RRT, EMT, NNP, other)
   Time call received
   Time vehicle called
   Ambulance/aircraft no.

Time and location of dispatch
  If air Outbound
        Departure to aircraft location (if off site)
        Take-off (airport/helipad and time)
        Landing (airport/helipad and time)
    Inbound
        Departure to aircraft location (if off site)
        Take-off (airport/helipad and time)
        Landing (airport/helipad and time)
Time of arrival at referring hospital
Referring facility
Referring physician
Time of departure from referring hospital
Time of arrival at destination facility
Destination facility (name, code, level of care)
Admitting physician at destination facility
Time of departure from destination facility
Time of arrival at home base facility/office
Special equipment needed (eg, nitric oxide)

III. **Clinical data**
Reason for transport
Type of case
  Medical
  Surgical
  Trauma (use pediatric trauma registry format)
  Neonate
  Cardiac
Intake diagnosis (for neonate multiples: twin A, triplet B)
Vital signs
Respiratory status (room air, FIO_2, NC, CPAP, intubated, ventilation)
Respiratory support (ventilator settings, $FIO2$, nitric oxide)
Transport team recommendations to referring team before
    transport team arrival
Transport team interventions/procedures
  Use *CPT* codes

Medications administered by transport team
    Grouped according to degree of medical control required
        (group 1, highest)
    Group 1: Resuscitation (eg, epinephrine, atropine, bicarbonate, airway control adjuncts, vasoactive infusions)
    Group 2: Drugs to treat neurologic emergencies and for gastro-intestinal decontamination, antidotes, analgesics, drugs to treat acute metabolic disturbances (eg, insulin, glucagon, hypertonic dextrose, polystyrene sulfonate [Kayexalate]), intravenous fluid administration for shock, surfactant
    Group 3: Routine therapy for acute but not life-threatening conditions, such as bronchodilator treatment, antibiotics, intravenous fluid therapy (except for shock)
Contact to transport team base/MCP
    No   Yes
    Time/name of MCP contacted

IV. **Adverse events before or during transport**
  1. Death
  2. Cardiac arrest
  3. Respiratory arrest (as defined by team)
  4. Hypotension (as defined by team)
  5. Unplanned extubation
  6. Obstructed, dysfunctional, or replaced endotracheal tube
  7. Air leak or pneumothorax
  8. Equipment failure
    a. Loss of oxygen
    b. Loss of suction
    c. Battery or power failure
    d. Ventilator malfunction
    e. Monitor malfunction
    f. Medication/IV infiltration
    g. Vehicle mishap
    h. Other

9. Delayed transport
   a. Ambulance, aircraft (reason)
   b. Personnel
   c. Multiple calls
   d. Elective/nonemergency
   e. Bed/staff availability
   f. Communications
   g. Weather
   h. Equipment
10. Aspiration
11. Dislodged catheter/line
12. Bradycardia/arrhythmia during transport
13. Worsening respiratory status
14. Medication error
15. Hypoxemia (eg, Spo_2 decreases by >10%)
16. Hypothermia (as defined by team)
17. Airway not cleared at time of admission (head positioning, mucus, poor mask control)
18. Patient's condition unstable on arrival at referring or receiving hospital
19. Referring physician
    a. Present on team arrival
    b. Present at any time but not on arrival
    c. Not present
20. Training of referring physician
    a. Pediatrics
    b. Pediatric emergency medicine
    c. Pediatric critical care
    d. Pediatric subspecialist
    e. Emergency medicine
    f. Neonatologist
    g. Family practice
    h. Other
21. Referring team (staff, nurses, respiratory therapists)
    a. Interactions
    b. Conflicts

22. Adverse events reporting
    a. Staff meeting
    b. Mortality/morbidity conference
    c. Legal affairs
    d. Debriefing/crisis management
    e. Human resources

V. **Diagnosis at transfer from ward, emergency department, intensive care, or neonatal intensive care**
    Medical
    Surgical
    Trauma
    Still hospitalized

VI. **Severity scoring**
    Systolic blood pressure: highest, lowest
    Diastolic blood pressure: highest, lowest
    Heart rate: highest, lowest
    PaO_2/FIO_2: lowest/highest
    PCO_2: highest
    pH: highest/lowest
    Pupillary reaction: normal, unequal or dilated, fixed and dilated
    Prothrombin time and control
    PTT/control ratio < 1.5 ☐ Yes ☐ No
    Bilirubin: highest
    Potassium: highest, lowest
    Calcium: highest, lowest
    Glucose: highest, lowest
    Bicarbonate: highest, lowest
    PRISM score from referring hospital
    PRISM score values within 24 hours after transport
    Pediatric trauma score
    Glasgow Coma Scale score
    Neonatal severity score (eg, SNAP)
    Apgar Score

VII. Disposition
Admitting unit at receiving hospital
a. NICU
b. PICU
c. Ward
d. Step-down unit
e. Burn unit
f. Emergency department
g. Operating room
h. Morgue/medical examiner
i. Date and time of disposition

VIII. Financial data
Third-party insurer preauthorization ☐ Yes ☐ No
Preauthorization contact
Reason for lack of preauthorization (if needed)
Team charge (date billed)
Reimbursement (date received)
Reason for denial
Code
If denied, appeal of denial ☐ Yes ☐ No
Appeal successful ☐ Yes ☐ No

*ECMO indicates extracorporeal membrane oxygenation; RN, registered nurse; RRT, registered respiratory therapist; EMT, emergency medical technician; NNP, neonatal nurse practitioner; FIO_2, fraction of inspired oxygen; NC, nasal cannula; CPAP, continuous positive airway pressure; CPT, Current Procedural Terminology; MCP, medical control physician; IV, intravenous; PTT, partial thromboplastin time; PRISM, Pediatric Risk of Mortality Score; SNAP, Score for Neonatal Acute Physiology; NICU, neonatal intensive care unit; and PICU, pediatric intensive care unit.

■ ■ ■ ■ ■ ■

■ **EMTALA Transfer Form Examples*** ■

1. Patient transfer checklist
2. Patient transfer order
3. Transfer form for use with medically indicated transfer or patient requested transfer[†]
4. EMTALA transfer acceptance or denial
5. Informed consent to refuse examination, treatment, or transfer

---

*From Bitterman RA. *Providing Emergency Care Under Federal Law: EMTALA.* Dallas, TX: American College of Emergency Physicians; 2000:261, 263, 269, 271. Used with permission.

†From Bitterman RA. *Supplement to Providing Emergency Care Under Federal Law: EMTALA.* Dallas, TX: American College of Emergency Physicians; 2004:S20. Available at: http://www2.acep.org/library/pdf/emtalaSupplement.pdf. Accessed February 14, 2006. Used with permission.

Patient Transfer Checklist

The following tasks must be completed before any patient is transferred from our facility to another acute care facility. Check off each task completed. Put the white copy of the completed checklist in the patient's medical record. Send the yellow copy to the receiving hospital with the patient. Send the pink copy to quality assurance.

A. EXAMINATION AND TREATMENT

☐ Medical screening examination (MSE) performed to the extent possible considering the emergency department's capabilities and ancillary services and/or on-call physicians available to determine if the patient has an emergency medical condition (MSE is only for emergency department cases), and/or

☐ Treatment provided, including any necessary stabilizing treatment, to the extent possible within the resources and physician personnel available to our facility.

B. INTERACTION WITH ACCEPTING FACILITY

☐ Transfer accepted by appropriate physician and documented on the Patient Transfer Order form.

☐ Transfer accepted by receiving facility.

☐ Receiving hospital has adequate space and qualified personnel to appropriately handle the patient's medical condition.

C. FORMS TO COMPLETE PRIOR TO TRANSFER (See Transfer Packet Instructions)

☐ If this is a **patient-requested** transfer:

  ☐ Complete the **Patient-Requested Transfer** form *and*

  ☐ Complete the **Patient Transfer Order** form

  or

☐ If this is a **medically indicated** transfer:

  ☐ Complete the **Medically Indicated Transfer** form *and*

  ☐ Complete the **Patient Transfer Order** form

D. TRANSFER PROCEDURE

☐ Arrange transfer of the patient through qualified personnel and transfer equipment as appropriate for the patient's condition.

☐ Send copies of pertinent patient medical records with the patient to the receiving facility.

☐ Tests: ___ Labs   ___ X-rays   ___ ECGs
          ___ Monitor strips   ___ ABGs   ___ Other _____

☐ Medical records

☐ Transfer forms

☐ Obtain the patient's vital signs and reassess the patient's medical condition *just prior to* the time of transport and document them in the patient's medical record.

☐ Give the nursing report to the receiving hospital.

☐ Send the patient's belongings with the patient.

☐ Notify the patient's family if desired and if available.

Signature _____ RN Print name _____

Date _____ Time _____

Patient Transfer Checklist		ADDRESSOGRAPH	Imprint patient's ID here
White/Patient Record	Yellow/Transfer With Patient Pink/QA		

Patient Transfer Order

To Be Completed by the Transferring Physician

Patient's Name _____

REASON FOR PATIENT TRANSFER (COMPLETE SECTION A OR B, BUT NOT BOTH.)

☐ **A. UNSTABLE PATIENT (Check either Box 1 or Box 2.)** | ☐ **B. STABLE PATIENT**

☐ 1. Patient requested transfer in writing after risks and benefits explained.

☐ 2. Transfer is medically indicated in the patient's best interest.

☐ Transfer is medically indicated.

☐ Patient requested transfer.

☐ HMO ☐ Private physician

☐ Other_____

If Box 2 is checked, then check either Box 2a or Box 2b.

☐ 2a. Our hospital has provided medical treatment within its capacity to minimize the risk to the individual's health and, in the case of a woman in labor, the health of the unborn child. The treating physician has certified that the medical benefits reasonably expected from the transfer outweigh the risks to the patient from effecting the transfer.

☐ 2b. Our hospital has not provided medical treatment within its capacity because an on-call physician has refused or failed to appear within a reasonable period of time to provide further examination or necessary stabilizing treatment. The treating physician has certified that, at this time, the medical benefits reasonably expected from the transfer outweigh the risks to the patient from effecting the transfer.

Name and address of on-call physician who refused/failed to appear _____

For the reasons listed above, I direct that the patient be transferred with the following instructions:

☐ 1. The receiving hospital/physician has agreed to accept this patient in transfer and has confirmed the availability of adequate space and qualified personnel necessary for the treatment of this individual.

Receiving hospital_____ Accepting physician_____

Date_____ Time_____

☐ 2. Copies of available medical records, tests, orders, consents, certification, and radiographs will accompany patient.

☐ 3. Mode of transfer: ☐ BLS ambulance ☐ ALS ambulance ☐ Neonatal transfer team ☐ Helicopter ☐ Car ☐ Other_____

☐ 4. Additional personnel, equipment, or life support services required to accompany patient:

_____

☐ 5. Medical orders _____

☐ 6. If radio on-line medical direction is necessary during transfer, control to be exercised by:

☐ This hospital ☐ Receiving hospital ☐ Other_____ ☐ None necessary

☐ 7. Physician's signature_____ Physician's name_____

Date_____ Time_____

TO BE COMPLETED BY HOSPITAL STAFF

Name of transfer agency _____ Person contacted _____

Contacted by _____ Date_____ Time_____

Time of arrival _____ Time of transfer _____

NOTES

Patient Transfer Order | ADDRESSOGRAPH | Imprint patient's ID here

White/Patient Record   Yellow/Transfer With Patient   Pink/QA

Emergency Medical Condition (EMC) Identified: *(Mark appropriate box(es), then go to Section II)*

I. MEDICAL CONDITION: Diagnosis _____

☐ **No Emergency Medical Condition Identified:** This patient has been examined and an EMC has not been identified.

☐ **Patient Stable** - The patient has been examined and any medical condition stabilized such that, within reasonable clinical confidence, no material deterioration of this patient's condition is likely to result from or occur during transfer.

☐ **Patient Unstable** - The patient has been examined, an EMC has been identified and patient is not stable, but the transfer is medically indicated and in the best interest of the patient.

I have examined this patient and based upon the reasonable risks and benefits described below and upon the information available to me, I certify that the medical benefits reasonably expected from the provision of appropriate medical treatment at another facility outweigh the increased risk to this patient's medical condition that may result from effecting this transfer.

II. REASON FOR TRANSFER: ☐ Medically Indicated   ☐ Patient Requested _____

  ☐ On-call physician refused or failed to respond within a reasonable period of time.

  Physician Name _____ Address _____

III. RISK AND BENEFIT FOR TRANSFER:

Medical Benefits:	Medical Risks:
☐ Obtain level of care / service NA at this facility.	☐ Deterioration of condition en route _____
Service _____	☐ Worsening of condition or death if you stay here.
☐ Benefits outweigh risks of transfer	There is always risk of traffic delay/accident resulting in condition deterioration.

IV. Mode/Support/Treatment During Transfer as Determined by Physician – (Complete Applicable Items):

  Mode of transportation for transfer: ☐ BLS   ☐ ALS   ☐ Helicopter   ☐ Neonatal Unit   ☐ Private Car   ☐ Other _____

  Agency _____ Name/Title accompany hospital employee _____

  Support/Treatment during transfer: ☐ Cardiac Monitor   ☐ Oxygen – (Liters) _____   ☐ Pulse Oximeter   ☐ IV Pump

  ☐ IV Fluid _____ Rate _____   ☐ Restraints – Type _____   ☐ Other _____   ☐ None

  Radio on-line medical oversight *(If necessary):* ☐ Transfer Hospital   ☐ Destination Hospital   ☐ Other

V. Receiving Facility and Individual: The receiving facility has the capability for the treatment of this patient (including adequate equipment and medical personnel) and has agreed to accept the transfer and provide appropriate medical treatment.

Receiving Facility / Person accepting transfer _____ Time _____

Receiving MD _____

Transferring Physician Signature _____ Date/Time _____

Per Dr. _____ by _____ RN/ Qualified Medical Personnel Date/Time _____

VI. ACCOMPANYING DOCUMENTATION – sent via: ☐ Patient/Responsible Party   ☐ Fax   ☐ Transporter

  ☐ Copy of Pertinent Medical Record   ☐ Lab/ EKG/ X-Ray   ☐ Copy of Transfer Form   ☐ Court Order

  ☐ Advance Directive   ☐ Other _____

  Report given (Person / title) _____

  Time of Transfer _____ Date _____ Nurse Signature _____ Unit _____

  Vital Signs Just Prior to Transfer T _____ Pulse _____ R _____ BP _____ Time _____

VII. PATIENT CONSENT TO "MEDICALLY INDICATED" OR "PATIENT REQUESTED" TRANSFER:

  ☐ I hereby **CONSENT TO TRANSFER** to another facility. I understand that it is the opinion of the physician responsible for my care that the benefits of transfer outweigh the risks of transfer. I have been informed of the risks and benefits upon which this transfer is being made.

  ☐ I hereby **REQUEST TRANSFER** to _____. I understand and have considered the hospital's responsibilities, the risks and benefits of transfer, and the physician's recommendation. I make this request upon my own suggestion and not that of the hospital, physician, or anyone associated with the hospital.

  The reason I request transfer is _____

Signature of ☐ Patient   ☐ Responsible Person _____ Relationship _____

  Witness _____   Witness _____

TRANSFER FORM

White: Receiving Facility; Yellow: Medical Record; Pink: QA

Patient Name:

Date of Birth:

Medical Record Number:

PHYSICIAN

NURSING

PATIENT

EMTALA Transfer Acceptance or Denial

Patient's Name _____ Age _____ Date _____ Time _____ AM/PM

Transferring Facility _____ Telephone _____ Person Calling _____

Patient's Problem or Diagnosis				

Vital Signs (if available)	T°	HR	RR	BP /	Oximetry %

Pertinent laboratory, diagnostic test results and treatment (if available and appropriate):

_____

Patient is: ☐ Stable   ☐ Unstable   (In the opinion of the transferring physician)

REASON FOR TRANSFER

☐ Needs specialized level of_____ care (eg, Level I trauma, neurosurgeon, NICU, etc.)

☐ Available capacity (bed space, equipment, personnel) not currently available at the transferring facility.

☐ Diagnostic testing only:_____ (eg, head CT, MRI, angiography, etc.)

☐ Continuity of care

☐ Lateral transfer for insurance reasons

☐ Patient requests transfer

☐ Patient's physician requests transfer

☐ On-call physician at transferring hospital is unavailable or refused to care for patient

☐ Other:_____

TRANSFER ACCEPTED	**TRANSFER NOT ACCEPTED**
Transfer by: ☐ BLS ☐ ALS ☐ Helicopter	**Reason for Not Accepting:**
☐ Private vehicle ☐ Other _____	☐ Lateral transfer for insurance reasons only
	☐ Not an emergency medical condition
ETA _____ AM/PM	☐ Does not require specialized care of this facility
Direct admission to (physician who accepted patient in transfer):	☐ Requires specialized care not available at this facility
	☐ Available capacity (bed space, equipment, personnel) not currently available at this facility:
_____	
Service: ☐ ICU ☐ CCU ☐ PICU ☐ Med/surg ☐ Ped	☐ Trauma closed ☐ No med/surg beds
	☐ No ICU/CCU/BICU/NICU
☐ Other _____	☐ ED over capacity and closed to EMS
ED to ED Transfer	☐ Other (explain): _____
To be seen by: ☐ Emergency physician ☐ Other_____	Requested reason for transfer not appropriate (explain):
Other information: _____	_____
	Other (explain): _____

_____

Signature (and ID#) of person taking the call and who decided to accept or reject the transfer on behalf of the hospital.

EMTALA Transfer Acceptance or Denial   Imprint patient's ID here

White/Patient Record   Yellow/Transfer With Patient   Pink/QA

ADDRESSOGRAPH

Informed Consent to Refuse Examination, Treatment, or Transfer

I understand that the hospital has offered (check all that apply):

A. ☐ To examine me (the patient) to determine whether I have an emergency medical condition, or

B. ☐ To provide medical treatment or to provide stabilizing treatment for my emergency condition, or

C. ☐ To provide a medically appropriate transfer to another medical facility.

The hospital and physician have informed me that the *risks* that might reasonably be expected from the offered services are:

_____

_____

and the *benefits* of the offered services are:

_____

_____

PHYSICIAN'S DOCUMENTATION

☐ The patient appears competent and capable of understanding risks and benefits.

☐ Alternative treatments have been discussed with the patient.

☐ The patient's family is involved.   ☐ Family members are not available.

☐ The patient does not want family members involved.

Physician's signature_____

I understand that if I refuse offered services, I am doing so against medical advice. I understand that my refusal may result in a worsening of my condition and could pose a threat to my life, health, and medical safety. I understand that I am welcome to return at any time. I choose to refuse the offered services.

Signature of patient or legally responsible person _____

Print name _____ Address _____

City_____ State/ZIP _____ Date _____ Time _____

Witness signature_____ Print name_____

The patient or a legally responsible person was offered but refused to sign this form after explanation of his or her rights and the risks and benefits of the services offered.

Hospital representative who witnessed refusal to sign _____

Date _____

Time _____

Informed Consent to Refuse Examination, Treatment, or Transfer

White/Patient Record   Yellow/Transfer With Patient   Pink/QA

ADDRESSOGRAPH

Imprint patient's ID here

Sample Transport Medicine Transfer Agreement

Parties: XYZ Transport Service (referred to as XYZ)
Address
ABC Hospital (referred to as ABC)
Address

Date: xx/xx/xx

This is an agreement between ABC and XYZ for the purposes of establishing terms, conditions, and limitations on the request for services by ABC and the provision of services by XYZ for air transport of patients to be transported to or received at ABC.

ABC represents that it is a licensed hospital operating under the laws of the State of [insert state] with locations at [insert location] and with designated helicopter landing sites at [insert location]. It is further understood that ABC from time to time requires the services of helicopter medical transport for patients being transferred to ABC or by ABC to other facilities on both scheduled and emergency bases.

XYZ represents that it operates a duly licensed transport service, including helicopters, for scheduled and emergency response for transfers between hospitals and from emergency scenes. XYZ further represents that all personnel responding with its service are duly licensed [paramedics] [flight nurses] [physicians] trained, qualified, and licensed/authorized to provide care within the State of [insert state].

XYZ agrees to respond to **accepted** requests for service from ABC with a helicopter equipped consistent with FAA and State requirements for transport vehicles and with an appropriately trained, qualified, and licensed/authorized medical crew and pilot on the following basis:

1. Response will be made to emergency requests by the nearest available aircraft with capabilities and crew appropriate to the nature of the request.
2. Nonemergency requests will be made at the time agreed between ABC and XYZ, subject to priority for emergency transports.
3. Responses are subject to availability of aircraft owing to prior use commitment, maintenance/repairs, flight-time restrictions, fuel, weather, or other safety or regulatory issues as determined by XYZ at its sole discretion.
4. Aircraft may be diverted for emergency or cases of greater need at the sole discretion of XYZ personnel. Rescue scene responses will be given greater priority than responses for patients currently in a hospital environment.
5. If a request is accepted, XYZ will provide an estimated time of arrival. XYZ will update ABC on estimated time of arrival in case any factor or change of circumstances occurs that appears will delay the estimated response time for a period of greater than 30 minutes. XYZ personnel will use their sole discretion in determining the reasonable possibility of delay.
6. If XYZ accepts a request, but the estimated response time or subsequent delays do not meet the reasonable needs of ABC, ABC may cancel the request at any time before arrival for transport from ABC or the sending hospital (in the case of transports to ABC).
7. XYZ may decline to transport any patient after accepting a request in which in its sole discretion such patient is not medically appropriate for transport; the transport would violate any XYZ, state, or federal rule or regulation; or aircraft safety or weather requires grounding or delay of flight.
8. XYZ agrees that all services for transport will be billed to the patient or the patient's third-party payer and not to ABC hospital, unless as agreed in writing in individual cases *or* if ABC fails to notify XYZ of a transport cancellation before arrival. A change in patient condition that prevents transport after arrival (whether determined by ABC or XYZ) will not result in a charge to ABC.
9. XYZ rates and charges are attached as Addendum 1.
10. XYZ agrees that it will accept custody of and transport patient medical records along with any patient being transported.

ABC understands and agrees that this is a nonexclusive agreement and that it is subject to availability, acceptance, diversion, and cancellation terms and conditions as stated above.

ABC further understands that all regulatory compliance requirements of state and federal law, including but not limited to EMTALA and HIPAA, are the responsibility of the hospital and that XYZ does not assume or agree to provide any compliance on behalf of the hospital.

ABC, its employees, and medical staff are responsible for providing any and all informed consents, explanations, and medical decisions to transport by transport vehicle consistent with EMTALA, including certification for transport. XYZ will be responsible for obtaining compliance documentation for its own purposes only.

Each party shall be responsible for maintaining professional liability insurance for its respective entity, employees, agents, and medical staff.

This agreement will remain in full force and effect until written notification by either party, with or without cause, with 7 days advance notice. This agreement is nonexclusive and does not limit either party from transacting similar services with other providers.

The parties agree to enter into reciprocal Business Associates Agreements for the purposes of HIPAA compliance, which agreements are separate and distinct from this agreement.

Approved: [date]

ABC

By _____

XYZ

By _____

Reference Card

Sample Contents for a Neonatal-Pediatric Emergency and Medication Reference Card*

Cardiac Arrest

1. Airway, Breathing, Circulation
2. 100% oxygen
3. Medications

■ Epinephrine
Newborn
0.1 mL/kg IV, ET (1:10,000)

Child
0.1 mL/kg IV, IO (1:10,000) every 3–5 min
0.1 mL/kg ET (1:1,000) every 3–5 min

Adult
Initially 1 mg IV every 3–5 min

■ *Atropine*
0.02 mg/kg IV, ET, IM
(minimum, 0.1 mg; maximum, 1.0 mg)

■ Dextrose
Newborn
$D_{10}W$ 2–4 mL/kg IV, IO

Child
D_{25} 2–4 mL/kg IV, IO

Adult
D_{50} 1 mL/kg IV, IO

■ Bicarbonate, 1 mEq/kg IV or (0.3 × kg × base deficit) (maximum, 50 mEq)

■ Defibrillate
Pediatric
2 J/kg, then 4 J/kg (asynchronous) (or eqivalent biphasic)

Adult
200 J, then 200–300 J, then 360 J (or eqivalent biphasic)

■ Cardioversion
0.5–1.0 J/kg (synchronous)

*The information provided is presented as a guide and should not be regarded as specific medical advice or direction. IV indicates intravenous; ET, endotracheal route; IO, intraosseous; IM, intramuscular; D, dextrose; W, water, NS, isotonic saline; SQ, subcutaneous; IVP, intravenous push; PR, per rectum; PE, phenytoin sodium equivalents; PO, by mouth; NG, nasogastric; and TDD, total digitalizing dose (to be divided 1/2, 1/4, 1/4 every 8 h).

Intubation: Endotracheal Tube (ETT) Selection:

Age	ETT Size (internal diameter)
<28 wk	2.5
28–38 wk	3.0
Newborn	3.5
6 mo to 1 y	4.0
>1 y	4 + (Age in Years) divided by 4 or (16 + Age in Years) divided by 4

Positioning Guidelines (centimeters at mandibular ridge)
0.5–4 kg: weight (kg) + 6
>4 kg, approximately 3 times ETT size

Glasgow Coma Scale

Standard   *Pediatric*

Eye opening
Spontaneous	4		Spontaneous
To voice	3		To speech
To pain	2		To pain
None	1		None

Verbal
Oriented	5		Coos and babbles
Confused	4		Irritable, cries
Inappropriate words	3		Cries (pain)
Incomprehensible	2		Moans (pain)
None	1		None

Motor
Obeys commands	6		Spontaneous movement
Purposeful (pain)	5		Withdraws (touch)
Withdraws (pain)	4		Withdraws (pain)
Flexion (pain)	3		Abnormal flexion
Extension (pain)	2		Abnormal extension
None	1		None

Total	(3–15)

Analgesia and Sedation
Morphine .... 0.1 mg/kg IV, IM
Meperidine .... 1 mg/kg IV, IM
Midazolam .... 0.05–0.1 mg/kg IV, IM
Fentanyl .... 1 mcg/kg IV
Ketamine .... 0.5–1 mg/kg IV

Reversal Agents
Naloxone .... 0.1 mg/kg IV, IM, ET (>20 kg = 2 mg)
Flumazenil .... 0.01 mg/kg IV (>20 kg = 0.2 mg)

Antibiotics

Acyclovir .... 10 mg/kg per dose
Ampicillin .... 25–100 mg/kg per dose
Ampicillin/sulbactam .... 80 mg/kg per dose
Cefazolin .... 20–30 mg/kg per dose
Cefotaxime .... 50 mg/kg per dose
Ceftazidime .... 30–50 mg/kg per dose
Ceftriaxone .... 25–75 mg/kg per dose
Cefuroxime .... 25–50 mg/kg per dose
Clindamycin .... 5–9 mg/kg per dose
Doxycycline .... 2 mg/kg per dose (maximum, 100 mg)
Gentamicin .... 1.7–2.5 mg/kg per dose
Oxacillin .... 25–40 mg/kg per dose
Vancomycin .... 10 mg/kg per dose

Asthma, Anaphylaxis, Stridor

Albuterol .... 0.15–0.25 mg/kg (maximum, 5 mg) in 3 mL NS (nebulized)
Terbutaline .... Load: 2–10 mcg/kg IV
                             Drip: 0.1–1.0 mcg/kg per min
                             SQ: 0.005–0.01 mg/kg per dose (maximum, 0.4 mg/dose)
Epinephrine .... 0.01 mg/kg = 0.01 mL/kg SQ (1:1,000)
                             (maximum, 0.5 mg = 0.5 mL)
Racemic epinephrine .... 0.25–1.0 mL in 3 mL NS (nebulized)
Methylprednisolone .... 1–2 mg/kg IV, IM
Dexamethasone .... 0.6–1 mg/kg IV, IM
Magnesium sulfate .... 40 mg/kg (maximum, 2 g) over 15 min
Diphenhydramine .... 1 mg/kg IV, IM

Cardiac

Adenosine .... 0.1 mg/kg rapid IVP
                             (maximum, 0.4 mg/kg or 12 mg)
Alprostadil
(prostaglandin E_1) .... 0.05–0.1 mcg/kg per min IV
Amiodarone .... 5 mg/kg (rate depends on clinical scenerio)
Calcium chloride 10% .... 20 mg/kg = 0.2 mL/kg slow IV
Dobutamine .... 2–20 mcg/kg per min IV
Dopamine .... 2–20 mcg/kg per min IV
Epinephrine .... 0.05–1 mcg/kg per min IV
Isoproterenol .... 0.05–2 mcg/kg per min IV
Furosemide .... 0.5–1 mg/kg IV
Lidocaine .... 1 mg/kg initial bolus
                             Drip: 20–50 mcg/kg per min
Magnesium sulfate .... 25–75 mg/kg IV over 20–30 min (maximum, 2 g)
Phenylephrine .... 5–20 mcg/kg per dose bolus
                             Drip: 0.1–0.5 mcg/kg per min
Procainamide .... 3–6 mg/kg over 5 min IV
                             (maximum, 100 mg per dose)
Propranolol .... 0.01–0.1 mg/kg IV slowly over 15 min; maximum dose,
                             1 mg (infants); 3 mg (children))

Cardiac, continued

Esmolol .... Load: 100–500 mcg/kg given over 1 min
Drip: Initial, 50 mcg/kg per min titrated by 50 mcg/kg per min to effect (maximum, 1,000 mcg/kg per min)

Endocrine

Glucose .... $D_{10}W$ 4 mL/kg IV, IO (neonates)
$D_{25}W$ 2 mL/kg IV, IO (children)

Glucagon .... 0.025–0.1 mg/kg IV, IM, SQ (maximum, 1 mg/dose)

Hydrocortisone .... (all IV, IM)	
Stress coverage	0.3–0.6 mg/kg per dose or 100 mg/meter^2
Acute adrenal insufficiency	1–2 mg/kg per dose (maximum, 100 mg)
Shock	50 mg/kg per dose

Drips (see above loading doses, as appropriate)

Alprostadil (prostaglandin E_1) .... 0.05–0.1 mcg/kg per min
Dobutamine .... 2–20 mcg/kg per min
Dopamine .... 2–20 mcg/kg per min
Epinephrine .... 0.05–1 mcg/kg per min
Insulin (regular) .... 0.1 units/kg per h
Isoproterenol .... 0.05–2 mcg/kg per min
Lidocaine .... 20–50 mcg/kg per min
Milrinone .... 0.25–0.75 mcg/kg per min
Nitroprusside .... 0.3–10 mcg/kg per min
Norepinephrine .... 0.05–2 mcg/kg per min
Phenylephrine .... Infusion: 0.1–0.5 mcg/kg per min
Terbutaline .... 0.08–0.4 mcg/kg per min
(titrate to maximum 6 mcg/kg per min)
Vasopressin
(gastrointestinal bleeding) .... Bolus 0.3 units/kg (maximum, 20 units) then 0.002–0.01 units/kg per min
Vasopressin (shock) .... Initial: 10–50 milliunits/kg per hour (0.15–0.8 milliunits/kg per min) titrate to effect

Hyperkalemia

Sodium polystyrene sulfonate
(Kayexalate) .... 1 g/kg PR, PO
Calcium chloride .... 20 mg/kg per dose = 0.2 mL/kg IV
Insulin (regular) .... 0.1 units/kg IV with glucose
Glucose (D_{25}) .... 0.5 g/kg = 2 mL/kg IV
Sodium bicarbonate .... 1–2 mEq/kg IV (maximum, 50 mEq)

Seizures

Lorazeparn .... 0.05–0.1 mg/kg IV
Diazepam .... 0.1 mg/kg IV
0.5 mg/kg PR
Phenobarbital .... 15–20 mg/kg IV at ≤1 mg/kg per min

Phenytoin .... 15–20 mg/kg IV in NS at ≤1 mg/kg per min
Fosphenytoin .... 15–20 mg PE/kg IV, IM

Increased Intracranial Pressure
100% oxygen
Mild hyperventilation with P_{CO_2}: 35 mm Hg
Keep head elevated, in midline position
Maintain adequate perfusion
Mannitol .... 0.25–0.5 g/kg IV or
Hypertonic saline .... 1–5 mL/kg (optimal concentration and dosage not established)
Lidocaine .... 1 mg/kg IV before intubation

Rapid-Sequence Intubation[†]
Oxygenate
Atropine, 0.02 mg/kg
Lidocaine, 1 mg/kg (if increased intracranial pressure or bronchospasm)
Sedation
Normotensive .... Thiopental, 2–5 mg/kg or
                                                                    Midazolam, 0.1–0.3 mg/kg or
                                                                    Etomidate, 0.3 mg/kg
Shock .... Etomidate, 0.3 mg/kg
Head injury .... Thiopental, 2–5 mg/kg
Status asthmaticus .... Ketamine, 0.5–2 mg/kg

Cricoid Pressure
Paralysis[‡]
Succinylcholine..................................... 1–2 mg/kg (do not use if potassium level increased or
                                                                    risk of malignant hyperthermia)
Rocuroniurn .... 0.6–0.8 mg/kg
Vecuronium .... 0.1–0.2 mg/kg
Pancuronium .... 0.1 mg/kg

Miscellaneous Drugs
Charcoal .... 1 g/kg PO or by NG tube (maximum, 50 g)
Digoxin (digitalization) .... <40 wk gestation: TDD* = 0.015–0.025 mg/kg IV
                                                                    Term–12 y: TDD* = 0.02–0.035 mg/kg IV
Diphenhydramine .... 1 mg/kg (IV, IM, PO)
Metoclopramide .... 0.5–2 mg/kg (antiemetic) IV, PO
Nifedipine .... 0.25 mg/kg (sublingual)
Methylprednisolone
    Status asthmaticus .... 2 mg/kg, then 1 mg/kg every 6 h IV, IM
    Spinal cord injury (blunt).............. 30 mg/kg over 15 min, then 5.4 mg/kg per hour for 23–48 h
Surfactant
    Beractant (Survanta) .... 4 mL/kg per dose, ET
    Colfosceril palmitatetyloxapol
    (Exosurf) .... 5 mL/kg per dose, ET
    Tolazoline .... 1–2 mg/kg over 10–15 min IV followed by
                                                                    0.2–0.5 mg/kg per hour

†Use cuffed tube after 8 years of age.

‡Neuromuscular blocking agents to be used only by staff trained and skilled in advanced airway monitoring and support.
Poison Center phone number: (800) 222-1222

■ ■ ■ ■ ■ ■

■ Sample Critical Care Transport ■ "Supply" Contents*

- ■ Neonatal transport supplies
- ■ Neonatal transport ambulance inventory
- ■ Infant transport medication inventory
- ■ Neonatal ambulance medication refrigeration daily log
- ■ Fixed-wing pediatric transport supplies

Neonatal Transport Supplies

Point-of-care testing

Glucometer (eg, One Touch) check strip 1
High and low test solutions .... 1 each
Pipettes 4
Glucometer (eg, One Touch) test strips 1
Pink and yellow lancets .... 4 each
Glucometer 1

IV and phlebotomy supplies

Alcohol and antiseptic (eg, Betadine [povidone
    iodine]) preps .... 6 each
Package of chlorhexidine preps 1
2 × 2 gauze pads 6
Adhesive bandages (eg, Band-Aids)
5-mL saline flush 4
Roll of 1" self adherent wrap (eg, Coban) 1

---

*These are samples of transport supplies carried by representative neonatal and fixed-wing
  pediatric transport teams. They are not meant to be all inclusive or directly applicable to
  all scenarios. Product and brand names are furnished for identification purposes only.
  No endorsement of the manufacturers or products listed is implied. Abbreviations are
  explained at the end of the document.

Small and large clear sterile dressing (eg, Tegaderm)............ 2 each
18-gauge IO needles 2
Umbilical bridge tapes.. 2
Adhesive (eg, Mastisol) and adhesive remover
   (eg, Detachol).. 1 each
Hypoallergenic tape (eg, Dermiform), clear plastic tape
   (eg, Transpore), or baby tape adhesive 1
Label tapes:
   PGE$_1$ (eg, prostaglandin E$_1$), arterial, maintenance,
   dopamine, dobutamine, morphine
23-gauge needles 4
19-gauge needles... 4
Filter needles 2
20-mL syringes.. 3
30-mL syringes.. 3
"Y" connectors (eg, Bifuse and Trifuse) .... 1 each
Stopcock.. 1

Syringes

60-mL.. 2
20-mL.. 2
10-mL.. 2
5-mL 3
3-mL 2
1-mL 3
Blood gas... 4

Tubes

Blank label 2
Heparin 2
Capillary + magnet.. 2
Catheter adapter... 1
Heparin lock 1
T extension piece.. 1
IV catheters:
     14 gauge, 16 gauge, 18 gauge, 20 gauge, and 22 gauge..... 1 each
     24-gauge intravenous catheters (eg, Angiocath)................. 4
     25-gauge and 23-gauge butterfly needles .... 2 each

IV arm board
Tourniquets: nonlatex and rubber band
IV pressure tubing 2
IV minivolume extension tubing 2
Aerobic blood culture bottle 1

Umbilical catheters

3.5F and 5F (also consider double lumen) .... 2 each
Instrument-procedure tray... 1
Umbilical twill tape.. 1
4-0 silk suture package
Povidone iodine swab sticks

Monitoring and general care supplies

Restraints .... 2 pairs
Neonatal-infant ECG leads... 1 set
Neonatal-infant oximeter probe 1
BP cuffs: sizes 1, 2, 3, and 4...................................... 1 each
Disposable blanket (eg, Mylar Silver Baby Swaddler)............ 1
Stockinette cap 1
Soft gel wedges... 2
Pacifier
Penlight
Marker (eg, Sharpie)
Tape measure
Thermometer

Airway supplies

Neonatal-infant resuscitation mask.................................. 1 each
0.5-L Anesthesia bag.. 1
0.5-L Self-inflating bag 1
Infant nasal cannula 1
Oropharyngeal airways: sizes 00, 0, 1, and 2
Intubation pack: laryngoscope with size 0 and 1 blades 1
ET tubes: sizes 2.0–8.0 .... 2 each
Laryngeal mask airways .... 1 each size
Bone cutter (if applicable) 1

Stylet 1
Yankauer suction catheter 1
Adhesive (eg, Mastisol) and adhesive remover
  (eg, Detachol) 1
End-tidal CO_2 detector (eg, Pedi-cap) 1
Surfactant adapters: 2.5, 3.0, 3.5, and 4.0 .... 1 each
Green oxygen tubing with manometer adapter 1
Humidity filter (eg, Humid-vent) 1
"O" ring 1
Skin dressing (eg, DuoDERM) 1
Multiaccess catheter (surfactant use): 2.5, 3.0, 3.5,
  and 4.0 .... 1 each
In-line suction catheters: 5F, 6F, 8F .... 2 each

Drainage or special equipment

Multilumen drainage catheters (eg, Replogle): 6F–14F .... 1 each
Sterile lubricant (eg, Surgilube)
8F feeding tube
Sterile specimen (bowel) bag
Chest tubes: 8F, 10F, and 12F .... 1 each
Chest drain valves (eg, Heimlich) 2

Soft gel wedge supports 2

Gloves: small, medium, and large .... 2 pairs each

Scissors and hemostat .... 1 each

Meningomyelocele dressing kit

Hot packs

Instant film pack (eg, Polaroid) 1

Neonatal Transport Ambulance Inventory (Ambulance Vendor Restocks Supplies)

NG Supplies	IV Supplies	IV Tubing	Respiratory Supplies
Catheter adapters, 2	Heparin lock caps, 2	Pressure tubing, 3	Self-inflating bag, 1
NG tubes: 6F and 8F, 1 each	Stopcocks, 2	Microbore tubing, 3	Anesthesia bag (0.5 L), 2
Multilumen drainage tube (eg, Replogle), 1 each	T piece, 2	Y adapters (eg, Bifuse), 2 Y adapter (eg, Trifuse), 1	Resuscitation masks, neonate-infant, 2 each
Surgilube, 2	Butterfly needles, 2 each	Arterial transducer, 1	Suction catheters, 2 each
Bowel bag, 1	Intravenous catheters (eg, Angiocath), 2 each		Isotonic saline, 3 mL, 5
	18-gauge IO needles, 2		Nebulizer kit, 1
	Tourniquets, 2		Intubation kit, 1
	Alcohol pads, 10		Pneumo kit, 1
	Steri wipes, 2		NCPAP circuit, 1
	2 × 2 gauze pads, 4		Ventilator circuit, 1
	Sterile dressing (eg, Tegaderm), 4		Sterile water (60 mL), 1
	IV Arm board		Adhesive (eg, Mastisol), 4
	Restraints, 1 pair		Adhesive remover (eg, Detachol), 4
	Needles, assorted		Yankauer suction, 1
	Syringes, assorted		

Neonatal Transport Ambulance Inventory (Ambulance Vendor Restocks Supplies), *continued*

Tape	Procedure Supplies	Patient Warming Supplies	Patient Supplies
Assorted tapes	Umbilical catheters: 3.5F and 5.0F	Port-A-Warm mattress	ECG leads, neonatal and infant, 2 each
Medication label tapes, 1	Cannula clamp, 1	Blanket (eg, Mylar), 1	BP cuffs, sizes 1–4, 1 each
Self-adherent wrap, 1	Suture kit and sutures, 1	Hats, 2	Stethoscope
Umbilical bridge tapes, 2	Sterile scissors, 1	Linen, assorted	Oximeter probes, 2
	Instrument tray	Heel warmers	Thermometer, 1
	Myelomeningocele kit		Diapers
	10F CT, 1		Pacifier
	Skin prep (eg, ChloraPrep), 2		Diaper wipes
	Gloves, assorted sizes		Penlight
	Pleural fluid receptacle (eg, Pleuravac)		Tape measure
	Sterile water, 1 L		

Neonatal Transport Ambulance Inventory (Ambulance Vendor Restocks Supplies), *continued*

Equipment	Manuals	Paperwork and Forms
ECG, BP, SpO$_2$, ETCO$_2$ cables	Transport policies and procedure	Consents for care in English and Spanish
Transilluminator	Infection control	Transport records
Monitor/defibrillator (eg, Lifepack)	Nursing policies and procedures	Medication worksheet
Suction buckets	Body substance exposure	Parent handbook
Oxygen flowmeter	I-Stat meter	Emergency type and crossmatch
Air flowmeter	Medical reference (eg, Neofax)	Death certificate; autopsy permits
Oxygen and air adapters	Hospital formulary	Maps and directions
Oxygen regulator		Spanish-translated forms
Sharps containers		Transport team flow sheet
Placenta cooler		Billing sheet
Breast milk cooler		Placenta pathology forms
Car seat		
Cleaning products		
Hand pump disinfectant (eg, Purell)		

Infant Transport Medication Inventory

Medication Bag Inventory	Quantity
Adenosine, 3 mg/mL, 2-mL vial	1
Albumin 5%, 50 mL	1
Albuterol inhaler, 2.5 mg/3 mL; ready to use	1
Ampicillin, 500-mg vial and 1 10-mL vial of nonbacterial water	2
Atropine, 0.1 mg/mL, 10-mL syringe	1
Calcium chloride, 100 mg/mL, 10-mL syringe	1
Calcium gluconate, 100 mg/mL, 10-mL vial	1
Clindamycin, 150 mg/mL, 2-mL vial	1
D_5W 100 mL	1
D_5W 250 mL	1
$D_{10}W$ 250 mL	1
Digoxin, 0.1 mg/mL, 1-mL ampule	1
Dobutamine, 12.5 mg/mL, 20-mL vial	1
Dopamine, 40 mg/mL, 5-mL vial	1
Epinephrine, 1:10,000, 10-mL syringe	2
Fentanyl, 0.05 mg/mL, 2-mL ampule	1
Gentamicin, 10 mg/mL, 2-mL vial	1
Heparin, 10 U/mL, 2-mL vial	1
Heparin, 1000 U/mL, 10-mL vial	1
Lactated Ringers, 500 mL	1
Morphine, 2-mg/mL syringe	2
Naloxone, 0.4 mg/mL, 1-mL ampule	2
Nonbacterial isotonic (normal) saline, 20-mL vial	2
Isotonic saline, 250 mL	1
Pancuronium, 1 mg/mL, 10-mL vial	1
Phenobarbital, 65 mg/mL, 1-mL vial	2
Phytonadione, 1 mg /0.5 mL, 0.5-mL syringe	2
Sodium bicarbonate, 0.5 mEq/mL, 10-mL syringe	2
Vecuronium, 1 mg/mL, 10-mg vial	1

Ambulance Refrigerator Medication Inventory	
Alprostadil, 500 µg, 1-mL ampule	1
Fosphenytoin, 100 mg/2 mL vial	1
Lorazepam, 2 mg/mL, 1-mL vial	2
Surfactant, 8-mL vial	2

Neonatal Ambulance Medication Refrigeration Daily Log

Check lock integrity after each transport, and complete information below. Medication refrigerator temperature: 3°C to 8°C for storage of medications in the ambulance. When medications are used, complete the patient charge sheet, cosign for controlled medications, exchange used medication pouch in pharmacy, return pouch to ambulance refrigerator.

Sun	Mon	Tue	Wed	Thu	Fri	Sat
1 Box # ___ Temp ___ Locked ___ Signature(s) ___	2 Box # ___ Temp ___ Locked ___	3 Box # ___ Temp ___ Locked ___	4 Box # ___ Temp ___ Locked ___	5 Box # ___ Temp ___ Locked ___	6 Box # ___ Temp ___ Locked ___	7 Box # ___ Temp ___ Locked ___
8 Box # ___ Temp ___ Locked ___ Signature(s) ___	9 Box # ___ Temp ___ Locked ___	10 Box # ___ Temp ___ Locked ___	11 Box # ___ Temp ___ Locked ___	12 Box # ___ Temp ___ Locked ___	13 Box # ___ Temp ___ Locked ___	14 Box # ___ Temp ___ Locked ___
15 Box # ___ Temp ___ Locked ___ Signature(s) ___	16 Box # ___ Temp ___ Locked ___	17 Box # ___ Temp ___ Locked ___	18 Box # ___ Temp ___ Locked ___	19 Box # ___ Temp ___ Locked ___	20 Box # ___ Temp ___ Locked ___	21 Box # ___ Temp ___ Locked ___
22 Box # ___ Temp ___ Locked ___ Signature(s) ___	23 Box # ___ Temp ___ Locked ___	24 Box # ___ Temp ___ Locked ___	25 Box # ___ Temp ___ Locked ___	26 Box # ___ Temp ___ Locked ___	27 Box # ___ Temp ___ Locked ___	28 Box # ___ Temp ___ Locked ___

Fixed-wing Pediatric Transport Supplies

Intubation kit

ET tubes: uncuffed, 2.5–4.0; cuffed, 4.0–8.0) .... 2 each
Pediatric McGill forceps
Laryngoscope handle
Straight laryngoscope blades (eg, Miller): No. 0, 1, 2, and 3
Curved laryngoscope blades (eg, Macintosh): No. 2 and 3
Stylets, pediatric and adult
Wound tape (eg, Elastoplast)
Adhesive (eg, Mastisol) and adhesive
    remover (eg, Detachol) .... 2 each
Xylocaine jelly
Trach tape
Spare bulbs
10-mL syringe
Oral airways... 6
Stethoscope
Pediatric nonrebreathing oxygen mask
Oxygen cannulas: infant and pediatric
Clear pediatric oxygen masks: infant, child, small
    youth, and small adult 4
0.5-L Pediatric anesthesia bag
1-L Pediatric anesthesia bag
Neonatal ETCO$_2$ adapter (for ET tube < 4.0)
Esophageal indicator detector (eg, EID bulb)

Cricoid kit

14-gauge intravenous catheter (eg, Angiocath) 1
Oxygen tubing with Y adapter
Alcohol and Betadine
10-mL Syringe
Instructions
Sterile gloves: sizes 6.5 and 7.5

Pediatric aerosol set with

Multidose nebulizer
"Cloudy step-down" adapter
T piece, 22 ID and 22 OD

6" Blue corrugated tubing
Pediatric aerosol mask
72" Oxygen connecting tubing
Albuterol bullets 9
Ipratropium bromide (eg, Atrovent) bullets 3
Racemic epinephrine packets 2
Isotonic saline bullets 4
Oxygen nipple adapter
Dosage card

IV Supplies
60-mL Luer-Lok syringe 1
Microdrip full sets 2
Microdrip half set 1
Dial-a-flows 2
Blood filter 1
Y blood sets (without vent) 1
3-way stopcocks 2
Dispensing pins 2
Pressure bags 2
22-gauge and 24-gauge Angiocaths .... 5 each
20-gauge Angiocaths 4
14-, 16-, and 18-gauge Angiocaths .... 2 each
Transilluminator (eg, Wee Sight) 1
15-gauge IO needles 2
3-mL syringes 2
T connectors 2
Gloves .... 2 pairs
Tourniquets: pediatric and adult
30-mL isotonic saline vial 1
Heparin lock flush vial 1
1" Clear tape with cotton balls
Clear dressings (eg, Tegaderm) 2
Adhesive (eg, Mastisol) and adhesive
    remover (eg, Detachol) .... 2 each
Alcohol and antiseptic (eg, Betadine) pads
Spinal needles (20 gauge and 22 gauge, 3")
Subdural instructions

Miscellaneous supplies

BP cuffs: No. 4 infant, child, small adult, and adult 5
Digital thermometer
Anderson tubes with clear dressing (eg, Tegaderm), and
    water-soluble lubricant (eg, KY Jelly): 10F and 16F 2
60-mL catheter-tip syringe
Foley catheters: 6F and 8F
Baby hat, pacifier, and bulb syringe
Ladder splint
Arm boards: neonatal, infant, pediatric, and large
Nonsterile gloves .... 2 pairs
Syringes: one 30 mL and 2 each 10 mL, 3 mL, and 1 mL
Glucometer and supplies
    Lancets
    Test strips
    High and low control solutions
    Alcohol pads
    Cotton balls
    Laboratory QA sheet

Fixed-wing Pediatric Supplies Bag

Chest tube pouch
    Chest tubes (12F, 16F, 20F, and 28F)
    Chest evaluation (eg, Heimlich) valves 2
    CT instrument kit
    Scalpels, No. 10 2
    Petroleum gauze (eg, Vaseline gauze) 2
    Antiseptic (eg, Betadine) swabs .... 2 packages
    Sterile gloves: sizes 6.5 and 7.5
    2-0 Silk suture
    Vial 1% lidocaine 1
    Elastoplast tape 1
Laryngeal mask airway pouch
    LMA sizes 1.0–5.0 .... 1 each
    30-mL Syringe and water-soluble lubricant (eg, KY Jelly)

██

Suction pouch

    Suction catheters: 5/6, 8, 10, and 14 .... 1 each

    Yankauer suction catheter

    Straight connector

    Isotonic saline bullets.. 4

    Self-inflating anesthesia bag with adult mask

Large drug bag

Heat pack

Transport manual and protocols

Cervical collars: sizes P-1, P-2, and P-3

    eg, NecLoc NL-300E, small; NecLoc NL-300E, medium

Pressure cables; 1 only in ground ALS bag 2

Transducers 2

Temperature probe.. 1

Temperature cable... 1

"C" batteries... 2

Towels... 2

Underpads (eg, Chux) 2

Clipboard

    Chart page 1 2

    Chart page 2 2

    Consent for transport 2

    QI report 2

    Map 2

    Emergency release of blood 2

    Ventilator sheet and e-tank information............................ 1

    Diabetic ketoacidosis chart

    Burn estimate and diagram

    Medication list

IO indicates intraosseous; ECG, electrocardiogram; BP, blood pressure; ET, endotracheal; NG, nasogastric; IV, intravenous; NCPAP, neonatal continuous positive airway pressure; CT, chest tube; ETco2, end-tidal carbon dioxide; AED, automatic external defibrillator; D, dextrose; W, water; ID, inner diameter; OD, outer diameter; QA, quality assurance; and QI, quality improvement.

Sample Neonatal and Pediatric Critical Care Respiratory Transport Supplies*

Alcohol wipes, 10
Centimeter measuring tape, 1
CPAP prongs: extra small, small, and large, 1 ea
Transport ventilator flow sensor, 1
Adhesive remover (Detachol), 2; Adhesive (Mastisol), 2;
    wound dressing (Replicare), 2
Endotracheal tubes: No. 2.0, 2.5, 3.0, 3.5, and 4.0 mm ID, 2 ea
Infant and pediatric laryngeal mask airways
ETT-NTT taping kit
Water-soluble lubricant, 3
Humid vents, 2
Infant stylet, 2
In-line suction catheters, 5/6.5F, blue, 1
Laryngoscope set (AA size) and laryngoscope (Miller) blades
    No. 0 and 1
Laryngoscope light bulb and batteries (2 size AA)
Multiaccess catheter for surfactant installation, 5F, No.4.0 adapter, 1
Multiaccess catheter, 5F, No.2.5, 3.0, and 3.5 adapters, 1 ea
Miscellaneous connectors and adapters: 15/22 mm, 22/22 mm,
    No. 8 Fortlite, 2; No. 6 Fortlite, 1
2" plastic tubing (Tygon) with 15-mm OD end
ETT holder, 1
Nonsterile gauze pads, 4 × 4, 5
Isotonic (normal) saline unit-dose vials, 8
Oxygen nasal cannula, infant, 1
CO_2 detector, 1

*CPAP indicates continuous positive airway pressure; ea, each; ID, inner diameter;
    ETT, endotracheal tube; NTT, nasotracheal tube; OD, outer diameter; ETco2, end-tidal
    carbon dioxide; and ECG, electrocardiogram.

ETco$_2$ sensors, 2
Scissors, 1
Suction catheters, 5F/6F, 2; 8F, 2; and 10F, 2
Tape, 1 roll
Tonsil tip suction, 1 infant size
Temperature port plug, 1
Umbilical clamp cutter, 1
ETT stabilizer(s)

Hardware and Cables Bag

E-Cylinder wrenches
Box end, 1
Socket type, 1
E-Cylinder washers, 4
Oxygen and air high-pressure quick connects
Isolette quick connects (round)
Medical air and oxygen quick connects (rectangular)
Point-of-care cartridges: No. 3 and No. 6, 3 ea
Hand sanitizer bottle
Calculator

Inside incubator

0.5-L Anesthesia bag
Blood pressure cuff
ECG leads
Infant and preemie resuscitation masks
Patient thermometer
Pulse oximeter sensor
Stethoscope

Lower incubator storage area

Stethoscope, 1
0.5-L Anesthesia bag, 1
Bubble tubing (4 lengths) and pressure "T," 1
Infant self-inflating resuscitation bags, 250 mL and 500 mL
Minispacer, 6" corrugated tube, 15 mm/22 mm adapter

CO_2 detector, 1
Instant camera

Assembled ventilator circuit bag

30" Extension set
30-mL Sterile water bottle
30-mL Syringe
Assembled ventilator circuit
Bubble tubing (4 lengths) and pressure T
Humidifier mounting bracket
Humidifier

Policies and Procedures

Outline

- Introduction and recommended policies
  - General policies, guidelines, and information
  - Safety and travel policies
  - Communication policies
  - Documentation policies
  - Human resources policies
  - Medical protocols and policies
- Policy examples
  - Stabilization of the unrepaired meningomyelocele lesion
  - Infant ground transport team intubation training
  - Infant ground transport nurse/respiratory therapist skills competency
  - Emergency lights and siren use during transport
  - Guidelines for selection of mode of transport

Policies and protocols are recommended for neonatal-pediatric transport teams. The following list is not exclusive or all inclusive of policies needed for any particular neonatal or pediatric transport team. Neonatal-pediatric transport teams should consider federal, state, and local regulations and current hospital policies when determining the additional policies needed.

General Policies, Guidelines, and Information

- Organizational chart
- Mission, vision, and value statements
- Scope of care
- Definition of line of authority for transport team members and contracted ground and air teams
- Press-release policy

- Confidentiality and security of patient care records, meeting minutes, and policies and procedures

Safety and Travel Policies

- Age parameters of patients to be transported
- Dress code
- Hearing protection, when appropriate for patient and/or team
- Seat belts and shoulder harnesses for patient and team
- Transport of twins and/or dual patient transport
- Helmet use by ground and/or air transport team personnel
- Interior modification of transport vehicles
- When to use alternative (backup) vehicles
- How to choose mode of transport (eg, ground, air, type of aircraft)
- Weight restrictions, density altitude (aircraft-related)
- Physical examinations and performance standards for weight, height, and lifting appropriate for service
- Annual tuberculosis testing
- Policy requiring immunization history (eg, tetanus, hepatitis B, measles, mumps, rubella)
- International transport policy, when appropriate
- International immunization history, when appropriate
- Passport requirements, when appropriate
- Use of medications (prescription and over-the-counter)
- Use indications and allowances for nonstandard personnel
- Minimum personnel configurations
- Medical control identification and backup
- Appropriate loading and unloading of patients
- Weight limit for each isolette and transport stretcher
- Refusal to transport patients (combative patient or family member)
- Screening family belongings for potential weapons or hazardous materials before flight
- Sharps disposal and disposal containers
- Securing equipment in transport vehicle
- Restraints, physical and chemical
- Cleaning and disinfecting transport vehicles, equipment, instruments, and uniforms

- Standard precautions and special precautions for identified or suspected infectious patients
- Infection control
- Process for identifying people at risk for exposure to infectious disease and communicating exposure to all affected personnel
- Occupational Safety and Health Administration (OSHA) exposure control plan for bloodborne pathogens and tuberculosis
- Hazardous materials
- Risk management
- Refueling (eg, with no patient on board, no crew members on board)
- Emergency procedures, method of exiting transport vehicle in a catastrophic event
- Emergency plan including the following:
  - List of personnel to be notified and order of notification
  - Communication with aircraft or ambulance
  - Process to initiate search and rescue
  - Plan to transport patient in case of an incident
  - Timeframe to activate emergency plan
  - Method of information dissemination and press release to ensure accuracy of information
  - Annual drill of emergency preparedness
- Policy stating the program will follow all Federal Aviation Regulations and Federal Communications Commission regulations
- Policy stating compliance with the Consolidated Omnibus Budget Reconciliation Act of 1986 (COBRA) and Emergency Medical Treatment and Active Labor Act (EMTALA) regulations
- Criteria and procedure for using lights and sirens
- Criteria for speed limitations
- Policy addressing security of aircraft and ambulance transport vehicles when unattended
- When nitric oxide or other inhaled gases are used, policies addressing:
  - Cylinder safety, monitoring, transportation regulations, weight, mounting, delivery of drug, emergency procedures, and occupational exposure
- Process for conditions causing delay of transport team (eg, weather, traffic, mechanical breakdown, deterioration in patient's condition)

Communication Policies

- Request for transport
- Identify authorized requestors, including "without discrimination" clause
- Process for admitting the patient, if applicable
- Process for monitoring transport (eg, time of departure, arrival, locations, and any necessary changes)
- Diversion criteria
- Weather and launch protocols
- Outline of location, distance, preferred transport arrangements, capabilities, and resources of receiving facility or facilities
- Cellular phone use
- Guidelines for timely notification of team for request for transport

Documentation Policies

- Record of patient care
  - Minimally including purpose of transport, treatments, medications, and patient's response to treatments and medications; transport facilities (referring and receiving hospitals); and who is receiving report

Human Resources Policies

- Disciplinary policies
- Written code of conduct
- Scheduling policies (addresses duty time to ensure adequate rest)
- Wellness programs (eg, smoking cessation, weight control)
- Preemployment and annual physical examinations or medical screening that includes history of chronic or acute illnesses and illnesses requiring use of medications that may cause drowsiness or affect judgment and coordination
- Duty status during pregnancy
- Duty status during acute illness
- Duty status while taking medication that may cause drowsiness
- Job requirements (education, training, licensing, experience level)
- Continuing education requirements

- Background checks of personnel and personnel carrying photo identification at all times
- Hours worked by transport personnel with minimum rest and duty times

Medical Protocols and Policies

- Diseases and injuries transported as dictated by scope of team mission (eg, neonatal diseases for neonatal teams, common injuries encountered when transporting to pediatric trauma center)
- Diseases affected by altitude as appropriate for flight teams
- Specification of certain specialty patients requiring prompt consultation
- Preparation for transport (eg, staff, equipment, supplies)
- Stating transfer of care is to higher level of care

Policy Examples

Examples of policies are provided and serve as examples of ways to write a policy. These are examples of policies used by established transport services and are not meant to be used as verbatum templates or specific standards of care. Individual hospital policies and procedures and team composition must be considered when drafting policies for each individual neonatal-pediatric transport team.

Stabilization of the Unrepaired Meningomyelocele Lesion*

I. Policy
    A. Transport and pre-operative stabilization of a meningomyelocele lesion will be done in a safe and consistent manner.
II. Purpose
    A. To protect an intact or ruptured lesion from sources of infection including airborne organisms and meconium, and reduce risk of mechanical trauma and drying out.
III. Procedure
    A. The lesion will be dressed using sterile technique (**NON-LATEX gloves** and mask) at time of delivery or by Transport Team.

---

*Used with permission: Patti Jason, BSN, CCRN. Children's Hospital and Regional Medical Center

■■■■■■■■■■■■■■■■■■■■■■■■■■■■■■■■

Meningomyelocele Dressing Supplies

2 rolls 2-¼" Kerlix (or pre-packaged
   sterilized Kerlix "donut" dressing)
1 2x3" Telfa dressing
1 2x2" occlusive dressing (Tegaderm)
6" strip #6 Bandnet dressing
Sterile scissors

1 8Fr feeding tube
1 5 mL syringe
5 mL sterile normal
  saline
1 steri drape
1 sterile towel

B. Using sterile technique, place supplies on open sterile towel.
If pre-packaged sterilized Kerlix "donut" dressing is unavailable,
unroll the 2-¼" roll of Kerlix, shaping it into a "donut," ensuring
the center hole will surround the lesion. Cut a 24" strip of
Kerlix and reinforce the donut shape.

C. Attach feeding tube to the Telfa using small occlusive dressing.
Draw 5 mL of normal saline into syringe, attach to feeding tube,
moisten Telfa pad with entire 5 mL of saline.

D. Place moistened Telfa pad over lesion.

E. Place "donut" on the skin surrounding the lesion to prevent
pressure on the protruding sac.

F. Cover dressing with a 4x4" piece of steri drape.

G. Secure entire "donut" and occlusive dressing using a 6" piece
of #6 Bandnet around infant's midsection.

H. Cut and apply steri drape as far caudal to the sac as possible,
but cephalad to the anus to keep expelled meconium from
irritating lesion.

I. Keep sterile dressing moist every 2 hours with 3-5 mL sterile
saline via feeding tube port.

J. No sterile linens are needed in isolette, but sterile **NON-LATEX
gloves** will be worn when handling the infant and lesion.

K. Cultures and antibiotic administration are not indicated unless
sepsis is suspected. (Surface culture of the lesion will be
obtained at Children's; vancomycin and gentamicin will be
given immediately pre-operatively.)

L. Infant will be kept in the prone position at all times during care.
During transport the patient seatbelts will be fastened at the
level of the axilla and thighs. Inpatient, immobilize the patient
as necessary, using supportive positioning.

M. Minimize latex exposure by using non-latex pacifier and supplies.

Infant Ground Transport Team Intubation Training*

I. **Purpose**

  A. Review and practice airway management skills with a focus on developing infant intubation skills for transport personnel.

II. **Policy**

  A. Intubation training proficiency will be based on completion of the requirements listed below. Medical control will provide oversight if intubation is necessary during transport.

III. **Intubation Training Requirements** *will include a literature review and "hands-on" practice with the following resources:*

  A. Literature Review & Written Test

  B. NRP Certification

  C. Ferret Lab & Case Scenario Review training sessions (4/year),

  1. Mega Code with SIM Baby. (2/year).

  D. Neonatal ICU Intubation Practice with medical oversight.

  E. OR Intubation Practice with medical oversight.

IV. **Intubation Procedure**

  A. Intubation guidelines will be followed in accordance with AHA-AAP NRP Manual; Lesson 5 (comprehensive format); LANG, 5th Ed., chapter 20 (concise format).

V. **Equipment Selection and Function Check**

  A. Select the correct size endotracheal tube:

  1.

Infant Size Kg	Gestation	ETT Size	Depth of Insertion
< 1000	< 28 wks	2.5 mm	6.5–7 cm
1000–2000 kg	28–34 wks	3.0 mm	7–8 cm
2000–3000 kg	34–38 wks	3.5 mm	8–9 cm
> 3000 kg	> 38 wks	3.5–4.0 mm	9–10 cm

  *Optional: cut ETT to 15cm mark and re-attach 15mm ETT adapter.
  *If used, position proximal end of stylet just short of Murphy hole.

  B. Select the correct laryngoscope blade and connect to the laryngoscope handle; ensure that the laryngoscope light is on and bright.

  1. Miller blades are preferred for infant sizes listed below:
  #0 < 3 kg   #1 > 3 kg

  C. Check that the Manual Resuscitation Bag and Mask is functional and capable of 100% oxygen administration.

*Used with permission: Patti Jason, BSN, CCRN. Children's Hospital and Regional Medical Center

D. Check wall suction function and set vacuum to 100 mmHg.
   1. Ensure that a tonsil tip suction catheter is well connected.
   2. Prepare tape and securing devices prior to intubation.
   3. Have an $ETCO_2$ adapter available for confirmation of intubation.
E. Ensure that the infant is connected to a cardiorespiratory monitor including SpO_2 with an audible pulse indicator and continuous blood pressure monitoring.
F. Locate ready to use and functional equipment within reach, next to the right side of the patient's head.
G. Call a "Time Out" to review the patient and procedure (CHRMC Clinical Policy/Procedure U—Universal Protocol for Ensuring Correct Patient, Correct Site and Correct Surgery or Procedure)
H. The RN will provide sedation and or paralysis if rapid sequence intubation is recommended by medical control. (CHRMC Clinical Policy/Procedure: S— Sedation With or Without Analgesia for Procedures).
I. Position the infant in the sniffing position (slightly extended).
J. Preoxygenate and assist ventilation with bag and mask as needed.
K. Suction infant's oral pharynx; suction residual gastric contents if suspected.
L. Monitor the infants HR, color and oxygen saturation.
M. Proceed with intubation by holding the laryngoscope handle in the left hand, inserting the blade into the right corner of the infant's mouth and sweeping the tongue toward the left side.
   1. Advance the blade a few centimeters, passing it anterior to the epiglottis (in the vallecula). Lift the blade vertically to elevate the epiglottis and visualize the glottis.
   2. To better visualize the vocal cords, have an assistant apply gentle pressure to the cricoid cartilage.
   3. With visualization of the vocal cords, insert the ETT tip approximately 2 cm past the cords.
      a. By holding the ETT tube at the location of the "insertion depth at the lips" while advancing the ETT through the cords, main stem intubation can be minimized.

N. Hold the ETT securely in place, remove the stylet and attach the $ETCO_2$ indicator:

1. Manually ventilate the patient and note the following responses to confirm tracheal intubation.
   a. Chest rise
   b, Bilateral breath sounds (absent insufflation sounds over epigastric area).
   c. Positive presence of $ETCO_2$ after 6–8 breaths.
   d. Positive presence of condensate within the ETT with manual breaths.
   e. Stable and/or improving vital signs.

O. Order a chest x-ray to confirm the proper ETT position (T2).

P. Secure the endotracheal tube according to guidelines: (CHRMC/RC P&P; Endo-or Nasotracheal Tube Care, pgs 45–47).

Q. Document the results of the intubation process, including failed attempts.

1. In the patient chart, document the ETT size and depth of insertion.
2. Note any complications or airway anomalies:
   a. Bleeding, inflammation; relative difficulty.
   b. Extreme anterior displacement of larynx, macroglossia, cleft palate, etc.
3. For the training proficiency record, successful and attempted intubations must be documented and placed in the transport file with the trainee's name, medical supervisor's name and patient's medical record number.
   a. Provide a date and time of the training intubation, the patient's weight, airway information (size, insertion depth), medication use specific to the procedure and a brief note describing the training session.

R. Intubation Practice in the Neonatal Intensive Care Unit at CHRMC

1. At the beginning of the shift, the Transport RCP or RN should let the neonatology attending know that they are available and in need of intubation practice for Transport Intubation Training.

a. A list of Transport Specialists requiring intubation practice in the NICU will be made available to the neonatal attending.

b. Didactic training, including literature reviews, ferret labs and infant mega-code attendance must be current.

S. The NICU Attending, Fellow or NNP will provide direct supervision on all intubations performed by the Infant Ground Transport team members.

1. Intubation procedures are to be reviewed prior to intubation.

2. An essential equipment inventory and function check is required.

3. Equipment and personnel must be located in an appropriate position relative to the patient prior to intubation.

4. A review of the intubation procedure will be discussed with the supervising provider, including the anticipated sequence of sedative and/or paralytic medications, and the effect on airway control.

5. During the intubation process, the practitioner in-training must verbalize anatomical landmarks (i.e., glottis, cords, etc.) and the details of the intubation process when performing training intubations.

T. Verbal critique by the attending/supervisor during the intubation process to include ongoing feedback with regard to technique and patient's condition.

U. Training intubations will be limited to 3 attempts per patient (or less if not well tolerated), at which time the supervising neonatologist, fellow, or NNP will perform the intubation.

V. Exclusion Criteria for Training Intubations include:

1. Patient is hemodynamically unstable,

2. Patients with difficult airways, typically requiring advanced skills to achieve intubation with minimal complications:

W. Special Consideration for Rapid Sequence Intubation on during transport would require oversight by Medical Control in administering Sedation and Paralysis.

1. The Transport RN will verify, draw up and administer intubation medications.

a. Refer to: CHRMC Clinical Policy/Procedure: **S**— Sedation With or Without Analgesia for Procedures; CHRMC Emergency Department Policy and Procedure Manual—ED Management of Patients with Upper airway Compromise.

b. The Transport RN and RCP will be trained in the onset, duration and possible side effects of the specific medications used for sedation and analgesia.

c. Airway and ventilation control must be demonstrated prior to elective pharmacologic neuromuscular control.

Infant Ground Transport Nurse/Respiratory Therapist Skills Competency*

I. *Purpose*

A. To establish guidelines for completion of yearly transport skills competency checklist.

II. *Procedure*

A. The transport nurse/respiratory therapist will complete an equipment checklist at the annual skills competency lab.

B. Staff will orally review and demonstrate back the skills required to operate the transport incubator and equipment according to the guidelines outlined in the annual competency review form.

C. A transport skills competency form is to be completed and signed by the Transport RN /RRT and filed in his/her personnel folder.

D. The yearly evaluation will include the following information:

1. Annual ICU RN/RRT competency skills summary sheet indicating transport hire date

2. Required ICU and Respiratory Care Department annual competency records completed in home department personnel file (ASC—Level III completed)

3. "Staff Initialed" copy of Infant Ground Transport RN or RRT Work Content Description

4. Biannual CPR, NRP certification

5. Transport Skills lab attendance date

6. Transport i-STAT competency

7. Transport equipment checklist

*Used with permission: Patti Jason, BSN, CCRN. Children's Hospital and Regional Medical Center

Emergency Lights and Siren Use During Transport*

I. *Policy Statement*
   A. Emergency lights and sirens will be used only in critical situations when ordered by the medical control physician.
II. *Supportive Data*
   A. The transport nurse or transport respiratory therapist will request an order from the medical control physician for use of emergency lights and sirens.
   B. The emergency medical technician (EMT) will be notified of the request.
   C. If possible, the family will be informed of emergency lights and sirens use. A parent or guardian may not ride on any transports ordered at departure to run with emergency lights and sirens.
   D. During emergency operation, the vehicle shall not exceed 10 mph over the posted speed limit. On Interstate highways, the maximum speed limit is 75 mph. All school zone speed limits must be adhered to at all times. Vehicle operators are required to drive at a speed that is safest for existing road and weather conditions, regardless of the posted speed limit.
III. *Documentation*
   A. The order for lights and sirens will be documented in the transport physician's orders. Use will also be documented in the transport notes.

Guidelines for Selection of Mode of Transport*

I. *Policy Statement*
   A. In selecting the mode of transport, the following criteria will be considered: referring physician's diagnosis, reported clinical condition of the patient, type and location of the referring health care facility, resources available at the referring health care facility, weather conditions, vehicle availability, personnel availability, personnel capabilities, road and traffic conditions, and time of day. Although selection of the most appropriate transport mode is the responsibility of the referring physician,

*Used with permission: All Children's Hospital, St. Petersburg, Flordia.

the transport medical control physician will ensure appropriateness of use of transport vehicles, personnel, and resources.

B. Responsibilities
1. Referring physician: Stabilizing the patient's condition and selecting the most appropriate mode of transport
2. Accepting physician: Notifying the transport team of requests for transport and, when known, specifying the mode of transport request
3. Transport nurse:
   a. Gathering demographic, vital sign, laboratory, and treatment data from the referring institution
   b. Assessing transport team availability for individual transport requests and communicating patient and team availability data to the medical control physician
   c. Communication of transport request denials or delays to the referring, accepting, and medical control physicians
4. Medical control physician:
   a. Ensuring appropriateness of use of transport team personnel and facilities for each transport request, given available referring physician's diagnosis, reported clinical condition of the patient, type and location of the referring health care facility, resources available at the referring health care facility, weather conditions,* vehicle availability, personnel availability, personnel capabilities, road and traffic conditions, and time of day, as well as other ongoing system demands
   b. Approving dispatch of each transport team before departure
   c. Assessing readiness for return according to given transport team's verbal report, available laboratory and treatment data, type and location of the referring health care facility, resources available at the referring health care facility, resources available in transit, resources available at receiving facility, weather conditions, vehicle type, personnel capabilities, road and traffic conditions, and time of day

---

*The pilot and driver will determine vehicle response based on weather.

d. Providing telephone advice for in-transit changes in patient condition

e. For neonates being transported to the neonatal intensive care unit, the medical control physician is the neonatologist on call. For any other patient being transported to any other area, the medical control physician is the pediatric intensivist on call.

II. *Supportive Data*

A. Ground transport

1. Ground transport should be used at the discretion of the referring physician with the approval of the medical control physician.

2. Patients transported by ground transport are generally in stable condition, may or may not require ongoing therapy, need basic or advanced monitoring, and may have little to high likelihood of deterioration in the condition in transit.

3. Ground transports beyond a 150-mile radius require approval of the transport program director.

B. Helicopter transport

1. Helicopter transport should be used at the discretion of the referring physician with the approval of the medical control physician.

2. Patients transported by helicopter transport are in potentially or actually unstable condition, may or may not require ongoing therapy, need advanced monitoring, and have a moderate to high likelihood of deterioration of their conditions in transit. The patient may meet one or more of the following criteria:

a) Neonate less than or equal to 28 days and/or less than 5 kg

b) Admission to an intensive care unit or emergency department

c) Intubated or requiring ongoing respiratory support

d) Cardiovascular instability

e) Neurological instability

   f) Unstable surgical or traumatic condition
   g) Any life- or limb-threatening condition
3. Referring hospital located more than 60 miles from receiving facility and meets all of the following criteria (flight for distance):
   a) Respiratory, cardiovascular, or neurologic dysfunction
   b) Period of high transport team or system demand
   c) Referring, accepting, and medical control physicians agree
   d) Parent or guardian consents
4. Helicopter transports beyond a 200-mile radius of Children's Hospital require approval of the transport program director.

C. Fixed-wing Transport
1. The use of a fixed-wing aircraft will be considered for transports beyond a 150-mile radius of the receiving facility.
2. Fixed-wing vendor selection will be based on Medicaid or insurance approval, aircraft availability, cost, vendor license, and safety record.
3. The type of aircraft selected will be based on diagnosis, distance, cost, aircraft availability, and amount and type of equipment required.
4. All fixed-wing transports require approval of the transport program director and administrator on call.
5. Parents and guardians will be notified of the mode of transport and, when applicable, will be included in the decision-making process.
6. One parent or legal guardian of the patient being transported may ride in the driver's compartment of the ground ambulance with approval of the transport team.
7. Parents or guardians may not ride in the helicopter owing to space and weight limitations.
8. Parents and guardians of the patient being transported may ride in the fixed-wing aircraft with the approval of the transport team, depending on the aircraft size and space limitations.

Selected Readings

American Heart Association and American Academy of Pediatrics. *Neonatal Resuscitation Program (NRP) Manual.* 4th ed. Dallas, TX and Elk Grove Village, IL: American Heart Association/American Academy of Pediatrics; 2000

Bishop MJ. Who Should Perform Intubations? *Respir Care.* 1999;44:750–755

Cochrane D, Aronyk K, Sawatzky B, Wilson D, Steinbok P. The effects of labor and delivery on spinal cord function and ambulation in patients with meningomyelocele. *Child Nervous System.* 1991;7:312–315

Commission on Accreditation of Medical Transport Systems. *Accreditation Standards.* 5th ed. Sandy Springs, SC: CAMTS; 2002

Cragan, Roberts HE, Edmonds LD, et al. Surveillance for ancephaly and spina bifida and the impact of prenatal diagnosis—United States 1985–1994. *MMWR CDC Surveill Summ.* 1995;44:1–13

Gomella TL. *LANGE Clinical Manual.* 5th ed. 2004;172–173

Gomella TL. *LANGE Clinical Manual.* 5th ed. 2004;595, 604, 608, 616, 622, 627

Hess DR. Indications for Translaryngeal Intubations. *Respir Care.* 1999;44:604–609

Hogge WA, Dungan JS, Brooks MP, et al. Diagnosis and management of prenatally detected myelomeningocele: a preliminary report. *Am J Obstet Gynecol.* 1990;163:1061–1065

Hurford WE. Orotracheal Intubation Outside the operating room: anatomic considerations and techniques. *Respir Care.* 1999;44:615–626

Luthy DA, Wardinsky T, Shurtleff DB, et al. Cesarean section before onset of labor and subsequent motor function in infants with meningomyelocele diagnosed antenatally. *New Engl J Med.* 1991;234:662–666

MacDonald MG. Umbilical artery catheterization. In: MacDonald MG, Fletcher MA, eds. *Atlas of Procedures in Neonatology.* 2nd ed. Philadelphia, PA: JB Lippincott Co; 1993:155–174

MacDonald M. Umbilical vein catheterization. In: MacDonald MG, Fletcher MA, eds. *Atlas of Procedures in Neonatology.* Philadelphia, PA: JB Lippincott Co; 1993:178–187

McEnery G, et al. The spinal cord in neurologically stable spina bifida: a clinical and MRI study. *Dev Med Child Neurol.* 1992;34:342–347

Shurtleff DA, Lemire RJ. Epidemiology, etiologic factors, and prenatal diagnosis of open spinal dysraphism. In: Pand D, ed. *Neurosurgery Clinics of North America.* Philadelphia, PA: WB Saunders Co; 1995:183–193

Shutleff DB, Luthy DA, Nyberg DA, Benedetti TJ, Mack LA. Meningomyelocele: management in utero and post natum. *Ciba Found Symp.* 1994;181:270–280

Thompson AE. Issues in airway management in infants and children. *Respir Care.* 1999;44:650–658

Tung BJ. The pediatric rescue airway. *Air Med J.* 2005;24/2:55–58

Watson CB. Prediction of a difficult intubation: methods for successful intubation. *Respir Care.* 1999;44:777–796

■ Transport Resources* ■

This appendix is divided into several sections on transport resources: The first section contains a listing of various organizations and Web sites offering information and educational opportunities on critical care and transport; the second contains information on journals that have published transport-related articles; the third section lists various training courses available that have served as training opportunities, documentation of skill level, or review opportunities for transport team members; the fourth section is a listing of programs offering ground, rotor-, and/or fixed-wing transport on a national and international level. Each of these sections has been reviewed extensively but will not be inclusive as new programs become available and existing programs merge or change their focus. Listing in these sections should not be interpreted as a recommendation or endorsement by the authors or the American Academy of Pediatrics.

1. **Transport Organizations and Web Sites**

   Aerospace Medical Association: This organization represents the fields of aviation, space, and environmental medicine. Its membership includes aerospace medicine specialists, scientists, flight nurses, physiologists, and researchers in the field. Most are with industry, the Federal Aviation Administration, National Aeronautics and Space Administration, Department of Defense, and universities. Approximately 25% of the membership is international. The organization publishes a monthly peer-reviewed journal entitled *Aviation, Space and Environmental Medicine*. It offers a yearly meeting to review information and latest research in the field of aviation medicine.

---

*EMS indicates emergency medical services.

ASMA
320 S Henry St
Alexandria, VA 22314-3579

Phone: (703) 739-2240
Fax: (703) 739-9652
http://www.asma.org

Air and Surface Transport Nurses Association: This nursing organization is composed of hospital-based, public service, military, and private providers of emergency and nonemergency patient air and ground transport. The majority of its members are employed by transport programs. Affiliate members, such as respiratory therapists, paramedics, pilots, aircraft vendors and operators, may also belong to the association. Its Web site offers specific information on air and ground transport. The organization publishes transport manuals and offers specific educational courses.

ASTNA
ASTNA National Office
9101 E Kenyon Ave
Suite 3000
Denver, CO 80237

Phone: (800) 897-6362
Fax: (303) 770-1812
http://www.astna.org

Air Medical Physician Association: This association seeks to attract physicians with an interest in air medical transport. Its mission is to offer opportunities to collectively study the impact of air transport on patients and to share expertise so that patients may receive the best care possible in the safest operating environment. Its Web site offers specific information on air transport and has links to the organization's published manual and membership list. Continuing medical education conferences are held yearly.

AMPA
383 F St
Salt Lake City, UT 84103

Phone: (801) 534-0829
Fax: (801) 534-0434
http://www.ampa.org

Air Medical Safety Advisory Council: Internet-based access to a variety of helicopter safety and accident information is provided.

http://www.amsac.org
http://www.safecopter.arc.nasa.gov

American Academy of Pediatrics, Section on Transport Medicine: The section facilitates interactions between members involved in pediatric interfacility transport for the purpose of improving care of infants, children, and adolescents who require transport. Membership is open to physician members of the American Academy of Pediatrics (AAP) and approved nonphysician Section affiliates who are actively involved in the study or practice of pediatric or neonatal transport. The section offers a biannual conference on transport medicine, and its Web site offers helpful links to other transport resources. It also publishes a transport newsletter and Guidelines for Air and Ground Transport of Neonatal and Pediatric Patients. A transport listserv is available through the section's Web site.

AAP—Section on Transport Medicine
National Headquarters
141 Northwest Point Blvd
Elk Grove Village, IL 60007-1098

Phone: (847) 434-4000
Fax: (847) 434-8000
http://www.aap.org/sections/transmed/

American Ambulance Association: This organization promotes health care policies that ensure excellence in the ambulance services industry and provides research, education, and communications programs to enable its members to effectively address the needs of the communities they serve. The Web site offers membership information, specifics on political legislation involved in ground transportation, and educational opportunities.

AAA

8201 Greensboro Dr
Suite 300
McLean, VA 22102

Phone: (703) 610-9018
        (800) 523-4447
Fax: (703) 610-9005
http://www.the-aaa.org

American Association of Critical-Care Nurses: A specialty nursing organization serving the needs of critical care nurses, AACN defines critical care nursing as that specialty within nursing that deals with human responses to life-threatening health problems. Its Web site offers specific information on educational opportunities, and its organization helps to publish 2 journals, the *American Journal of Critical Care* and *Critical Care Nurse.*

AACN
101 Columbia
Aliso Viejo, CA 92656-4109

Phone: (800) 899-2226
        (949) 362-2000
Fax: (949) 362-2020
http://www.aacn.org

American Association for Respiratory Care: This is an association for respiratory therapists with subspecialty interests including air and ground transport. Its Web site offers a variety of critical care links and educational and employment opportunities.

AARC
9425 N MacArthur Blvd
Suite 100
Irving, TX 75063-4706

Phone: (972) 243-2272
Fax: (972) 484-2720
      (972) 484-6010
http://www.aarc.org

American College of Emergency Physicians: This national organization represents emergency physicians with a number of subspecialty interests, including pediatrics and transport. Its Web site offers specific topics of interest to emergency physicians in addition to educational and employment opportunities.

ACEP

National Headquarters
1125 Executive Circle
Irving, TX 75038-2522

PO Box 619911
Dallas, TX 75261-9911

Phone: (800) 798-1822
      (972) 550-0911
Fax: (972) 580-2816
http://www.acep.org

Washington DC Office
2121 K St, NW
Suite 325
Washington, DC 20037

Phone: (800) 320-0610
      (202) 728-0610
Fax: (202) 728-0617

Association of Air Medical Services: This international association is a voluntary nonprofit organization that serves air and surface medical transport providers. It encourages and supports its members in maintaining a standard of performance reflecting safe operations and efficient, high-quality patient care. Its Web site provides specific information about the organization, a list of individual members, and an annual resource guide.

AAMS
AAMS National Office
526 King St, Suite 415
Alexandria, VA 22314-3143

Phone: (703) 836-8732
Fax: (703) 836-8920
http://www.aams.org

Atlas and Database of Air Medical Services (ADAMS): This compilation of information on air medical service providers who respond to emergency medical and trauma scenes, implemented in a geographic information system, can be accessed via its Web site.

http://www.ADAMSairmed.org

Board of Certification for Emergency Nursing: This organization certifies nurses who provide emergency services across the health care continuum, including flight nurses. Its Web site contains information on the various certifications offered and how and where they can be obtained.

BCEN
915 Lee St
Des Plaines, IL 60016

Phone: (800) 900-9659, extension 2630
        (847) 460-2630
Fax: (847) 460-2631
http://www.ena.org/bcen/
e-mail: bcen@ena.org

The Comcare Alliance: The Alliance is a coalition of organizations that includes nurses, physicians, emergency medical technicians, 911 directors, wireless companies, public safety and health officials, law enforcement groups, automobile companies, consumer organizations, telematics suppliers, safety groups, and others working to encourage the deployment of lifesaving wireless communications networks and technologies. Its Web site offers a newsletter and a list and status of its projects.

888 17th St, NW 12th Floor
Washington, DC 20006
Phone: (202) 429-0574
http://www.comcare.org

Commission on Accreditation of Medical Transport Systems: This organization supports a program of voluntary evaluation of compliance with accreditation standards for air-medical or ground interfacility transport. The Web site offers a list of accredited programs and publishes a set of accreditation standards.

CAMTS
PO Box 1305
Anderson, SC 29622

Phone: (864) 287-4177
Fax: (864) 287-4251
http://www.camts.org

Emergency Medical Services for Children: This program supports 2 resource centers—the EMSC National Resource Center (NRC), located in Washington, DC, and the National EMSC Data Analysis Resource Center (NEDARC), located in Salt Lake City, UT. NRC provides support and assistance to states on a variety of topics, operates a clearinghouse, and provides information to professionals and the public. NEDARC specializes in providing assistance on data collection and analysis. The Web site provides links to various EMS programs and offers updates on research and legislation before congress.

EMSC

EMSC National Resource Center
111 Michigan Ave, NW
Washington, DC 20010

Phone: (202) 884-4927
Fax: (202) 884-6845
http://www.ems-c.org

National EMSC Data Analysis
   Resource Center
(NEDARC)
University of Utah
615 Arapeen Dr, Suite 202
Salt Lake City, UT 84108

Phone: (801) 581-6410
Fax: (801) 581-8686
http://www.ems-c.org

Emergency Nurses Association: The ENA is a national association for nurses dedicated to the advancement of emergency nursing practice. Its Web site offers information on annual meetings and educational and employment opportunities. Transport interests are represented via subspecialty interest groups.

ENA
915 Lee St
Des Plaines, IL 60016-6569

Phone: (800) 900-9659
http://www.ena.org

EMS Web Site: This Web site focuses on individuals with an interest in rescue and EMS services. It offers various links to other EMS services and offers educational and employment opportunities.

http://http://www.fireemsrescue.com

Flight Nursing: This Internet resource focuses on educational opportunities specifically for flight-based nursing.

http://http://flightnursing.com

Flight Web: The primary goal of the site is to provide timely news, information, and resources. In addition, communications between the various specialties (air medical professionals around the world, including EMS pilots, flight nurses, medics, respiratory therapists, physicians, communication specialists, maintenance, administration, and others) are facilitated by hosting forums such as the Flight Med mailing list (http://www.flightweb.com/static-pages/index.php?page = flightmed).

http://www.flightweb.com

Helicopter Association International (HAI): HAI is a not-for-profit, professional trade association of 1350-plus member organizations in more than 70 nations. It is dedicated to promoting the helicopter as a safe and efficient method of transportation and to the advancement of the civil helicopter industry.

HAI
1635 Prince St
Alexandria, VA 22314

Phone: (703) 638-4646
Fax: (703) 683-4754
http://www.rotor.com

International Association of Emergency Managers (IAEM): This is an international organization whose goals are to promote the saving of lives and protection of property during emergencies and disasters. Its Web site offers lists of educational opportunities, job resources, and a list server.

IAEM
201 Park Washington Ct
Falls Church, VA 22046-4527

Phone: (703) 538-1795
Fax: (703) 241-5603
e-mail: info@iaem.com

The International Trauma Anesthesia and Critical Care Society:
Also operating under the name Trauma Care International, this nonprofit, international multidisciplinary society is dedicated to improving the care of trauma patients. Its Web site offers information on meetings, course listings, and various clinical and basic research awards. It publishes a quarterly peer-reviewed journal, and pediatric trauma is represented through a subcommittee.

ITACCS
ITACCS World Headquarters
PO Box 4826
Baltimore, MD 21211

Fax: (410) 235-8084
e-mail: info@nwas.org

National Air Transportation Association: An association of aviation business service providers, its mission is to be the leading national trade association representing the business interests of general aviation service companies on legislative and regulatory matters at the federal level. The association sponsors an annual trade show, and its Web site offers information and links to various aviation interests.

NATA
4226 King St
Alexandria, VA 22302

Phone: (800) 808-6282
        (703) 845-9000
Fax: (730) 845-8176
http://www.nata.aero

▪▪▪▪▪▪▪▪▪▪▪▪▪▪▪▪▪▪▪▪▪▪▪▪▪▪▪▪▪▪▪▪▪▪▪▪

National Association of Air Medical Communication Specialists: This organization's mission is to represent the air medical communication specialist on a national level through education, standardization, and recognition. The membership consists of active communications specialists and administrative managers. Air-medical flight programs and others associated with or interested in communications can join as associate members. Its Web site offers information on continuing education and job opportunities. The organization publishes a manual for training air-medical communications specialists.

NAACS
PO Box 28
Otis Orchards, WA 99027-0028

Phone: (877) 396-2227
http://www.naacs.org

National Association of EMS Physicians: The National Association of EMS Physicians is an organization of physicians and other professionals partnering to provide leadership and foster excellence in out-of-hospital emergency medical services. The Web site contains general and specific educational opportunities and offers annual continuing education activities.

NAEMSP
PO Box 15945-281
Lenexa, KS 66285-5945

Phone: (913) 492-5858
　　　　(800) 228-3677
Fax: (913) 599-5340
http://www.naemsp.org/
e-mail: info-naemsp@goAMP.com

National Association of Neonatal Nurses: This organization represents the community of neonatal nurses that provides evidence-based care to high-risk neonatal patients. Within the organization are special interest groups that include critical care transport. The Web site contains general and specific education opportunities and offers annual continuing education activities.

NANN
4700 W Lake Ave
Glenview, IL 60025-1485

Phone: (800) 451-3795
   (847) 375-3660
Fax: (888) 477-6266
International Fax: (732) 380-3640
http://www.nann.org

National Association of State EMS Directors: This organization supports its members by providing leadership in the development and improvement of EMS systems and national EMS policy. The organization participates in all the states and territories and acts as a resource for EMS information and policy. Its Web site offers information about itself, EMS news, educational opportunities and Web links.

NASEMSD
201 Park Washington Ct
Falls Church, VA 22046-4527

Phone: (703) 538-1799
Fax: (703) 241-5603
http://www.nasemsd.org

National EMS Pilots Association: The association serves pilots involved in emergency medical services, including helicopter and fixed-wing pilots in EMS. Its Web site offers information on job and educational opportunities. Pilot and vendor databases are available.

NEMSPA
526 King St
Suite 415
Alexandria, VA 22314-3143

Phone: (703) 836-8930
Fax: (703) 836-8920
http://www.nemspa.org

National Flight Nurses Association
Now the Air and Surface Transport Nurses Association

http://http://www.nfna.org

National Flight Paramedic Association: Members are involved in transporting critical care patients by airplane, helicopter, and ground ambulance. Most members are flight paramedics, but this is not a requirement. There are also associate memberships for anybody with an interest in the paramedical profession. The Web site offers specific information on job and educational opportunities within the industry.

NFPA
951 E Montana Vista
Salt Lake City, UT 84124

Phone: (801) 266-6372
Fax: (801) 534-0434
http://www.flightparamedic.org

Pediatric Critical Care Medicine: This is a multidisciplinary resource on the Internet for pediatric critical care. The Web site provides specific reviews of current literature, research, funding, and professional opportunities in pediatric critical care.

http://www.pedsccm.org

Pem-Database.Org: This Web-based database platform for professionals practicing pediatric emergency medicine (PEM) is sponsored by a not-for-profit organization dedicated to the advancement of PEM through the application of information technology.

http://www.pemdatabase.org

Pediatric Transport Listserv: PEDTPT-L is an international forum for professionals interested in interhospital transport of children. PEDTPT-L is a listserv offering access to people regarding pediatric interfacility transport. It is available to people with an interest in transport medicine and can be accessed by free subscription by using the following information:

LISTSERV@LISTSERV.BROWN.EDU
With the message: Subscribe PEDTPT-L

Outside the United States

Australian Nursing Council: ANC sets and regulates nursing national standards with a state or territory nurse regulatory authority. This includes the flight nurses. Its Web site lists several publications and educational opportunities.

ANC
PO Box 873
20 Challis St
Dickson ACT 2602

Phone: +612 6257 7960
Fax: +612 6257 7955
http://www.anc.org.au
e-mail: anc@anc.org.au

Flight Nurses of Australia: This organization for Australian flight nurses promotes their subspecialty. Its Web site lists contact numbers for various committee members and publishes a standard for flight nursing practice.

PO Box 346
Rockdale, NSW 2216

Phone: +08 8383 6196

In-Flight Nurses Association: This is a representative forum of flight nurses within the Royal College of Nursing. Its Web site offers some clinical and educational information and links to other members.

IFNA
http://www.ntlworld.com/gerpaul/ifna/RCN aaaIFNA/rcn ifna.html
e-mail: ifna.uk@ntlworld.com

International Society of Air Medical Services (Australasia)

ISAS (Australasia)
PO Box 843
Niddire Victoria 3042
Australia

http://www.isas.org.au

New Zealand Nurses Organization: The organization represents nursing and nurse midwifery throughout New Zealand. The New Zealand Flight Association is a subspecialty group that promotes excellence in flight nursing. The organization publishes a monthly journal, and its Web site offers information on educational and job opportunities.

National Office
Level 3, Willbank Ct
57 Willis St PO Box 2128
Wellington

Phone: 0800028 38 48
Fax: 04 382 9993
http://www.nzno.org.nz

NurseScribe: This Web site lists various links to nursing organizations, national and international, including several transport organizations.

http://www.enursescribe.com

NSW Newborn and Paediatric Emergency Transport Service (NETS)

Phone: +61 1300 36 2500
Fax: +61 1300 36 2498
http://www.nets.org.au
e-mail: consultATnets.org.au

Royal Flying Doctor Service of Australia: This is an organization of medical transport and service providers serving a large proportion of Australia. Its Web site describes the range of services offered.

RFGS Central Operations
8-10 Stuart Terr
Alice Springs NT 0870
Australia

Phone: +61 8 8238 3333
Fax: +61 8 8234 5640
http://www.rfds.org.au/central/default.htm
e-mail: enquiries@flyingdoctor.net

2. **Journals With a Previous Published Interest in Neonatal and Pediatric Transport**

Air Medical Journal: The official journal of the Air and Surface Transport Nurses Association, Air Medical Physician Association, Association of Air Medical Services, National EMS Pilots Association, and National Flight Paramedics Association. The journal is published monthly and contains original research, collective reviews, case studies, editorials, and letters to the editor concerning clinical practice, laboratory and clinical research, education, planning, and administration of medical care by air-medical professionals. It also contains selected academic articles examining the management, flight operations, and safety aspects of the aviation component of air medical services.

Manuscripts are submitted, in the appropriate format to: *Air Medical Journal,* 10801 Executive Center Dr, Suite 509, Little Rock, AR 72211; phone: (501) 223-0183; e-mail: d.drennan@elsevier.com.

Emergency Medicine Journal: (formerly *Journal of Accident and Emergency Medicine*) is published bimonthly by the BMJ publishing group. It is the journal of the British Association for Accident & Emergency Medicine and the official journal of the British Association for Immediate Care and the Faculty of Prehospital Care of the Royal College of Surgeons of Edinburgh. It focuses on developments and advances in emergency medicine and critical care and represents all specialties involved in emergency and prehospital care. Articles included consist of editorials, reviews, original articles, short reports, research series, and best evidence topic reports. Articles are submitted online using submission protocols.

Critical Care Medicine: A monthly publication focusing on all aspects of acute and emergency care for the critically ill or injured patient. It is the official journal for the Society of Critical Care Medicine. Submitted manuscripts are peer reviewed and submitted to the editor: Critical Care Medicine, 701 Lee St, Suite 200, Des Plaines, IL 60016; phone: (847) 827-6869; e-mail: journals@sccm.org. The publisher is Lippincott Williams & Wilkins.

Pediatrics: The official journal of the American Academy of Pediatrics. It publishes articles on original research or observations and special feature articles in the field of pediatrics as broadly defined. Articles pertinent to pediatrics are also included from related fields such as nutrition, surgery, dentistry, public health, child health services, human genetics, animal studies, psychology, psychiatry, education, sociology, and nursing. Committee statements and guidelines also are published regularly. It is owned and controlled by the American Academy of Pediatrics and is published monthly by the American Academy of Pediatrics, PO Box 927, Elk Grove Village, IL 60009-0927.

Journal of Pediatrics: Publishes original research articles, clinical and laboratory observations, reviews of medical progress in pediatrics and related fields, grand rounds and clinicopathologic conferences, and special articles. The journal is published by Elsevier, Inc, and articles can be submitted to the editor: The Journal of Pediatrics, Children's Hospital Medical Center 3333 Burnet Ave, MLC 3021 Cincinnati, OH 45229-3039; Alice Landwehr, managing editor; phone: (513) 636-7140; fax: (513) 636-7141; e-mail: journal.pediatrics@cchmc.org. The journal also accepts electronically submitted articles at http://jpeds.edmgr.com.

Pediatric Critical Care: The official journal of the Society of Critical Care Medicine, the World Federation of Pediatric Intensive and Critical Care Societies, the Paediatric Intensive Care Society UK, and the Latin American Society of Pediatric Intensive Care. It is written for pediatricians, neonatologists, respiratory therapists, nurses, and others who deal with pediatric patients who are critically ill. The journal includes a full range of scientific content, including clinical articles, scientific investigations, solicited reviews, and abstracts from pediatric critical care meetings. It also includes abstracts of selected articles published in Chinese, French, Italian, Japanese, Portuguese, and Spanish. The journal is published by Lippincott Williams & Wilkins. Articles for submission are forwarded to the editor at: Society of Critical Care Medicine, 701 Lee St, Suite 200, Des Plaines, IL 60016; phone: (847) 827-6869, e-mail: journals@sccm.org.

Pediatric Emergency Care: A monthly publication that presents information for emergency physicians, pediatricians, and allied health professionals who provide care for acutely ill or injured children and adolescents. The journal addresses most immediate acute care management problems, with articles on topics such as transport, pediatric airway management, acute trauma, sharp object ingestion, and toxicology. The journal is published by Lippincott Williams & Wilkins, and articles are submitted to the editor with a cover letter to Room 2011, The Children's Hospital of Philadelphia, 34th St & Civic Center Blvd, Philadelphia, PA 19104; fax: (215) 590-2768; e-mail: ludwig@email.chop.edu.

Prehospital Emergency Care: The official journal of the National Association of EMS Physicians, National Association of State EMS Directors, and the National Association of EMS Educators. It is published quarterly with clinical and research information on advances in medical care in the out-of-hospital setting. The journal is published by Elsevier, and articles are submitted to the editor: James J. Menegazzi, PhD, Editor-in-Chief, Prehospital Emergency Care, 230 McKee Pl, Suite 500, Pittsburgh, PA 15213; phone: (412) 647-7992; fax: (412) 647-4670; e-mail: menegazz + @pitt.edu

Trauma Care Journal: The official journal of the International Trauma Anesthesia and Critical Care Society, which also operates under the name Trauma Care International. It is a quarterly journal on prehospital trauma care and anesthesia issues. Articles are submitted to the managing editor, Linda J. Kesseling, MS, ELS, Trauma Care, ITACCS, PO Box 4826, Baltimore, MD 21211.

3. **Pediatric and Neonatal Transport-related Certification Courses (see also chapters 2, 3, 8, 14, and 23)**

Basic Life Support (BLS): Noninvasive assessments and interventions used to treat victims of respiratory and/or cardiovascular emergencies and stroke. This term has become synonymous with cardiopulmonary resuscitation (CPR) and includes automated external defibrillation.

http://www.americanheart.org

Neonatal Resuscitation Program (NRP): Designed to teach an evidence-based approach to resuscitation of neonates using teaching modules. The causes, prevention, and management of mild to severe neonatal asphyxia are explained so that health care professionals develop optimal knowledge and skill in resuscitation. Specific skills and special situations are addressed. Program information can be accessed at: American Academy of Pediatrics Division of Life Support Programs, 141 Northwest Point Blvd, Elk Grove Village, IL 60007; phone: (847) 434-4798; fax: (847) 228-1350; http://www.aap.org/nrp/nrpmain.html.

S.T.A.B.L.E.: An educational program designed to address the pretransport stabilization and postresuscitation care of sick neonates in the community hospital setting. It has been developed for maternal-child health care providers (including nurses, physicians, respiratory therapists, and other prehospital care providers) and consists of several modules, including a learner, instructor, and cardiac module. Program information can be found at http://www.stableprogram.org.

Advanced Cardiac Life Support (ACLS) Course: Medical interventions used to treat victims of respiratory and/or cardiac emergencies and stroke, including invasive techniques such as intubation and administration of drugs. Developed by the American Heart Association for the resuscitation of patients in cardiac arrest or prearrest states. The ACLS course provides a basic level of information combined with skill development, providing participants with the skills and knowledge to manage an adult cardiac arrest situation. http://www.americanheart.org

Advanced Pediatric Life Support (APLS): The fourth edition of *APLS: The Pediatric Emergency Medicine Resource* represents quantum leaps in the content and scope of the course. Originally conceived as a course in the basic elements of pediatric emergency medicine for physicians who did not regularly care for ill or injured children, the course now attempts to be the definitive resource in pediatric emergency medicine education for physicians and physician extenders in training and in practice. The expanded horizon of the fourth edition is neatly captured in the mission statement adopted by the APLS Steering Committee.

http://www.aap.org/profed/nrp/aplsmain.htm

Advanced Trauma Care for Nurses (ATCN): ATCN is an advanced course designed for registered nurses interested in increasing knowledge in the management of multiple trauma patients. The course is taught in concert with the ATLS (Advanced Trauma Life Support) course for physicians. The nurse participants audit the ATLS course. During the ATLS skill and testing stations, the nurses are separated from the physician group and directed through interactive, hands-on, scenario-based ATCN skill stations.

http://www.traumanursesoc.org/edu_atcn.html

Course in Advanced Trauma Nursing (CATN II): The course is designed to expand trauma nursing knowledge and enhance complex decision-making skills. Advanced trauma nursing is based on the physiologic principles and human responses to injury and illness. The nurse applies critical decision making to optimally affect the outcome of critically injured or ill patients. CATN II concepts correlate broad psychophysiologic and pathophysiologic processes to specific clinical problems.

http://www.ena.org/catn_enpc_tncc/catn/

Emergency Nursing Pediatric Course (ENPC): A 16-hour course designed to provide core-level pediatric knowledge and psychomotor skills needed to care for pediatric patients in the emergency setting. The course presents a systematic assessment model; integrates the associated anatomy, physiology, and pathophysiology; and identifies appropriate interventions. Triage categorization and prevention strategies are included in the course content. ENPC is taught using a variety of formats, including lectures, videotapes, and skill stations that encourage participants to integrate their psychomotor abilities into a patient situation in a risk-free setting.

http://www.ena.org/catn_enpc_tncc/enpc/

Pediatric Advanced Life Support (PALS): A joint project of the American Academy of Pediatrics and the American Heart Association, the PALS course provides knowledge and skill sessions to improve participant performance during a pediatric resuscitation. The goal of PALS is to provide the learner with advanced assessment skills to recognize infants and children at risk for cardiopulmonary arrest. Information and strategies needed to prevent cardiopulmonary arrest in infants and children are addressed, as are the cognitive and psychomotor skills needed to resuscitate infants and children and stabilize their conditions, including advanced airway management and administration of medication.

http://www.americanheart.org

Pediatric Education for Prehospital Professionals (PEPP): PEPP is a curriculum developed by the American Academy of Pediatrics to provide core pediatric education for prehospital providers. Pediatric assessment skills are stressed throughout the course that has separate ALS and BLS curricula or can be taught to mixed audiences. http://www.peppsite.com/

The Transport Nurse Advanced Trauma Course (TNATC): Formally known as the Flight Nurse Advanced Trauma Course, is a 3-day educational experience focused on care of trauma patients during initial resuscitation and transport. Information concerning locations and course offerings can be obtained by calling The Air and Surface Transport Nurses Association at (800) 897-NFNA (6362); fax: (303) 770-1812; e-mail: astna@gwami.com.

Trauma Nursing Core Curriculum (TNCC): This course is sponsored by the Emergency Nursing Association. Currently in the fifth edition (2000) (6th edition scheduled for 2006), this course is designed to provide nurses (emergency department and inpatient and critical care areas) with core trauma knowledge through lectures and integration of skills stations. The goal of the course is to decrease the overall morbidity and mortality of trauma patients by increasing the level of nursing care provided in a variety of settings.

http://www.ena.org/catn_enpc_tncc/tncc/

4. Programs and Service Organizations Performing International Transport

Following is a brief listing of programs and organizations that report or advertise experience or availability in the transport of patients internationally and in other parts of the world. It is by no means complete. Listing in this section does not imply endorsement by the authors or the American Academy of Pediatrics. Other similar programs can be accessed through a variety of Web sites, such as http://www.combose.com/ Health/Public_Health_and_Safety/Emergency_Services/Medical/ Air_Ambulance/.

The AAP Section on Transport Medicine also maintains a database that includes many of the transport programs in the United States. Although not currently specifically designed to identify programs with international experience, contact names and numbers for the individual systems are included (http://www.aap.org/sections/transmed/database.pdf).

US- and Canada-based Companies

National Air Ambulance
Fort Lauderdale, FL
Phone: (800) 327-3710; (954) 359-9900
e-mail: inquiry@nationaljets.com

Air Ambulance Professionals
1535 Perimeter Rd, Hangar 36B
Fort Lauderdale, FL 33909
Phone: (800) 752-4195; (954) 481-0555
e-mail: info@airambulanceprof.com

Care Flight International
Clearwater, FL
Phone: (800) 282-6878; (813) 530-7972

AAA Air Ambulance America
PO Box 4051
Austin, TX 78765-4051
Phone: (800) 222-3564; (512) 479-8000
e-mail: admin@airambulance.com

Skyservice Lifeguard
Montreal, Quebec, Canada
Phone: (800) 463-3482 (North America); (514) 497-7000
   (worldwide)
Fax: (514) 636-0096
e-mail: lifeguard@skyservice.com

Aeromedical Services International
Las Vegas, NV
Phone: (800) 222-9993; (702) 798-4600

Air Ambulance Incorporated
San Carlos, CA
Phone: (800) 982-5806; (702) 798-4600

Critical Air Medicine
San Diego, CA
Phone: (800) 247-8326; (619) 571-0482

Schaefer's Air Service
Van Nuys, CA
Phone: (800) 247-3355; (818) 786-8713

AEA International/SOS
Seattle, WA and Singapore
Phone: (800) 468-5232; (206) 340-6000
AEA International/SOS
Philadelphia, PA 31685
Phone: (800) 523-8930
Note: AEA International acquired SOS International in 1998.

Travel Care International, Inc
Phone: (800) 524-7633 (United States); (715) 479-8881
   (outside the United States)

Air MD
4707 140th Ave
Suite 204
Clearwater, FL 33762
Phone: (800) 282-6878
e-mail: info@airmed.net

US Air Ambulance
5919 Approach Rd
PO Box 18718
Sarasota, FL 34270

Caribbean, Mexico, and Latin America

Bohlke Aviation International
Alexander Hamilton Airport
St Croix, US Virgin Islands
Phone: (809) 778-9177

Emergencia Aera Nacional
Mexico City
Phone: [52] (5)-655-3644 or [52] (5)-573-2100

Vuelo de Vida (Life Flight)
Caracas, Venezuela
Phone: [58] (2) 919-054 or (2) 351-143

United Kingdom and Europe

Aeromed 365 Ltd
Suite 66
Worth Business Centre
Worth Corner
Phone: + 44 (0) 8709-596999
Fax: + 44 (0) 8707 559 599

Air Ambulance International
Box 1044
Magnolia, TX 77355
Phone: (800) 513-5192 (in the United States); (832) 934-2390
Fax: (832) 934-2395

■■■■■■■■■■■■■■■■■■■■■■■■■■■■■■■

Austrian Air Ambulance
Vienna, Austria
Phone: [43] (1)-401-44

Compagnie Generale de Secours
Paris, France
Phone: [33] (0) 1-4747-6666

Euro-Flite Ltd
Helsinki International Airport
Vantaa, Finland
Phone: [358] (0) 1-174-655

German Air Rescue
Stuttgart, West Germany
Phone: [49] (711)-701-070

Jet Flite
Helsinki International Airport
Vantaa, Finland
Phone: [358] (0)-822-766

MEDIC'AIR International
35, rue Jules Ferry
93170 Bagnolea
Paris, France
Phone: [33] (0) 1-4172-1414

Swiss Air Ambulance
Zurich, Switzerland
Phone: [41] (1)-383-1111
Transport operations in Europe, Russia, Africa, and the
    Middle East

Trans Care International
London, England
Phone: [44] (181)-993-6151

The Wings Medical Group of Companies
WINGS
238 Broomhill Rd
Brislington, Bristol BS4 5RG

Phone: +44 (0) 117 9719333
Fax: +44 (0) 117 3007000
http://www.wings-medical-group.co.uk
e-mail: admin@wings-medical-group.co.uk

UK London Heathrow
PO Box 279, Iver Bucks
SLO 0BQ10X
Phone: +44 (0) 208-897-6185; +44 (0) 1753 651 511

Middle East

Herzliya Medical Center
Tel Aviv
Phone: [972] (9)-592-555
Air transport for the Middle East and Eastern Mediterranean

M.A.R.M.
Izmir (Smyrna)
Phone: [90] (51)-633-322 or (51)-219-556

Africa

Flying Doctors Society
Nairobi, Kenya
Transport service through East Africa
Phone: [254] (2)-501-280 or (2)-336-886

Medical Air Rescue Service, Ltd
Belgravia, Harare, Zimbabwe
Phone: [263] (0)-73-45-13/14/15

Medical Rescue International
Johannesburg, SA
Phone: [27] (11)-403-7080
Transport network covering sub-Saharan Africa

EuroAssistance
Johannesburg, South Africa
Phone: [27] (11)-315-3999

Medical Rescue International
Aukland Park, South Africa
Phone: [27] (11)-403-7080

India

East West Rescue
New Delhi, India
Phone: [91]-11-2469 8865; [91]-11-2462 3738; [91]-11-2469 9229;
   [91]-11-2469 0429
Transports throughout Indian subcontinent and adjacent islands

Southeast Asia

AEA International
(Asia Emergency Assistance)
Singapore
Phone: [65] 338-2311 or 338-7800
Transport from Hong Kong, China, Far East Asia, Pacific Rim,
   and westernmost Pacific islands

Heng-Gref Medical Services
Singapore
Phone: [65] 272-6028
Transport from South East Asia and Indonesia

Index